ESSENTIALS OF
NURSING LEADERSHIP
& MANAGEMENT

Patricia Kelly-Heidenthal, RN, MSN

Professor Emerita
Purdue University Calumet
Hammond, Indiana

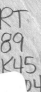

THOMSON
✦
DELMAR LEARNING

Australia   Canada   Mexico   Singapore   Spain   United   Kingdom   United   States

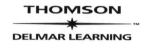

Essentials of Nursing Leadership & Management
by
Patricia Kelly-Heidenthal, RN, MSN

Vice President, Health Care Business Unit:
William Brottmiller

Editorial Director:
Cathy L. Esperti

Acquisitions Editor:
Matthew Filimonov

Senior Developmental Editor:
Elisabeth F. Williams

Editorial Assistant:
Patricia Osborn

Marketing Director:
Jennifer McAvey

Marketing Channel Manager:
Tamara Caruso

Marketing Coordinator:
Karen Summerlin

Production Editors:
Mary Colleen Liburdi
James Zayicek

Library of Congress Cataloging-in-Publication Data:

Kelly-Heidenthal, Patricia.
  Essentials of nursing leadership & management / Patricia Kelly-Heidenthal.
    p. cm.
Includes bibliographical references and index.
  ISBN 1-4018-3017-X
  1. Nursing services—Administration. 2. Leadership. I. Title: Essentials of nursing leadership and management. II. Title.

RT89.K45 2004
362.17'3'068—dc22

2003060626

NOTICE TO THE READER

CONTENTS

CHAPTER 5

Delegation / 91

CHAPTER 6

Staffing / 117

CONTRIBUTORS

Rinda Alexander, PhD, RN, CS
Professor of Nursing
Purdue University Calumet
Hammond, Indiana
and
Professor of Nursing
University of Florida
College of Nursing
Gainesville, Florida

Margaret M. Anderson, EdD, RN, CNAA
Professor and Chair
Department of Nursing and Health Professions
Northern Kentucky University
Highland Heights, Kentucky

Ida M. Androwich, PhD, RN-C, FAAN
Professor
Community, Mental Health,
and Administrative Nursing
Niehoff School of Nursing
Loyola University Chicago
Chicago, Illinois

Anne Bernat, RN, BSN, MSN, CNAA
Vice President for Nursing
Southern Maryland Hospital
Clinton, Maryland

Sister Kathleen Cain, OSF, JD
Attorney
Franciscan Legal Services
Baton Rouge, Louisiana

Corinne Haviley, RN, MS
Director, Ambulatory Care Services
Northwestern Memorial Hospital
Chicago, Illinois

Paul Heidenthal, MS
Consultant
Austin, Texas

Karen Houston, RN, MS
Director of Quality and Continuum of Care
Albany Medical Center
Albany, New York

Mary Anne Jadlos, MS, ACNP-CS, CWOCN
Acute Care Nurse Practitioner
Wound, Skin, Ostomy Service
Northeast Health Acute Care Division
Troy, New York

Stephen Jones, MS, RN-C, PNP, ET
Pediatric Clinical Nurse Specialist/Nurse
Practitioner
The Children's Hospital at Albany Medical Center
Albany, New York
and
Founder and Principal
Pediatric Concepts
Averill Park, New York

Glenda Kelman, PhD, ACNP-CS
Chair, Division of Nursing
The Sage Colleges
Troy, New York
and
Acute Care Nurse Practitioner
Wound, Skin, Ostomy Service
Northeast Health Acute Care Division
Troy, New York

Mary Elaine Koren, RN, DNSc
Assistant Professor
School of Nursing
Northern Illinois University
DeKalb, Illinois

Lyn LaBarre, MS, RN, CEN
Administrator, Emergency Services
Albany Medical Center
Albany, New York

Linda Searle Leach, PhD, RN, CNAA
Assistant Professor of Nursing
California State University
Fullerton, California

Camille B. Little, RN, MS
Instructional Assistant Professor
Mennonite College of Nursing
Illinois State University
Normal, Illinois

Sharon Little-Stoetzel, RN, MS
Assistant Professor of Nursing
Graceland University
Independence, Missouri

Patsy L. Maloney, RN-C, MSN, EdD, CNAA
Associate Professor and Director of Continuing
Nursing Education
School of Nursing
Pacific Lutheran University
Tacoma, Washington

Maureen T. Marthaler, RN, MS
Assistant Professor
Purdue University Calumet
Hammond, Indiana

Judith W. Martin, RN, JD
Attorney
Franciscan Legal Services
Baton Rouge, Louisiana

Mary McLaughlin, RN, MBA
Project Specialist
Albany Medical Center
Albany, New York

Terry W. Miller, PhD, RN
Dean and Professor
School of Nursing
Pacific Lutheran University
Tacoma, Washington
and
Professor Emeritus
San Jose State University
San Jose, California

Leslie H. Nicoll, PhD, MBA, RN
Principal and Owner, Maine Desk
Editor in Chief, CIN, Computers, Informatics,
Nursing
and
Editor in Chief, *Journal of Hospice
and Palliative Nursing*
Portland, Maine

Laura J. Nosek, PhD, RN
Adjunct Associate Professor of Nursing
Frances Payne Bolton School of Nursing
Case Western Reserve University
Cleveland, Ohio
and
Marcella Nichoff School of Nursing
Loyola University
Chicago, Illinois
and
Consultant in Nursing Administration
Excelsior College (formerly Regents College)
Albany, New York

Amy Androwich O'Malley, RN, MSN
Director of Nursing Resources
Children's Memorial Hospital
Chicago, Illinois

Karin Polifko-Harris, PhD, RN, CNAA
Principal/Owner
KPH Consulting
Naples, Florida

Robyn D. Pozza, JD
Attorney
Austin, Texas

Jacklyn L. Ruthman, PhD, RN
Assistant Professor
Bradley University
Peoria, Illinois

Patricia M. Lentsch Schoon, MPH, RN
Assistant Professor
College of St. Catherine
St. Paul, Minnesota

Kathleen Fischer Sellers, PhD, RN
Assistant Professor
SUNY Institute of Technology
Utica, New York

REVIEWERS

Connie J. Boerst, RN, MSN
Assistant Professor of Nursing
Bellin College of Nursing
Green Bay, Wisconsin

Mary Meg Brown, MSN, APRN, CNAA
Instructor of Nursing
Alcorn State University
Natchez, Mississippi

Karen Edmondson, RN, MN
Instructor of Nursing
University of South Carolina, Spartanburg
Spartanburg, South Carolina

Donna Molyneaux, RN, BSN, MSN, DNSc
Associate Professor of Nursing
Gwynedd Mercy College School of Nursing
Gwynedd Valley, Pennsylvania

Kathy Pearson, RN, MSN
Instructor of Nursing
Temple College
Temple, Texas

Kathleen Poindexter, RN, MSN
Associate Professor of Nursing
Ferris State University
Big Rapids, Michigan

Marsha Purtee, RN, MS
Instructor of Nursing
Kettering College of Medical Arts
Kettering, Ohio

Bruce Wilson, RN, PhD
Associate Professor of Nursing
University of Texas Pan American
Edinburg, Texas

PREFACE

The National Academy of Sciences, Institute of Medicine (IOM) Report, April 2003, *Health Professions Education: A Bridge to Quality,* states that all programs that educate and train health professionals should adopt five core competencies: embrace the ability to deliver patient-centered care, work as a member of an interdisciplinary team, engage in evidence-based practice, apply quality improvement approaches, and use information technology. See **http://www.nap.edu**. These core competencies are essential for the health professional of the future.

Essentials of Nursing Leadership & Management is designed to help beginning nurse leaders and managers develop the knowledge and skill to lead and manage nursing care delivery for patients. The text addresses the topics mentioned in the IOM Report and prepares the beginning nurse leader and manager to move into modern day health care. The contributors to this edition include educators, nursing faculty, clinical nurse specialists, lawyers, nurse practitioners, wound and ostomy care nurses, nurse entrepreneurs, and many other specialists. These contributors are from various areas of the U.S., thus allowing them to offer a broad view of nursing leadership and management.

Each chapter of *Essentials of Nursing Leadership & Management* discusses the latest theories relevant to its specific topic. Various points of view are presented through case studies and interviews with staff nurses, nurse practitioners, nursing administrators, nursing risk managers, nursing faculty, doctors, patients, and a hospital administrator. Also included are many interviews with nursing leaders and managers.

ORGANIZATION

Essentials of Nursing Leadership & Management consists of seventeen chapters arranged in five units. These chapters provide beginning nurse leaders and managers with the knowledge needed in today's health care environment.

- **Unit I** introduces essential concepts of leadership and management and then discusses contemporary nursing and team building.
- **Unit II** discusses managing nursing care. Planning care in organizations, delegation, staffing, budgeting, and performance and quality improvement are all explored.
- **Unit III** covers leadership in nursing. Power, change, and conflict resolution, decision making and critical thinking, and time management are discussed in detail.
- **Unit IV** discusses professional issues. The legal and ethical aspects of patient care are explored, as are cultural diversity and spirituality.
- **Unit V** investigates preparation for professional nursing practice. NCLEX preparation, your first job, career planning, and achieving life balance are all discussed.

Discussion of timely topics such as nurse-sensitive outcomes, evidence based practice, information technology, HIPAA, magnet hospitals, interdisciplinary team work, quality and performance improvement, and population based care is included throughout the chapters. The real world of nursing is also embraced by presenting a variety of different views on some topics.

The textbook uses graphics and photographs to engage learners and enhance their learning. Photographs provide visual reinforcement of concepts such as teamwork and the changes occurring in health care settings today while adding visual interest. Figures and tables depict concepts and activities described in the text. Highlights are used consistently throughout the text to help the reader identify the various chapter elements.

FEATURES

Each chapter includes several creative features that provide the learner with a consistent format for learning and an assortment of resources for understanding and applying the knowledge presented. Pedagogical features include:

- An opening quote and scenario that begin each chapter and establish the background for the reader's approach to the chapter.
- Objectives that state the chapter's learning goals.
- An introduction to each chapter that briefly describes the purpose and scope of the chapter.
- A bulleted summary and multiple choice review questions at the end of each chapter, which assist the reader in remembering and using the material presented.
- Key terms, which appear in a Glossary and also appear in bold type in each chapter. They are designed to encourage understanding of new terms presented in the chapter.
- References, which are the key for readers to find sources of the material presented in each chapter.
- Suggested readings, which help the readers find additional information concerning the topics covered in each chapter.

Special features are used throughout the text to emphasize key points and to provide specific types of information. These include:

- Stop and think exercises, which encourage critical thinking about topics covered in the chapter.
- Real world interviews with staff nurses, nurse practitioners, nursing administrators, nursing risk managers, nursing faculty, doctors, patients, and a hospital administrator, which are sprinkled throughout the chapters to illustrate various points of view. Interviews with nursing leaders and managers are also included.
- Literature applications, which illustrate the applicability of current literature for practice.
- Exploring the Web exercises, which guide the reader to the Internet and give Internet addresses for the latest information related to the chapter content.
- Review activities, which encourage students to think critically about how to apply chapter content to the work place and other "real world" situations. They provide reinforcement of key leadership and management skills. Exercises are numbered in each chapter to facilitate using them as assignments or activities.
- A case study that provides a "real-world" illustration of the chapter's topic.
- Tables and figures, which appear throughout the text and provide convenient capsules of information for the student's reference.

ACKNOWLEDGMENTS

A book such as this requires great effort and the coordination of many people with various areas of expertise. A special huge thank you goes to my husband and best friend, Paul, for helping me with every stage of the book, i.e., editing, organizing my computer efforts, and just supporting me every step of the way. I would like to thank all of the contributors for their time and effort in sharing their knowledge gained through years of experience in both the clinical and academic setting. All of the contributing authors worked within tight time frames to accomplish their work. A special thanks goes to Robyn Pozza, Attorney, for the new legal charts and many contributions to the legal chapter.

I thank the reviewers for their time spent critically reviewing the manuscript and providing the valuable comments that have added to this text. Special thanks also go to my Dad and Mom, Ed and Jean Kelly, my sisters, Tessie Dybel and Kathy Milch, Aunt Verna and Uncle Archie Payne, Aunt Pat and Uncle Bill Kelly, to my nieces and nephew and grand nephew, to my dear friends, Patricia Wojcik, Florence Lebryk, and Lee McGuan, who have supported me through this book and most of my life. Special thanks to my wonderful nursing friends, Zenaida Corpuz, Dr. Mary Elaine Koren, Dr. Barbara Mudloff, Dr. Patricia Padjen, and Jane McKeon, and especially to Gerri Kane, Janice Klepitch, Sylvia Komyatte, and Julie Martini, as well as Anna Fizer, Judy Ilijanich, Trudy Keilman, Judy Rau, and Lillian Rau, who have supported me throughout this book and during our 40 years together as nurses. Special thanks to my faculty mentors, Dr. Imogene King, Dr. Joyce Ellis, and Nancy Weber.

I would like to acknowledge and sincerely thank the team at Delmar Learning who have worked to make this textbook a reality. Matt Filomonov, Acquisitions Editor, and Beth Williams, Senior Developmental Editor, are great people who have worked tirelessly. They brought knowledge, guidance, humor, and attention to help keep me motivated and on track throughout the project. Thanks to Patricia Osborn, Editorial Assistant, who offered much support along the way.

Thanks also go to many RNs in Austin, Texas, for their reviews and feedback, on an ongoing basis. These nurses include Deloris Armstrong, Joyce Batcheller, Jan Costly, Mark Dorward, Constance S. Faircloth, Lorraine Flatt, Lisa Lilly, Jan Robinson, Bonnie Clipper Salzberg, Kit Thompson, Sue Thompson, Karen Woodard, and Ana Zeletz.

Thanks to Richard Komyatte, Edward P. Robinson, Matt Zaucha, and many others for their help on this project. Thanks to all who helped with reference, editorial and office support, including Ramona Hamilton, Sheila Berlin, and Constance Abney.

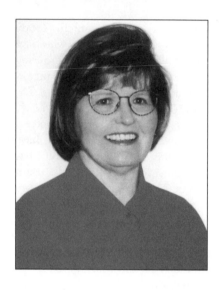

Patricia Kelly-Heidenthal earned a Diploma in Nursing from St. Margaret Hospital School of Nursing, Hammond, Indiana; a Baccalaureate in Nursing from DePaul University in Chicago, Illinois; and a Master's Degree in Nursing from Loyola University in Chicago, Illinois. She has worked as a staff nurse, school nurse, and a nurse educator, and has traveled extensively nationwide and in Canada and Puerto Rico, teaching conferences for the Joint Commission on Accreditation of HealthCare Organizations, Resource Applications, Pediatric Concepts, Kaplan, and Health Education Systems, Inc (HESI). Pat was Director of Quality Improvement at the University of Chicago Hospitals and Clinics in Chicago, Illinois. She has taught at Wesley-Passavant School of Nursing, Chicago State University, and Purdue University Calumet in Hammond Indiana. She is Professor Emeritus, Purdue University Calumet, Hammond Indiana. Pat has taught fundamentals of nursing, adult nursing, nursing leadership and management, nursing issues, nursing trends, quality improvement, and legal aspects of nursing. Pat is a member of Sigma Theta Tau and the Texas and American Nurses Association. She is listed in Who's Who in American Nursing, 2000 Notable American Women, and the Inter-national Who's Who of Professional and Business Women.

Pat has served on the Board of Directors of Tri City Mental Health Center, St. Anthony's Home, and Quality Connection. She is the author of *Nursing Leadership & Management,* Delmar Learning, 2003, and she contributed a chapter on "Preparing the Under-graduate Student and Faculty to Use Quality Improve-ment in Practice" to *Improving Quality,* Second Edition, by Claire Gavin Meisenheimer. Pat has written several articles, including Chest X-Ray Interpretation and many articles on Quality Improvement. Pat is a Disaster Volunteer for the American Red Cross and a volunteer at an Austin, Texas, church food pantry. Throughout most of her career, she has taught Nursing at the University level. She continues to work part time as a staff nurse in an Emergency Department in Austin, Texas. Pat may be contacted at patkh1@aol.com.

DEDICATION

This book is dedicated to my wonderful husband, Paul, my loving Dad and Mom, Ed and Jean Kelly, to my super sisters, Tessie Dybel and Kathy Milch, to my dear aunts and uncles, Aunt Verna and Uncle Archie Payne and Aunt Pat and Uncle Bill Kelly, to my nieces, Natalie Bevil, Melissa Milch, and Stacey Milch, and nephew, John Milch, and grand nephew, Brock Bevil, as well as to my dear friends, Patricia Wojcik, Florence Lebryk, and Lee McGuan, to my nursing mentors, Dr. Imogene King, Dr. Joyce Ellis, and Nancy Weber, and to my wonderful nursing friends, Zenaida Corpuz, Dr. Mary Elaine Koren, Dr. Barbara Mudloff, Dr. Patricia Padjen, Jane McKeon, and especially to Gerri Kane, Janice Klepitch, Sylvia Komyatte, and Julie Martini, as well as Anna Fizer, Judy Ilijanich, Trudy Keilman, Judy Rau, and Lillian Rau, who have supported me throughout this book and during our 40 years together as nurses. Finally, I dedicate this book to future generations of RNs including two in my family, Kerrie Ellingsen and Diane Stoddard.

HOW TO USE THIS BOOK

Never doubt that a small group of thoughtful, committed citizens can change the world; indeed, it's the only thing that ever has. (Margaret Mead)

Quote A nursing or health care theorist quote gives a professional's perspective regarding the topic at hand; read this as you begin each new chapter and see whether your opinion matches or differs, or whether you are in need of further information.

Chapter Objectives These goals indicate to you the performance-based, measurable objectives that are targeted for mastery upon completion of the chapter.

OBJECTIVES

Upon completion of this chapter, the reader should be able to:

1. Discuss traditional theories of change.
2. Discuss chaos theory and the concept of the learning organization.
3. Apply strategies for implementation of change.
4. Identify common responses to change.
5. Discuss conflict.
6. Review conflict resolution.
7. Identify strategies to facilitate conflict resolution.

You are a new nurse on a medical-surgical unit and have just come from a unit meeting. At the meeting, your nurse manager reported the results of the patient satisfaction survey from the previous year. Patient satisfaction has steadily declined, and for the past 3 months, only 20% of patients were satisfied. The manager selected a task force to investigate potential solutions to this problem and appointed you to the committee. The survey identified some reasons for the dissatisfaction: long waiting periods after pushing the nurse call light, not being informed about tests and procedures being performed, and being treated in an impersonal manner.

What should be the first step of the task force?

How can critical thinking and the decision-making process help the group solve the situation?

Opening Scenario This mini case study with related critical thinking questions should be read prior to delving into the chapter; it sets the tone for the material to come and helps you identify your knowledge base and perspective.

Case Study These short cases with related questions present a beginning clinical nursing management situation calling for judgment, decision making, or analysis in solving an open-ended problem. Familiarize yourself with the types of situations and settings you will later encounter in practice, and challenge yourself to devise solutions that will result in the best outcomes for all parties, within the boundaries of legal and ethical nursing practice.

Literature Application Study these key findings from nursing and health care research, theory, and literature, and ask yourself how they will influence your practice. Do you see ways in which your nursing could be affected by these literature findings and research results? Do you agree with the conclusions drawn by the author?

Stop and Think Ethical, cultural, spiritual, legal, delegation, and performance improvement considerations are highlighted in these boxes. Before beginning a new chapter, page through and read the Stop and Think sections and jot down your comments or reactions, then see whether your perspective changes after you complete the chapter.

STOP AND THINK

Ask yourself the critical thinking questions inspired by Table 11-1 when you are making decisions at every step of the nursing process. Have I gathered the best, most up-to-date research and evidence to help with the decision? Is my assessment accurate and complete? Is the nursing diagnosis logical and clear? Is the plan of care relevant and complete? Is the implementation consistent? Is the evaluation adequate? Have I been fair in working with my patient? Have I avoided being vague, inaccurate, inconsistent, and illogical? Have I tried to think in new "out of the box" ways to solve my patient's problems? Continue to apply the critical thinking questions and to review the research and best evidence at each step.

REAL WORLD INTERVIEW

I graduated from a diploma nursing program in 1962. I worked for 5 years and then was home for 15 years raising my children. I wanted to return to nursing and took a refresher course. It was very hard. So much had changed. I made it, though. I think that with the shortage of nurses now, hospitals would be smart to try to make it easier for nurses who have left nursing to return by offering reasonable, supportive refresher courses. I stayed at the hospital I went back to and later retired with just short of 19 years of service. When I retired, I was shocked to find out what my pension was going to be. It was $425 a month—this after almost 19 years of service. If it wasn't for my husband's pension, who, with a high school education, gets almost 10 times what I get, I would never be able to retire. My husband worked through a union. I understand that teachers who work through unions often get 75% of their salary when they retire. Some nurses who are single or divorced would like to retire but simply can't afford to do so. You keep hearing about the poor pay for teachers, and while I agree it should be better, at least they can afford to retire. Who thinks about nurses? It seems to me that more and more of the doctors' work is being given to the nurses and yet a survey I read said that the gap between the doctors' and nurses' pay is greater than what it was at the end of World War II. New nurses should start thinking about retirement benefits when they look for their first job. I know my 40 years as a nurse went fast.

Gerri Kane, RN
Retired Staff Nurse

Real World Interviews RWI Interviews with well-known nursing leaders, such as Dr. Loretta Ford, Dr. Tim Porter O'Grady, and others are included as well as interviews with nurses, doctors, hospital administrators, staff, patients, and family members. As you read these, ask yourself whether you had ever considered that individual's point of view on the given topic. How would knowing another person's perspective affect the care your deliver?

Key Concepts This bulleted list serves as a review and study tool for you as you complete each chapter.

KEY CONCEPTS

- Patient care needs should drive improvement opportunities.
- Decisions should be driven by data.
- Improvement initiatives should be linked to the organization's mission, vision, and values.
- Organizational goals and objectives should be communicated up and down the organization.
- There should be a balance in improvement goals focused on patient clinical and functional status, access, cost, and patient satisfaction outcomes.
- The University of Colorado Hospital model is an example of a multidisciplinary evidence-based practice model for using different sources of information to change or support your practice.
- The Model for Improvement and FOCUS-PDSA can be applied to a system or an individual.

Key Terms Study this list prior to reading the chapter, then again as you complete a chapter, to test your true understanding of the terms and concepts covered. Make a study list of terms you need to focus on to thoroughly appreciate the material of the chapter.

KEY TERMS

benchmarking	quality assurance
outcome elements of quality	sentinel event
performance improvement	structure elements of quality
process elements of quality	

Review Questions These questions will challenge your comprehension of objectives and concepts presented in the chapter and will allow you to demonstrate content mastery, build critical thinking skills, and achieve integration of the concepts.

REVIEW QUESTIONS

1. Which of the following describes the benchmarking process?
   A. Reviewing your own unit's data for opportunities
   B. Collecting data on an individual patient
   C. Reviewing data in the literature

Review Activities These thought-provoking activities at the close of a chapter invite you to approach a problem or scenario critically and apply the knowledge you have gained.

REVIEW ACTIVITIES

1. Risk management, infection control practitioners, and a benchmark study have revealed that your unit's utilization of indwelling catheters is above average. Brainstorm reasons why this may be occurring. Creating a fishbone (root cause) diagram may help.
2. Think about your last clinical rotation experience. Identify one process that you believe could be improved and describe how you would begin improving the process. Use the FOCUS methodology.

Exploring the Web Internet activities encourage you to use your computer and reasoning skills to search the Web for additional information on quality and nursing leadership and management.

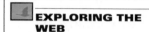

EXPLORING THE WEB

- What site would you access to find out about the history of collective bargaining? *http://www.nlrb.gov*
- Which sites can you visit for information on nursing leaders, women, and nursing history? *http://members.tripod.com* and *http://www.members.aol.com*
- What site has a funny, not scholarly, synopsis of nursing power? *http://www.nursing-power.net*
- What site supports political power for patients? *http://www.healthcareform.net*
- Find two nurses identified on the following site: *http://dbois@distinguishedwomen.com*

References Evidence-based research, theory, and general literature, as well as nursing, medical, and health care sources, are included in these lists; refer to them as you read the chapter and verify your research.

REFERENCES

American Nurses Association. (n.d.). Mission statement. Retrieved March 2, 2000, from http://www. nursingworld.org Charatan, F. (1999).

American Nurses Association. (1995). *Nursing's social policy statement.* Washington, DC: American Nurses Publishing.

Bower, F. L. (2000). *Nurses taking the lead: Personal qualities of effective leadership.* Philadelphia: Saunders.

Brown, L. D. (1996) *Health policy in the United States: Issues and options.* New York: the Ford Foundation.

DuBrin, A. J. (2000). *The active manager.* South Western College Publisher.

Fagin, C. (1998). Nursing research and the erosion of care. *Nursing Outlook, 46*(6), 259–261.

Suggested Readings These entries invite you to pursue additional topics, articles, and information in related resources.

SUGGESTED READINGS

American Nurses Credentialing Center. (2001). *Informatics nurse certification. Basic eligibility requirements.* Retrieved July 19, 2001, from http://www.nursing world.org

Ball, M. J., Hannah, K. J., & Douglas, J. (2000). Nursing and informatics. In M. Ball, K. Hannah, S. Newbold, & J. Douglas (Eds.), *Nursing informatics: Where caring and technology meet* (3rd ed., pp. 6–14). New York: Springer-Verlag.

Bard, M. R. (2000). The future of e-health. *Cybercitizen Health, 1*(1), 1–13.

Jenkins, S. (2000). Nurses' responsibilities in the implementation of information systems. In M. J. Ball, K. J. Hannah, S. Newbold, & J. Douglas (Eds.), *Nursing informatics: Where caring and technology meet* (pp. 207–223). New York: Springer-Verlag.

CHAPTER 1

> Leadership is the essence of professionalism and should be considered an essential component of all nurse and other professional roles.
> (Joyce Clifford, PhD, RN, FAAN)

Essential Concepts of Leadership and Management

OBJECTIVES

Upon completion of this chapter, the reader should be able to:

1. Define management.
2. Discuss Benner's model of novice to expert.
3. Discuss management roles.
4. Discuss organizational management theories.
5. Discuss motivation theories.
6. Discuss characteristics and theories of leadership.

People's Choice Hospital is the largest hospital in your community. It has over 1,000 professional, technical, administrative, and clerical staff and 10 patient care units. It is owned by a large foundation that has 10 other hospitals in surrounding communities and sponsors charitable, educational, and research activities. You have just been hired as a beginning staff nurse on one of the units.

How will the organization's management affect patient care and your nursing role?

Is it necessary to develop nursing leadership skills in your role?

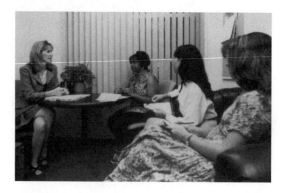

Nursing professionals use their expertise and specialized knowledge to perform management and leadership roles. Many people think leaders are corporate executives, political representatives, military generals, or those who head organizations. Alfred DeCrane Jr., chairman of the board and chief executive officer of Texaco and a trustee of the University of Notre Dame, reminds us that this occurs because these leaders are in highly visible and high-profile positions. He says that we need leadership not just at the top of our organizations but across and throughout all levels (DeCrane, 1996). The Pew Health Professions Commission (1995) recommends that leadership be considered a competency for health professions and calls for leadership development as part of the preparation of health care providers.

Nurses make a critical difference every day in managing the care of their patients and patients' families, yet nurses believe those accomplishments are part of their ordinary work. Beginning nurses manage the care of individual patients or small groups of patients, adding to their ability to manage the nursing care of additional patients as they develop their skill and judgment. All nurses can demonstrate leadership when they influence their patients and other members of the health care team and community to move toward their health care goals. This is true whether they are working with an individual patient or whether they are managing a patient care unit or an entire nursing department. Nurses manage and lead patient care and by doing so provide caring that is extraordinary. This chapter discusses management and leadership theories. Theories of motivation also are discussed.

DEFINITION OF MANAGEMENT

Management can be defined as a process of planning, organizing and staffing, leading, and controlling actions to achieve goals. Planning involves setting goals and identifying ways to meet them. Organizing and staffing is the process of ensuring that the necessary human and physical resources are available to achieve the planning goals. Organizing also involves assigning work to the right person or group and specifying who has the authority to accomplish certain tasks. Leading is influencing others to achieve the organization's goals and involves energizing, directing, and persuading others to achieve those goals. Finally, controlling is comparing actual performance to a standard and revising the original plan as needed to achieve the goals (DuBrin, 2000).

Each of these elements of management may be used more or less, depending on whether the nurse manager is a beginning nurse, the nurse manager of a patient care unit, or the nurse manager of an entire health care facility.

The beginning nurse uses the nursing process to plan patient care and selects interventions to achieve patient goals. Whether working alone or with others, the nurse then organizes care and, as needed, works with or plans for additional staff to achieve patient goals. This often involves leading or influencing other staff to achieve these patient care goals. These other staff may be nursing practitioners, nursing managers, physicians, and staff from other health care departments such as dietary, physical therapy, pharmacy, and so on. The beginning nurse evaluates or controls patient care given by themself and others to ensure that the patient's goals are met. Beginning nurses often have limited organizing and staffing responsibilities other than organizing their own work and sometimes helping to organize the work of unlicensed staff who report to them. Nurse managers of patient care units have many more responsibilities for organizing and staffing a unit.

Nurse managers often seem to work at a hectic pace and sustain that effort through long hours, frequently working without breaks.

Nurses need management skills whether they are managing the care of a small group of patients, a group of patients on an entire unit, or all the patients in the entire facility. Nurses need to possess technical, interpersonal, conceptual, diagnostic, and political skills to achieve their goals. These skills can be learned (DuBrin, 2000). Beginning nurses develop these management skills as they work with individual patients or small groups of patients. As beginning nurses develop their technical clinical expertise, their ability to use interpersonal, conceptual, diagnostic, and political skills to work with patients and health care staff both on the patient care unit and off the unit grows as well. The experienced nurse is one who has developed the ability to see the big picture and use all of these skills to achieve patient care goals.

Yukl (1998) says that people in management become adept at continuously seeking information and are constantly engaged in interactions with others who need information, help, guidance, or approval. This is true for the beginning nurse manager who is constantly handling patient, staff, organizational, and other practitioner concerns. It is also true for the more experienced nurse manager.

The typical manager is on the go. Research by McCall, Morrison, and Hanman (1978) showed that the daily activities of managers are diverse and fast paced with regular interruptions. Priority activities are integrated among inconsequential ones. In the scope of one morning, a nurse manager may engage in serious decisions about patient care, respond to a patient complaint, problem-solve a staff sick call, and participate in a celebration for an employee. Managerial work is driven by problems that emerge in random order and that have a range of importance and urgency. These circumstances create an image of the nurse manager as a "firefighter" involved in immediate and operational concerns. A significant proportion of a nurse manager's time is spent in interaction with others, and more of the work is concerned with handling information than in making decisions (McCall, Morrison, & Hanman, 1978).

If the nurse progresses from being a staff nurse to being a nurse manager of a unit and, later, of an entire nursing facility, more and more time is spent on the planning aspects of the management process.

Benner's Model of Novice to Expert

Benner's (1984) model of novice to expert provides a framework that can facilitate professional staff development by building on the skill sets and experience of each practitioner. Benner's model acknowledges that there are tasks, competencies, and outcomes that practitioners can be expected to have acquired based on five levels of experience.

Benner's model of novice to expert is based on the Dreyfus and Dreyfus (1980) model of skill acquisition applied to nursing. There are five stages of Benner's model: novice, advanced beginner, competent, proficient, and expert. See Table 1-1.

TABLE 1-1
BENNER'S MODEL: NOVICE TO EXPERT

Novice nurses are recognized as being task oriented and focused on the rules. They tend to see nursing as a list of tasks to do rather than seeing the big picture of patient care needed to meet patient care goals. Once novices have mastered most tasks required to perform their ascribed roles, they move on to the phase of advanced beginner.

The advanced beginner is the nurse who can demonstrate marginally acceptable independent performance. This nurse still focuses on the rules and is more experienced though may still need help identifying priorities.

Competent nurses have been in their role for 2 to 3 years. These nurses have developed the ability to see their actions as part of the long-range goals set for their patients. They lack the speed of the proficient nurse, but they are able to manage most aspects of clinical care.

Proficient nurses characteristically perceive the whole situation rather than a series of tasks. They have often been on the job for 3 to 5 years. They develop a plan of care and then guide the patient from point A to point B. They draw on their past experiences and know that in a typical situation, a patient must exhibit specific behaviors to meet specific goals. They realize that if those behaviors are not demonstrated within a certain time frame, then the plan needs to be changed.

Expert nurses are those nurses who intuitively know what is going on with their patients. Their expertise is so embedded in their practice that they have been heard to say, "There is something wrong with this patient. I'm not sure what is going on, but you had better come and evaluate them." Not heeding the call derived from the intuitive sense of an expert nurse has resulted in a patient's proceeding to a cardiac arrest. These expert nurses often seek advanced education.

Compiled with information from Benner, P., 1984. *From Novice to Expert*. Menlo Park, CA, Addison Wesley.

Management Roles

A frequently referenced taxonomy of managerial roles is from an in-depth, month-long study of five chief executives by Henry Mintzberg. A taxonomy is a system that groups or classifies principles. Mintzberg's observations led to the identification of three categories of managerial roles: (1) information processing roles, (2) interpersonal roles, and (3) decision-making roles (Mintzberg, 1973). A role includes behaviors, expectations, and recurrent activities within a pattern that is part of the organization's structure (Katz & Kahn, 1978).

The information processing roles identified by Mintzberg (1973) are those of monitor, disseminator, and spokesperson and are used to manage people's information needs. The interpersonal roles consist of figurehead, leader, and liaison, and each of these is used to manage relationships with people. The decision roles are entrepreneur, disturbance handler, allocator of resources, and negotiator. Nurse managers take on these roles when they manage care.

More recently, Yukl (1998) and colleagues (Kim & Yukl, 1995; Yukl, Wall, & Lepsinger, 1990) described 13 managerial role functions for managing the work and for managing relationships. The role functions for managing the work are planning and organizing, problem solving, clarifying roles and objectives, informing, monitoring, consulting, and delegating. The role functions for managing relationships are networking, supporting, developing and mentoring, managing conflict and team building, motivating and inspiring, and recognizing and rewarding.

The amount of time a nurse manager spends in each of these role functions varies by the level of the nurse manager's position in an organization. The staff nurse may spend a large part of time both giving care and monitoring a few others as they deliver care as well as monitoring the outcomes of care given. The next highest percentage of this nurse's time is spent in planning care, with other responsibilities such as coordinating, evaluating, negotiating, and serving as a multispecialist and generalist taking less than 10% each of this nurse's time.

In contrast, the middle-level nurse manager, such as the nurse manager of critical care nursing, may spend less time in direct care and more time in each of the other functions, particularly planning, monitoring, and coordinating. At the highest level of the organization, usually described as the nurse executive level, planning and being a generalist are a greatly expanded role function, whereas direct patient care monitoring is not as primary a role function as it is in the other two levels. Nurses in executive-level roles in health care organizations often have the title of chief nurse executive or vice president of patient care services.

Use of Resources

Nurse managers use four types of resources to accomplish their purpose (DuBrin, 2000). This is true for the beginning nurse as well as for nurse managers of a unit or a nursing department. Nurse managers use human resources, such as

the right staff on the health care team, to complete various assignments. They use financial resources wisely to help achieve organizational goals. Nurse managers also use physical resources, such as patient care equipment, wisely to complete their work. Finally, nurse managers use information resources to stay up-to-date in delivering care to their patients.

ORGANIZATIONAL MANAGEMENT THEORIES

Much of our current understanding of management is based on the classical theories of management that were introduced in the 1800s during the industrial age as factories developed. Since then many other theories have emerged (Shortell & Kaluzny, 2000). See Table 1-2.

MOTIVATION THEORIES

The human relations perspective in management theory grew from the conclusion that worker output was greater when the worker was treated humanistically. This spawned a human resources point of view and a focus on the individual as a source of motivation. Motivation is not explicitly demonstrated by people but rather is interpreted from their behavior. **Motivation** is whatever influences our choices and creates direction, intensity, and persistence in our behavior (Hughes, Ginnett, & Curphy, 1999; Kanfer, 1990). Motivation is a process that occurs internally to influence and direct our behavior in order to satisfy needs (Lussier, 1999). Motivation theories are not management theories per se; however, they are frequently discussed with management theories.

Motivation theories are useful because they help explain why people act the way they do and how a nurse manager can relate to individuals as human beings and workers. When you are

TABLE 1-2
MAJOR PERSPECTIVES VIEW OF THE SITUATION IN OPENING SCENARIO

Perspective	Key Contributions	Effect on Opening Scenario
Scientific Management	Focuses on productivity; organization is a machine to be run efficiently to increase production	Staffing and equipment needs are met efficiently on the unit
	Manager has limited span of number of workers they control	
	Workers must have proper tools and equipment to work efficiently	
	Uses time and motion studies to make the work efficient	
Bureaucratic	Focuses on superior-subordinate communication transmitted from top to bottom via a clear chain of command	Care delivery and staffing are structured for efficient performance
	Uses rational, impersonal management	
	Uses merit and skill as bases for promotion/reward	
	Uses rules and regulations, focuses on exacting work processes and technical competence	
	Career service, salaried managers	
Human Relations	Focuses on the individual worker as the source of control, motivation, and productivity in organizations	Organization uses participatory problem solving with staff and managers
	Hawthorne studies at Western Electric plant in Chicago led to the belief that human relations between workers and managers and among workers were main determinants of efficiency	

(continues)

Table 1-2 *(continued)*

Perspective	Key Contributions	Effect on Opening Scenario
	The Hawthorne effect refers to change in behavior as a result of being watched	
	Participatory decision making increased worker autonomy and training to improve work	
Contingency	Organizational structure depends on the environment, task, technology, and the contingencies facing each unit	Uses flexible approach. Emphasizes that there is no one best way to manage people or work. It encourages managers to study individuals and the situation before adapting efforts and deciding on a course of action to meet the requirements of the situation
Resource Dependence	Emphasizes the need to secure necessary resources	Demonstrates the value of resources used by providing reliable and valid data on patient care processes and outcomes
Strategic Management	Achieves fit or alignment among the organization's strategy, external environment, and internal structure and capabilities	Links quality improvement efforts to core strategies and capabilities of the organization to meet patient and community needs
Population Ecology	External environmental pressures are primary determinant of success. There is little managers and staff can do if action is not tolerable to external environment	Highlights powerful role played by the external environment. Quality improvement efforts alone may not be sufficient if the organization is not well positioned for success in the environment

(continues)

Table 1-2 *(continued)*

Perspective	Key Contributions	Effect on Opening Scenario
Institutional	External norms, rules, and requirements cause organizations to conform in order to receive legitimacy. Organizations in a similar institutional environment come to resemble each other	Quality improvement efforts must take into account regulatory and accreditation pressures from local, state, and federal agencies and the Joint Commission on Accreditation of Healthcare Organizations (JCAHO), as well as taking into account public expectations
Learning Organization	Organization is always adapting and learning from the environment	Organization and staff maintain ongoing education
Management Science	Uses mathematical, statistical, and computer techniques to help with management decisions	Staff use computers for decisions and have more access to information
Systems Approach	Emphasizes that an organization is a system of interrelated parts and if a manager adjusts one part of a system, then other parts will be affected automatically. Emphasizes that the organization is an open system that constantly interacts with its environment	Encourages staff to look at their activities on one unit as part of a larger picture that may affect other units

Compiled with information from Shortell & Kaluzny, 2000.

STOP AND THINK

Review Table 1-2. Could any of these management perspectives help you to manage nursing care of a small group of patients on a clinical unit? How would a nurse manager of an entire nursing department apply any of these theories? Do you see any of Yukl's 13 managerial role functions illustrated by staff nurses on a clinical unit where you practice?

interested in creating change, influencing others, and managing performance and outcomes, it is helpful to understand the motivation that is reflected in a person's behavior. Motivation is a critical part of leadership because we need to understand each other in order to be good leaders and good followers.

There are process motivation theories and content motivation theories (Lussier, 1999). The process motivation theories are expectancy theory and equity theory. The content motivation theories include Maslow's need hierarchy, Aldefer's expectancy-relatedness-growth (ERG) theory, Herzberg's two-factor theory, and McClelland's manifest needs theory. Selected motivation theories are presented in Table 1-3.

DEFINITION OF LEADERSHIP

Leadership is commonly defined as a process of interaction in which the leader influences others toward goal achievement (Yukl, 1998).

TABLE 1-3
SELECTED MOTIVATION THEORIES

Main Contributors	Key Aspects
Abraham Maslow Hierarchy of Needs (1908–1970)	Motivation occurs when needs are not met. Certain needs have to be satisfied first, beginning with physiological needs then safety and security then social needs, followed by self-esteem needs and then self-actualization needs. Needs at one level must be satisfied before one is motivated by needs at the next higher level. See Figure 1-1.
Frederick Herzberg (1968) Two-factor theory	Hygiene maintenance factors include adequate salary, job security, and safe and tolerable working conditions. When these factors are absent, people are dissatisfied; when they are present, job dissatisfaction can be avoided. However, these factors alone will not motivate people.
	Motivation factors include satisfying and meaningful work, development and advancement opportunities, responsibility, and recognition. When these factors are present, people are motivated and satisfied with the job. When they are absent, people have a neutral attitude about the organization.
Douglas McGregor (1906-1964) Theory X	Theory X: leaders must direct and control as motivation results from reward and punishment. Employees prefer security, direction, and minimal responsibility and need coercion and threats to get the job done.
Theory Y	Theory Y: leaders must remove obstacles as workers have self-control, self-discipline; their reward is their involvement in work and in their opportunity to be creative.
William Ouchi (1981) Theory Z	Theory Z: collective decision making, long-term employment, mentoring, holistic concern, and use of quality circles to manage service and quality; a humanistic style of motivation based on Japanese organizations.

LITERATURE APPLICATION

Citation: Laborde, A. S., & Lee, J. A. (2000). Skills needed for promotion in the nursing profession. *Journal of Nursing Administration, 30*(9), 432-439.

Discussion: This research was designed to identify skills (interpersonal versus technical) needed for job promotion within the nursing field. As a nurse changes positions from primarily clinical practice to management, interpersonal skills seem to be more important than technical ones to move up the organizational ladder. Even though technical skills are necessary for those who supervise nurses, interpersonal skills become more important as tools to influence and lead others.

The hypotheses were as follows: more interpersonal skills would be important for promotion to upper-level management positions, whereas more technical skills would be important for promotion to lower-level management; a significant difference would exist between decision makers' perceptions of the importance of the skills and the skills' objective importance to promotion decisions. A stratified random sample of 219 nurse administrators was obtained from a large hospital in the southeastern United States. Sixty scenarios with hypothetical candidates were used to approximate the promotion situations. Hypothetical candidates were described in terms of their interpersonal and technical skills, and the participants were asked to decide how likely they would be to recommend this candidate for a promotion by using a Likert-type 5-point scale in which 1 was definitely not promote and 5 was definitely promote. No significant differences were found between the position and the number of interpersonal skills used. However, at the lower-level management position of clinical nurse 3 (CN3), a greater number of technical skills influenced promotion decisions more than for the middle management position.

Implications for Practice: The findings suggest that technical skills are more important for clinical nurse promotions than for nurse manager positions. The skills needed for success change as one moves from clinical practice to a managerial position. Several strategies were proposed to increase managerial effectiveness. A dual career ladder would provide a mechanism for retaining technical skills. It would give the employee a choice between developing technical skills and pursuing management. Succession planning may reduce the political influences and personal bias in the promotion process. Mentoring programs could provide valuable insights for new managers. Providing realistic job previews and complete job descriptions can clarify misunderstandings and reduce managerial burnout and turnover. Additional research is needed to improve management development programs for nurses and to evaluate designs for how managers are selected.

Influence is an instrumental part of leadership and means that leaders affect others, often by inspiring, enlivening, and engaging others to participate. The process of leadership involves the leader and the follower in interaction. This implies that leadership is a reciprocal relationship. Leadership can occur between the leader and another individual; between the leader and a group; or between a leader and an organization, a community, or a society. Defining leadership as a process helps us to understand more about leadership than the traditional view of a leader being in a position of authority, exerting command, control, and power over subordi-

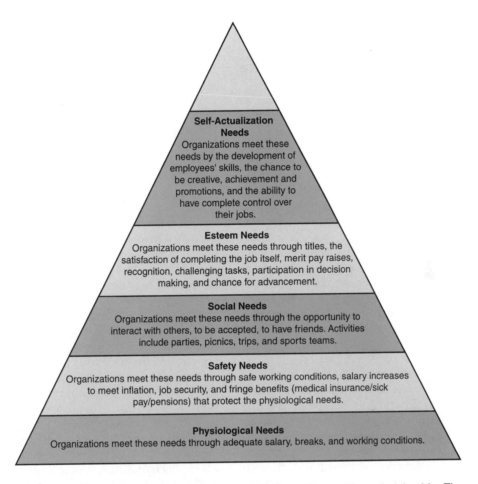

Self-Actualization Needs
Organizations meet these needs by the development of employees' skills, the chance to be creative, achievement and promotions, and the ability to have complete control over their jobs.

Esteem Needs
Organizations meet these needs through titles, the satisfaction of completing the job itself, merit pay raises, recognition, challenging tasks, participation in decision making, and chance for advancement.

Social Needs
Organizations meet these needs through the opportunity to interact with others, to be accepted, to have friends. Activities include parties, picnics, trips, and sports teams.

Safety Needs
Organizations meet these needs through safe working conditions, salary increases to meet inflation, job security, and fringe benefits (medical insurance/sick pay/pensions) that protect the physiological needs.

Physiological Needs
Organizations meet these needs through adequate salary, breaks, and working conditions.

Figure 1-1 How Organizations Motivate with Hierarchy of Needs Theory (From *Leadership: Theory, Application, Skill Building* [p. 81], by R. N. Lussier and C. F. Achua, 2001, Cincinnati, OH: South-Western College)

nates. What this means for nurses as professionals is that they function as leaders when they influence others toward goal achievement. Nurses are leaders. There are many more leaders in organizations than those who are in positions of authority. Each person has the potential to serve as a leader.

Today's nurse must know how to lead. Recall that leading is one of the four managerial functions along with planning, organizing and staffing, and controlling. Whereas management is more formal and relies on tools such as plan-

ning, budgeting, and controlling, leading involves having a vision and goals for what the organization can become, and then getting the cooperation and teamwork from others to achieve those goals (DuBrin, 2000).

As mentioned earlier, a beginning nurse uses less of the planning function when managing care for a small group of patients than does the experienced nurse manager of the unit or department. So, too, leadership ability grows in the beginning nurse who may demonstrate some leadership in working with other staff; for example, the new nurse speaks up about the need for improvement in an element of care delivery. Leadership ability often grows as the nurse becomes more confident and experienced in working with others.

Leadership can be formal leadership, as when a person is in a position of authority or in a sanctioned, assigned role within an organization that connotes influence, such as a clinical nurse specialist (Northouse, 2001). An informal leader is an individual who demonstrates leadership outside the scope of a formal leadership role or as a member of a group rather than as the head or leader of the group. Staff nurses demonstrate leadership when they advocate for patient needs or when they take action to improve health care. Nurses also demonstrate leadership when they speak up to improve quality of care.

Not all leaders are managers. Bennis's work on managers and leaders popularized the phrase, "Managers are people who do things right and leaders are people who do the right thing" (Bennis & Nanus, 1985, p. 21).

Kotter (1990a) describes the differences between leadership and management in the following way: Leadership is about creating change, and management is about controlling complexity in an effort to bring order and consistency. He says that leading change involves establishing a direction, aligning people through empowerment, and motivating and inspiring them toward producing useful change and achieving the vision, whereas management is defined as planning and budgeting, organizing and staffing, problem solving and controlling complexity to produce predictability and order (Kotter, 1990b).

Leadership Characteristics

According to Bennis and Nanus (1985), there are three fundamental qualities that effective leaders share. The first quality is a guiding vision. Leaders focus on a professional and purposeful vision that provides direction toward the pre-

ferred future. The second quality is passion. Passion expressed by the leader involves the ability to inspire and align people toward the promises of life. The third quality is integrity that is based on knowledge of self, honesty, and maturity that is developed through experience and growth. McCall (1998) describes how self-awareness—knowing our strengths and weaknesses—can allow us to use feedback and learn from our mistakes. Daring and curiosity are also basic ingredients of leadership from which leaders draw on to take risks, learning from what works as much as from what does not (Bennis & Nanus, 1985).

Certain characteristics are commonly attributed to leaders. These traits are considered desirable and seem to contribute to the perception of being a leader. They include intelligence, self-confidence, determination, integrity, and sociability (Stodgill, 1948, 1974). Research among 46 hospitals designated as magnet hospitals for their success in attracting and retaining registered nurses emphasized the value of leaders who are visionary and enthusiastic, are supportive and knowledgeable, have high standards and expectations, value education and professional development, demonstrate power and status in the organization, are visible and responsive, communicate openly, and are active in professional associations (Scott, Sochalski, & Aiken, 1999; McClure, Poulin, Sovie, & Wandelt, 1983; Kramer & Schmalenberg, 1988). Research findings from studies on nurses revealed that caring, respectability, trustworthiness, and flexibility were the leader characteristics most valued. In one study, nurse leaders identified managing the dream, mastering change, designing organization structure, learning, and taking initiative as leadership characteristics (Murphy & DeBack, 1991). Research by Kirkpatrick and Locke (1991) concluded that leaders are different from nonleaders across six traits: drive, the desire to lead, honesty and integrity, self-confidence, cognitive ability, and knowledge of the business. It is important to remember that there is no set of traits that is definitive and reliable in determining who is a leader and who is not and that leadership can be learned.

Leadership Theories

The major leadership theories can be classified according to the following approaches: behavioral, contingency, and contemporary.

Behavioral Approach

Leadership studies from the 1930s by Kurt Lewin and colleagues at Iowa State University conveyed information about three leadership styles that are still widely recognized today. The three styles are autocratic, democratic, and laissez-faire leadership (Lewin, 1939; Lewin & Lippitt, 1938; Lewin, Lippitt, & White, 1939).

Autocratic, Democratic, and Laissez-faire Leadership. Autocratic leadership involves centralized decision making, with the leader making decisions and using power to command and control others. The *autocratic* style is used by the leader in situations in which (1) the task or outcome is relatively simple (e.g., telling the unlicensed assistive personnel (UAP) to take a temperature); (2) most team members would agree with the decision and provide consensus; and (3) a decision has to be made promptly.

Democratic leadership is participatory, with authority often delegated to others. To be influential, the democratic leader uses expert power and the power base afforded by having close, personal relationships. In the *democratic* style, the leader will ask the opinions of the entire team, but the final decision usually lies with the leader, or there may be mutual decision making by both team members and the leader, with everyone having an equal vote. This process encourages everyone to fully accept the team's conclusion. This mutual style may be the most creative because all have the opportunity to provide input and differing perspectives into the decision.

The third style, laissez-faire leadership, is passive and permissive and the leader defers decision making. Lewin (1939) contrasted these styles and concluded that autocratic leaders were associated with high-performing groups but that close supervision was necessary and feelings of hostility were often present. Democratic leaders engendered positive feelings in their groups and performance was strong whether or not the leader was present. Low productivity and feelings of frustration were associated with laissez-faire leaders.

Employee-Centered and Job Centered Leaders. Behavioral leadership studies from the University of Michigan and from Ohio State University led to the identification of two basic leader behaviors: job-centered and employee-centered behaviors. Effective leadership was described as having a focus on the human needs of subordinates and was called employee-centered leadership (Moorhead & Griffin, 2001). Job-centered leaders were seen as less effective because of their focus on schedules, costs, and efficiency, resulting in a lack of attention to developing work groups and high-performance goals (Moorhead & Griffin, 2001).

The researchers at Ohio State focused their efforts on two dimensions of leader behavior: initiating structure and consideration. Initiating structure involves an emphasis on the work to be done, a focus on the task and production. Leaders who focus on initiating structure are concerned with how work is organized and on the achievement of goals. Leader behavior includes planning, directing others, and establishing deadlines and details of how work is to be done. For example, a nurse demonstrating the leader behavior of initiating structure could be a nurse who, at the beginning of a shift, makes out a patient assignment delegating care to the UAP.

The dimension of consideration involves activities that focus on the employee and emphasize relating and getting along with people. Leader behavior focuses on the well-being of others. The leader is involved in creating a relationship that fosters communication and trust as a basis for respecting other people and their potential contribution. A staff nurse demonstrating consideration behavior will take the time to talk with coworkers, be empathetic, and show an interest in them as people.

CASE STUDY 1-1

Among the individuals commonly identified as leaders (Table 1-4), can you identify a set of traits that they all possess or traits that are associated with them?

Table 1-4 Leaders Among Us: Past and Present

Mother Theresa	Martin Luther King
Imogene King	John F. Kennedy
Hildegard Peplau	Sister Callista Roy
Joyce Ellis	Franklin Delano Roosevelt
Rosa Parks	Dorothea Orem
John Adams	Florence Nightingale
Colin Powell	Betty Neuman
Pope John Paul II	George Washington
Myra Levine	Virginia Henderson
Clara Barton	Martha Rogers
Margaret Thatcher	Alexander the Great
Dorothy Johnson	Zenaida Corpuz
Winston Churchill	Lydia Hall

Now divide your class into groups. Have each group identify a nurse or someone who they see as a leader. Describe the leader's characteristics and then have the groups share with the class who the leaders are and their characteristics. Are the leaders identified also managers? How are managers and leaders different? When you work on the clinical unit, do you see any staff nurses displaying management and/or leadership actions? How can you develop these skills in yourself?

The leader behaviors of initiating structure and consideration define leadership style. The styles are nurses who use:

- Low initiating structure, low consideration
- High initiating structure, low consideration
- High initiating structure, high consideration
- Low initiating structure, high consideration

The Ohio State University studies associate the high initiating structure–high consideration leader behaviors with better performance and satisfaction outcomes than the other styles.

Nurses who use high initiating structure and high consideration leader behaviors will initiate and develop clear, well-structured assignments and work considerately with their staff to achieve quality outcomes.

Another model based on these two dimensions is the managerial grid developed by Blake, Mouton, and McCanse (2001). Five styles identify the extent of structure, called concern for production, and consideration, called concern for people, demonstrated by the leader. The five leader styles are impoverished leader (1,1) for low production and people concern; authority compliance leader (9,1) for high production concern and low people concern; country club leader (1,9) for high people concern but low production concern; middle-of-the-road leader (5,5) for moderate concern in both dimensions; and team leader (9,9) for high production and people concern. Figure 1-2 shows the Leadership Grid with the dimensions of people and production from low to high on a scale from 1 to 9. Team leader (9,9) is usually an effective leadership approach because it emphasizes both concern for people and concern for production.

Contingency Approaches

Another approach to leadership is **contingency theory**. Contingency theory acknowledges that different leader behavior patterns will be effective in different situations (Fielder, 1967; Hersey & Blanchard, 2000; House, 1971; Kerr & Jermier, 1978). Contingency approaches emphasize the need for nurses to demonstrate leadership and change their approach to situations by evaluating the needs of patients, the environment, and the staff on an ongoing basis. Nurse leaders adjust their leadership approach to meet the needs of the situation.

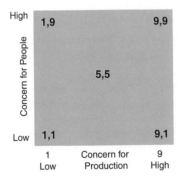

Figure 1-2 Blake, Mouton, and McCanse Leadership Grid (From *Leadership: Theory Application, Skill Building* [p. 75], by R.N. Lussier and C.F. Achua, 2001, Cincinnati, OH: South-Western College)

Follower Readiness. Hersey and Blanchard consider follower readiness as a factor in determining leadership style and examine *task behavior* and *relationship behavior*.

High task behavior and low relationship behavior are called a telling leadership style. A high task, high relationship style is called a selling leadership style. A low task and high relationship style is called a participating leadership style. A low task and low relationship style is called a delegating leadership style.

Follower readiness, called maturity, is assessed in order to select one of the four leadership styles for a situation. For example, groups with low maturity whose members are unable or unwilling to participate or are unsure need a leader to use a telling leadership style to provide direction and close supervision. For example, the nurse who tells the newly certified UAP to take a patient's temperature *now* is using a telling style.

The selling leadership style is a match for groups with low to moderate maturity who are unable but willing and confident and need clear direction and supportive feedback to get the task done. For example, the charge nurse who tells a new nurse to pass medications and then remains available to help with the medications, as needed, is using a selling style.

Participating is the leadership style recommended for groups with moderate to high maturity who are able but unwilling or are unsure and who need support and encouragement. For example, the charge nurse who asks staff to help decide the best ways to do a task is using a participating style.

The leader should use a delegating style with groups of followers with high maturity who are able and ready to participate and can engage in the task without direction or support. For example, the charge nurse who asks the experienced nurse to pass medication without help is using a delegating style.

An additional aspect of this approach is the idea that the leader not only changes leadership style according to followers' needs but also develops followers over time to increase their level of maturity (Lussier & Achua, 2001).

Contemporary Approaches

Contemporary approaches to leadership address the leadership functions necessary to develop learning organizations and lead the process of transforming change. These approaches include charismatic leadership and transformational leadership theory.

Charismatic Theory. A charismatic leader has an inspirational quality that promotes an emotional connection from followers. House (1977) developed a theory of charismatic leadership that described how charismatic leaders behave as well as distinguishing characteristics and situations in which such leaders would be effective. Charismatic leaders display self-confidence, strength in their convictions, and communicate high expectations and their confidence in others. They have been described as emerging during a crisis, communicating vision, and using personal power and unconventional strategies (Conger & Kanungo, 1987). One consequence of this type of leadership is a belief in the charismatic leader that is so strong it takes on an almost supernatural purpose and the leader is worshipped as if superhuman. Examples of charismatic leaders include Winston Churchill and Lee Iacocca, former chief executive officer (CEO) of Chrysler Corporation. Charisma seems to be a special and valuable quality that some people have and some people do not.

Transformational Leadership Theory. Burns (1978) defined transformational leadership as a process in which "leaders and followers raise one another to higher levels of motivation and morality" (p. 21). Transformational leadership theory is based on the idea of empowering others to engage in pursuing a collective purpose by working together to achieve a vision of a preferred future. This kind of leadership can influence both the leader and the follower to a higher level of conduct and achievement that transforms them both (Burns, 1978). Burns maintained that there are two types of leaders: the traditional manager concerned with day-to-day operations, called the transactional leader, and the leader who is committed to a vision that empowers others, called the transformational leader.

Transformational leaders motivate others by behaving in accordance with values, providing a vision that reflects mutual values, and empowering others to contribute. Bennis and Nanus (1985) describe this new leader as a leader who "commits people to action, who converts followers into leaders, and who converts leaders into agents of change" (p. 3). According to research by Tichy and Devanna (1986), effective transformational leaders identify themselves as change agents; are courageous; believe in people; are value driven; are lifelong learners; have the ability to deal with complexity, ambiguity, and uncertainty; and are visionaries. Yet transformational leadership may be demonstrated by anyone in an organization regardless of position

STOP AND THINK

As the nurse enters the room of a new postoperative patient with a laryngectomy, the patient begins to bleed from his neck incision. The nurse applies direct pressure with one hand and calls for assistance. Help arrives and the patient is taken to surgery with the nurse still maintaining pressure on the bleeding site. The patient lives and goes home a few days later.

How does good management on a patient care unit ensure good patient care in an emergency?

How can you develop good management skills to improve your ability to care for a group of patients?

(Burns, 1978). The interaction that occurs between individuals can be transformational and motivate both to a higher level of performance (Bass, 1985).

Transformational leadership at the organizational level is about innovation and change. The transformational leader uses vision based on shared values to align people and inspire growth and advancement. It is both the inspiration and the empowerment aspects of transformational leadership that lead to commitment beyond self-interest, commitment to a vision, and commitment to action that creates change. Transformational leadership theory suggests that the relationship between the leader and the follower inspires and empowers an individual toward commitment to the organization.

Nurse researchers have described nurse executives according to transformational leadership theory and have used this theory to measure leadership behavior among nurse executives and nurse managers (Leach, 2000; McNeese-Smith, 1995; Dunham-Taylor, 1995, 2000; Trofino, 1995; Wolf, Boland, & Aukerman, 1994; McDaniel & Wolf, 1992; Young, 1992; Dunham & Klafehn, 1990). Additionally, transformational leadership theory has been the basis for nursing administration curriculum and for investigation of relationships such as between a nurse's commitment to an organization and productivity in a hospital setting (Leach, 2000; McNeese-Smith, 1997; Searle, 1996). Cassidy and Koroll (1998) explored the ethical aspects of transformational leadership, and Barker (1990) comprehensively discussed nursing in terms of transformational leadership theory.

FUTURE DIRECTIONS

The organizations that nurses are a part of are changing. They reflect the advance and the promise of the technology that enables us to perform our work. Peter Drucker (1994) identifies the organization of the future as a knowledge organization composed of knowledge workers. Knowledge workers are those who bring specialized, expert knowledge to an organization.

They are valued for what they know. The knowledge organization will share, provide, and grow the information necessary to work efficiently and effectively. Drucker says that knowledge organizations, in which the knowledge worker is at the front lines with the expertise and the information to act, will be the dominant organizational type (Drucker, 1994; Helgesen, 1995). In organizations such as these, the ideas of leadership at the top and leadership equated with the power of a position are obsolete notions. Workers with the expertise and information to act are the organization's leaders. They provide the service, interact with the customer, represent the organization, and accomplish its goals. Leadership is needed at all levels within such an organization, not just at the top and not just with certain positions in the organization. Every nurse plays a role in fulfilling the purpose of the organization and in so doing is both a leader and a follower.

Chaos, Complexity, and Self-Organizing Systems

Margaret Wheatley, in *Leadership and the New Science* (1992), says, "There is a simpler way to lead organizations, one that requires less effort and produces less stress than the current practices" (p. 3). She presents us with a new view of leadership, one encompassing connectedness and self-organizing systems that follow a natural order of both chaos and uncertainty, which is different from a linear order in a hierarchy. The leader's function is to guide an organization using vision, to make choices based on mutual values, and to engage in the culture to provide meaning and coherence. This type of leadership fosters growth within each of us as individuals and as members of a group. The notion of connection within a self-organizing system optimizes autonomy at all levels because the relationships between the individual and the whole are strong (Wheatley, 1992). The nurse in a self-organizing system takes personal responsibility for growth and for assisting others to grow in their ability to function in a health care system.

REAL WORLD INTERVIEW

Leadership in nursing is probably one of the more personal forms of leadership. Nursing is one of the most intimate leadership relationships because of the vulnerability the patient brings to the relationship. With patients who are dying or in terrible situations, the nurse provides them with two vital leadership characteristics: optimism and courage. With patients who have lost their courage, it is the nurse who shows courage and strength that supports a patient and their family. Optimism and courage are the trademarks of great leaders. Nurses lead the patient, their family, their nurse colleagues, and other health care providers. They have the courage to care in the face of fear and uncertainly, and in the face of disability or in death. Caring, hope, and support are a source of optimism that nurses provide. There are very few professions where you touch an individual's life so profoundly.

Jay Conger, PhD
Author, Learning to Lead

KEY CONCEPTS

- Nurses are leaders and make a difference to health care organizations through their contributions of expert knowledge and leadership. Leadership development is a necessary component of preparation as a health care provider.
- Management is a process used to achieve organizational goals. It involves the management functions of planning, organizing and staffing, leading and controlling. There are many theories of management.
- Motivation is an internal process that contributes to our behavior in an effort to satisfy our needs. Maslow's hierarchy of needs reflects the belief that the needs that motivate us have an order, and lower-level needs have to be satisfied first or we will not be motivated to address higher-level needs. Herzberg's two-factor theory of motivation identifies maintenance factors, such as security and salary, that are needed to prevent job dissatisfaction, and motivators, such as development and opportunities to advance, that contribute to job satisfaction.
- Leadership is a process of influence in which the leader influences others toward goal achievement. Leadership can be formal and informal, occurring by being in a position of authority in an organization, such as manager, or leadership can occur outside the scope of a formal role, such as demonstrating leadership to achieve a patient's goals.
- Leadership and management are different.
- Nursing leadership in the future will be needed at all levels within an organization, not just at the top. Every knowledge worker, with specialized knowledge and expertise, will be both a leader and a follower in knowledge organizations.
- Organizations are viewed as self-organizing systems in which, initially, what looks like chaos and uncertainty is indeed part of a larger coherence and a natural order.

KEY TERMS

autocratic leadership
consideration
contingency theory
democratic
  leadership
employee-centered
  leadership
formal leadership
informal leader
initiating structure

job-centered leaders
knowledge workers
laissez-faire
  leadership
leadership
management
motivation
role
transactional leader
transformational
  leader

REVIEW QUESTIONS

1. Why is leadership important for nurses if they are not in a management position?
   A. It is not really important for nurses.
   B. Leadership is important at all levels in an organization because nurses have expert knowledge and are interacting with and influencing the customer.
   C. Nurse leaders leave their jobs sooner for other positions.
   D. Nurses who lead are less satisfied in their jobs.

2. Management as a process that is used today by nurses in health care organizations is best described as
   A. scientific management.
   B. decision making.
   C. commanding and controlling others using hierarchical authority.
   D. planning, organizing and staffing, leading, and controlling.

3. Motivation is whatever influences our choices. What factors did Herzberg say would motivate workers and lead to job satisfaction?
   A. Being offered a substantial bonus when being hired

B. Realizing that no one ever gets fired from the organization and that job security is high
   C. Having good relationships with colleagues and supervisors
   D. Being offered opportunities for development and advancement

4. Leadership is defined as
   A. being in a leadership position with authority to exert control and power over subordinates.
   B. a process of interaction in which the leader influences others toward goal achievement.
   C. managing complexity.
   D. being self-confident and democratic.

REVIEW ACTIVITIES

1. Take the opportunity to learn about yourself by reflecting on five predominant factors identified as being influential in a nurse's leadership development: self-confidence, innate leader qualities/tendencies, progression of experiences and success, influence of significant others, and personal life factors. Consider what reinforces your confidence in yourself. What innate qualities or tendencies do you have that contribute to your development as a nurse leader? Consider what professional experiences, mentors, and personal experiences or events can help you develop your leadership ability. How can you provide these experiences?

2. Describe the type of manager you want to be as a staff nurse in a health care organization. Identify specific behaviors you plan to use to manage a patient's care. How will you plan, organize and staff, lead, and control patient care?

3. Rate each of these 12 job factors that contribute to job satisfaction by placing a number from 1 to 5 on the line before each factor.

Very important		Somewhat important		Not important
5	4	3	2	1

_____ 1. An interesting job I enjoy doing

_____ 2. A good manager who treats people fairly

_____ 3. Getting praise and other recognition and appreciation for the work I do

_____ 4. A satisfying personal life at the job

_____ 5. The opportunity for advancement

_____ 6. A prestigious or status job

_____ 7. Job responsibility that gives me freedom to do things my way

_____ 8. Good working conditions (safe environment, nice office, cafeteria)

_____ 9. The opportunity to learn new things

_____10. Sensible company rules, regulations, procedures, and policies

_____11. A job I can do well and succeed at

_____12. Job security and benefits

Write the number from 1 to 5 that you selected for each factor. Total each column for a score between 6 and 30 points. The closer to 30 your score is, the more important the factor (motivating or maintenance) is to you.

Motivating factors		Maintenance factors	
1.	_____	2.	_____
3.	_____	4.	_____
5.	_____	6.	_____
7.	_____	8.	_____
9.	_____	10.	_____
11.	_____	12.	_____
Totals	_____		_____

From *Leadership: Theory, Application, Skill Development* (pp. 15–16), by R. N. Lussier and C. F. Achua, 2001, Cincinnati, OH: South-Western College Publishing.

EXPLORING THE WEB

Search the Web, checking the following sites.

- Emerging Leader:
  http://www.emergingleader.com
- Leadership Directories: Who's who in the leadership of the United States:
  http://www.leadershipdirectories.com
- Health Leadership Associates:
  http://www.healthleadership.com
- Population Leadership Program:
  http://www.popldr.org
- Leadership Knowledge Base: Information to Improve Your Leadership Skills:
  http://www.sonic.net

REFERENCES

Barker, A. (1990). *Transformational nursing leadership: A vision for the future*. Baltimore: Williams & Wilkins.

Bass, B. (1985). *Leadership and performance beyond expectations*. New York: Free Press.

Benner, P. (1984). *From Novice to Expert*. Menlo Park, CA: Addison Wesley.

Bennis, W., & Nanus, B. (1985). *Leaders: The strategies for taking charge*. New York: Harper & Row.

Blake, R. R., Mouton, J. S., & McCanse. From Leadership, Theory, Application and Skill Development, 1st Edition by Lussier/Achua © 2001. South Western, a division of Thomson Learning.

Burns, J. M. (1978). *Leadership*. New York: Harper & Row.

Cassidy, V., & Koroll, C. (1998). Ethical aspects of transformational leadership. In E. Hein (Ed.), *Contemporary leadership behavior:*

Selected readings (5th ed., pp. 79–82). Philadelphia: Lippincott.

Conger, J., & Kanungo, R. (1987). Toward a behavioral theory of charismatic leadership in organizational settings. *Academy of Management Review, 12*, 637–647.

DeCrane, A., Jr. (1996). A constitutional model of leadership. In F. Hesselbein, M. Goldsmith, & R. Beckhard (Eds.), *The leader of the future: New visions, strategies, and practices for the next era* (pp. 249–256). San Francisco: Jossey-Bass.

Dreyfus, S. E., & Dreyfus, H. L. (1980). *A five stage model of the mental activities involved in direct skill acquisition.* Unpublished report supported by the Air Force Office of Scientific Research USAF (Contract F49620-79-C-0063). University of California at Berkeley.

Drucker, P. F. (1994). *The post-capitalist society.* New York: Harper & Row.

Dubrin, A. J. (2000). *The Active Manager.* Cincinatti, OH: South Western College Publishing.

Dunham, J., & Klafehn, K. A. (1990). Transformational leadership and the nurse executive. *Journal of Nursing Administration, 20*(4), 28–34.

Dunham-Taylor, J. (1995). Identifying the best in nurse executive leadership: Part 2, interview results. *Journal of Nursing Administration, 25*(7/8), 24–31.

Dunham-Taylor, J. (2000). Nurse executive transformational leadership found in participative organizations. *Journal of Nursing Administration, 30*(5), 241–250.

Fielder, F. (1967). *A theory of leadership effectiveness.* New York: McGraw-Hill.

Helgesen, S. (1995). *The web of inclusion: A new architecture for building organizations.* New York: Doubleday Currency.

Hersey, P., & Blanchard, K. (2000). *Management of organizational behavior* (8th ed.). Englewood Cliffs, NJ: Prentice Hall.

Herzberg, F. (1968, January/February). One more time: How do you motivate employees? Harvard Business Review, 53–62.

House, R. H. (1971). A path-goal theory of leader effectiveness. *Administrative Science Quarterly, 16*, 321–338.

House, R. H. (1977). A 1976 theory of charismatic leadership. In J. Hunt & L. Larson (Eds.), *Leadership: The cutting edge* (pp. 21–26). Carbondale, IL: Southern Illinois University Press.

Hughes, R. L., Ginnett, R. C., & Curphy, G. J. (1999). *Leadership: Enhancing the lessons of experience* (3rd ed.). San Francisco: Irwin McGraw-Hill.

Kanfer, R. (1990). Motivation theory in industrial and organizational psychology. In M. D. Dunnette & L. M. Hough (Eds.), *Handbook of industrial and organizational psychology: Vol. 1* (pp. 53–68). Palo Alto, CA: Consulting Psychologists Press.

Katz, D., & Kahn, R. L. (1978). *The social psychology of organizations* (2nd ed.). New York: John Wiley.

Kerr, S., & Jermier, J. (1978). Substitutes for leadership: Their meaning and measurement. *Organizational Behavior and Human Performance, 22*, 374–403.

Kim, H., & Yukl, G. (1995). Relationships of self-reported and subordinate-reported leadership behaviors to managerial effectiveness and advancement. *Leadership Quarterly, 6*, 361–377.

Kirkpatrick, S. A., & Locke, E. A. (1991). Leadership: Do traits matter? *The Executive, 5*, 48–60.

Kotter, J. (1990a). *A force for change: How leadership differs from management.* Glencoe, IL: Free Press.

Kotter, J. (1990b). What leaders really do. *Harvard Business Review, 68*, 104.

Kramer, M., & Schmalenberg, C. (1988). Magnet hospitals: Part II institutions of excellence. *Journal of Nursing Administration, 18*(2), (pp. 11–19).

Laborde, A. S., & Lee, J. A. (2000). Skills needed for promotion in the nursing profession. *Journal of Nursing Administration, 30*(9), 432–439.

Leach, L. S. (2000). *Nurse executive leadership and the relationship to organizational commitment among nurses.* Unpublished doctoral dissertation, University of Southern California, Los Angeles.

Lewin, K. (1939). Field theory and experiment in social psychology: Concepts and methods. *Journal of Sociology, 44,* 868–896.

Lewin, K., & Lippitt, R. (1938). An experimental approach to the study of autocracy and democracy: A preliminary note. *Sociometry, 1,* 292–300.

Lewin, K., Lippitt, R., & White, R. (1939). Patterns of aggressive behavior in experimentally created social climates. *Journal of Social Psychology, 10,* 271–299.

Lussier, R. N. (1999). *Human relations in organizations: Applications and skill building* (4th ed.). San Francisco: Irwin McGraw-Hill.

Lussier, R. N., & Achua, C. F. (2001). *Leadership: Theory, application, skill development.* Cincinnati, OH: South-Western College.

Maslow, A. (1970). *Motivation and personality* (2nd ed.). New York: Harper & Row.

McCall, M. W., Jr. (1998). *High flyers: Developing the next generation of leaders.* Boston: Harvard Business School Press.

McCall, M. W., Jr., Morrison, A. M., & Hanman, R. L. (1978). *Studies of managerial work: Results and methods* (Tech. Rep.). Greensboro, NC: Center for Creative Leadership.

McClure, M., Poulin, M., Sovie, M., & Wandelt, M. (1983). *Magnet hospitals: Attraction and retention of professional nurses.* Kansas City, MO: American Nurses Association.

McDaniel, C., & Wolf, G. (1992). Transformational leadership in nursing service. *Journal of Nursing Administration,12*(4), 204–207.

McGregor, D. (1960). *The human side of enterprise.* New York: McGraw-Hill.

McNeese-Smith, D. (1995). Job satisfaction, productivity, and organizational commitment: The result of leadership. *Journal of Nursing Administration, 25*(9), 17–26.

McNeese-Smith, D. (1997). The influences of manager behavior on nurses' job satisfaction, productivity, and commitment. *Journal of Nursing Administration, 27*(9), 47–55.

Mintzberg, H. (1973). *The nature of managerial work.* New York: Harper & Row.

Moorhead, G., & Griffin, R. W. (2001). *Organizational behavior: Managing people in organizations* (6th ed.). Boston: Houghton Mifflin.

Murphy, M., & DeBack, V. (1991). Today's nursing leaders: Creating the vision. *Nursing Administration Quarterly, 16*(1), 71–80.

Northouse, P. (2001). *Leadership: Theory and practice* (2nd ed.). Thousand Oaks, CA: Sage.

Ouchi, W. (1981). *Theory Z: How American business can meet the Japanese challenge.* Reading, MA: Addison-Wesley.

Pew Health Professions Commission. (1995). *Critical challenges: Revitalizing the health professions for the 21st century.* San Francisco: UCSF Center for the Health Professions.

Scott, J. G., Sochalski, J., & Aiken, L. (1999). Review of magnet hospital research: Findings and implications for professional nursing practice. *Journal of Nursing Administration 29*(1), 9–19.

Searle, L. (1996, January). 21st century leadership for nurse administrators. *Aspen's advisor for nurse executives, 11*(4), 1, 4–6.

Shortell, S. M., & Kaluzny, A. D. (1997). *Essentials of Health Care Management.* Clifton Park, NY: Delmar Learning.

Shortell, S. M., & Kaluzny, A. D. (2000). *Health Care Management.* Clifton Park, NY: Delmar Learning.

Stodgill, R. M. (1948). Personal factors associated with leadership: A survey of the literature. *Journal of Psychology, 25,* 35–71.

Stodgill, R. M. (1974). *Handbook of leadership: A survey of theory and research.* New York: Free Press.

Tichy, N., & Devanna, D. (1986). *Transformational leadership.* New York: Wiley.

Trofino, J. (1995). Transformational leadership in health care. *Nursing Management, 26*(8), 42–47.

Wheatley, M. J. (1992). *Leadership and the new science: Learning about organization from an orderly universe.* San Francisco: Berrett-Koehler.

Wolf, G., Boland, S., & Aukerman, M. (1994). A transformational model for the practice of professional nursing. Part 1. *Journal of Nursing Administration, 24*(4), 51–57.

Young, S. (1992). Educational experiences of transformational nurse leaders. *Nursing Administration Quarterly, 17*(1), 25–33.

Yukl, G. (1998). *Leadership in organizations* (4th ed.). Upper Saddle River, NJ: Prentice Hall.

Yukl, G., Wall, S., & Lepsinger, R. (1990). Preliminary report on validation of the managerial practices survey. In K. E. Clarke & M. B. Clark (Eds.), *Measures of leadership* (pp. 223–238). West Orange, NJ: Leadership Library of America.

SUGGESTED READINGS

Avolio, B. (1999). *Full leadership development: Building the vital forces in organizations.* Thousand Oaks, CA: Sage.

Bass, B. (1998). *Transformational leadership: Industrial, military, and educational impact.* Mahwah, NJ: Erlbaum.

Bower, F. L. (2000). *Nurses taking the lead: Personal qualities of effective leadership.* Philadelphia: Saunders.

Buerhaus, P. I. (2000). Implications of an aging registered nurse workforce. *Journal of the American Medical Association, 283,* 2948–2954.

Conger, J., & Spreitzer, G. (Eds). (1992). *Learning to Lead.* San Francisco: Jossey Bass.

Cronin, S. N., & Bechere, D. (1999). Recognition of staff nurse job performance and achievements: Staff and manager perceptions. *Journal of Nursing Administration, 29*(1), 26–31.

Kanges, S., Kee, C. C., & McKee-Waddle, R. (1999). Organizational factors, nurses' job satisfaction and patient satisfaction with nursing care. *Journal of Nursing Administration, 29*(1), 32–42.

Levi, P. (1999). Sustainability of healthcare environments. *Image: Journal of Nursing Scholarship, 31*(4), 395–398.

Likert, R. (1967). *The human organization: Its management and value.* New York: McGraw-Hill.

O'Neil, E., & Coffman, J. (Eds.). (1998). *Strategies for the future of nursing: Changing roles, responsibilities, and employment patterns of registered nurses.* San Francisco: Jossey-Bass.

Parse, R. (1997). Leadership: The essentials. *Nursing Science Quarterly, 10*(3), 109.

Santos, S. R., & Cox, K. (2000). Workplace adjustment and intergenerational differences between matures, boomers, and Xers. *Nursing Economic$, 18*(1), 7–13.

Senge, P. (1990, Fall). The leader's new work: Building learning organizations. *Sloan Management Review,* 7–22.

Urwick, L. (1944). *The elements of administration.* New York: Harper & Row.

Vroom, V. H. (1964). *Work and motivation.* New York: McGraw-Hill.

Zalenik, K. A. (1977). Managers and leaders: Are they different? *Harvard Business Review, 55*(5), 67–80.

CHAPTER 2

Nursing Today

> For us who Nurse, our Nursing is a thing, which, unless in it we are making progress every year, every month, every week, take my word for it, we are going back. (Florence Nightingale, 1872)

OBJECTIVES

Upon completion of this chapter, the reader should be able to:

1. Identify the role of nursing today.
2. Discuss the Pew Health Professions Commission's Report.
3. Discuss evidence-based practice.
4. Discuss use of research in nursing today.
5. Discuss health care variation.
6. Identify health care stakeholders.
7. Review major subcultures of health care professionals.
8. Review the movement toward population-based health care.
9. Review Joint Commission on Accreditation of Healthcare Organizations (JCAHO) accreditation standards.

You stop to eat at a local restaurant and see an old friend and her husband. They tell you they had to take their 2-year-old boy to the Emergency Department that past week for a temperature of 104°. Though the boy is better now, they are worried about the hospital bill. They are both working but have not been able to afford health insurance. This scene occurs over and over again in today's health care environment as Americans struggle to find a way to ensure access to cost-effective, quality care for all.

What are your thoughts about this situation?

What advice do you have for your friend?

How can nursing today improve and advocate for better health care for patients?

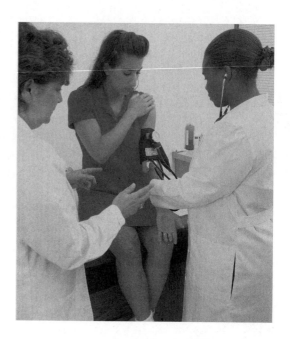

Health care delivery in the United States is a combination of public and private initiatives organized to provide citizens with access to cost-effective, quality health care. Most Americans are in good health, but many citizens are children, elderly, sick, disabled, or otherwise in need of access to quality health care services at a reasonable cost. The need for access, quality, and cost-effectiveness has driven various initiatives to improve health care in the past and present.

Nurses must be prepared to deal with these health care initiatives both today and in the future. The Pew Health Professions Commission has identified 21 competencies that health care practitioners of the future must have in order to continue to meet patient needs. This chapter addresses some of these competencies. Evidence-based care, population-based care, and health care variation are discussed. Leaders in nursing, the role of health care stakeholders, including the Joint Commission on Accreditation of Healthcare Organizations (JCAHO), and other forces influencing health care delivery today also are discussed.

NURSING TODAY

Nursing is recognized as a profession in most circles today, although in the late 1990s, many nurses still reported "knowing the right thing to do and having no support or authority to carry it out" (Aroskar, 1998). In order to continue to grow as a profession in the 21st century, the PEW Health Professions Competencies (O'Neil & the Pew Health Professions Commission, 1998) offers guidance. See Table 2-1. Several of the competencies identified are discussed in this chapter.

Transdisciplinary Nursing

Health needs of the future will require a professional nurse who can demonstrate caring, competency, and practice in a transdisciplinary fashion. Transdisciplinary practice brings nurses to the table with more-equal footing and diminishes the notion that the team needs a captain to function. With each discipline bringing its unique talents to the job of providing care for a patient and that patient's family, transdisciplinary practice removes the gatekeeper and allows patients access to all caregivers based on what expertise is needed. Success in transdisciplinary practice will depend on each profession maintaining the

TABLE 2-1
PEW HEALTH PROFESSIONS 21 COMPETENCIES

1. Embrace a personal ethic of social responsibility and service.
2. Exhibit ethical behavior in all professional activities.
3. Provide evidence-based clinically competent care.
4. Incorporate the multiple determinants of health in clinical care.
5. Apply knowledge of the new sciences.
6. Demonstrate critical thinking, reflection, and problem-solving skills.
7. Understand the role of primary care.
8. Rigorously practice preventive health care.
9. Integrate population-based care and services into practices.
10. Improve access to health care for those with unmet health needs.
11. Practice relationship-centered care with individuals and families.
12. Provide culturally sensitive care to a diverse society.
13. Partner with communities in health care decisions.
14. Use communication and information technology effectively and appropriately.
15. Work in interdisciplinary teams.
16. Ensure care that balances individual, professional, system, and societal needs.
17. Practice leadership.
18. Take responsibility for quality of care and health outcomes at all levels.
19. Contribute to continuous improvement of the health care system.
20. Advocate for public policy that promotes and protects the health of the public.
21. Continue to learn and help others learn.

O'Neil, E. H., and the Pew Health Professions Commission, *Twenty-One Competencies for the Twenty-First Century.* San Francisco, CA: Pew Health Professions Commission. December, 1998.

highest standards, including expectations of advanced education, some sort of certification, and requirements for continuing education to maintain competency (Carroll-Johnson, 2001). Transdisciplinary practice also requires that nurses utilize current research and evidence in improving care delivery for their patients.

Evidence-Based Practice

Evidence-based practice (EBP) is defined as the conscientious, explicit, and judicious use of current best evidence in making decisions about the care of individual patients (Sackett, Rosenberg, Gray, Haynes, & Richardson, 1996). EBP uses outcomes research and other current research findings to guide the development of appropriate strategies to deliver quality, cost-effective care. Outcomes provide evidence about benefits, risks, and results of treatments so individuals can make informed decisions and choices to improve their quality of life.

Nursing-oriented sources for EBP include the *Online Journal of Knowledge Synthesis for Nursing* from Sigma Theta Tau International, a journal from the United Kingdom called *Evidence-Based Nursing: Linking Research to Practice*, *Nursing Research, Evidence Based Nursing, Clinical Effectiveness in Nursing, Internet Journal of Advanced Nursing Practice, Journal of American Academy of Nurse Practitioners*, and the *Journal of Evidence-Based Nursing*, to name just a few. Nurses seeking to increase the use of evidence in their clinical practice may want to apply the model developed by the University of Colorado. See Figure 2-1. The model highlights the elements of EBP.

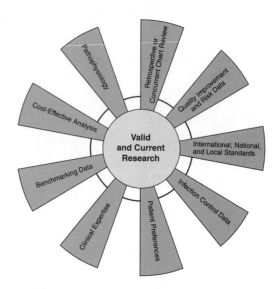

Figure 2-1 University of Colorado Hospital Evidence-Based Multidisciplinary Practice Model. (By permission of University of Colorado Hospital Research Council, Denver, CO)

LITERATURE APPLICATION

Citation: Soukup, S. M. (2000). Preface to section on evidence-based nursing practice. *Nursing Clinics of North America, 35*(2), xvii-xviii.

Discussion: Author discusses a nurse's response to queries as to whether she has integrated evidence-based practice. The nurse responds, "Yes, I practice state-of-the-art nursing. My education and professional practice experiences have prepared me to care for more than 700 chronically ill patients annually, in the past 5 years. These patients have an average reported expected pain rating of 6.9 (using a scale of 1 to 10, with 10 being severe pain), and my pain management interventions have kept these patients, during my hours of care, at a reported actual pain rating of 4. Also, as a team member, these patients have not had any known pressure ulcers, skin tears, or catheter-related infections. On two occasions, for patients who were dying, I created a humanizing environment for these patients and their families when they were rapidly transferred from the critical care unit. My documentation has met organizational standards during monthly peer reviews; I have provided leadership for emergencies with positive outcomes; and physician and patient satisfaction rating for clinical practice on our unit is 9.5 on a scale of 10, with 10 being the highest. Our unit-based team has not had a needle-stick-related or back-related injury during the past 2 years. This has contributed to a significant cost avoidance and benefit to the organization.

Implications for Practice: Nurses practicing in the 21st century must embrace the principles of evidence-based practice as an approach to clinical care and professional accountability.

Nursing Research Nurses today review current literature and the best available evidence from research and clinical practice in order to improve patient care. Nurses also may participate in the implementation of a nursing research project. Observations of the patient and changing techniques are important to nursing research as are designing a study and computing statistical analysis. If nursing research is of interest, the staff nurse should seek additional course work in research and statistics. Continuing education conferences on nursing research are often offered by professional organizations on both local and national levels.

Nursing Data Sets and Classification Systems
In order to gather data about the practice of nursing, a **Nursing Minimum Data Set** (NMDS) has been developed (ANA, 1995). The NMDS uses a common language of nursing that can be used for research and outcomes assessment. Some of the elements included in the NMDS are the patient's nursing diagnosis, nursing interventions, and nursing outcomes. Using the NMDS allows nurses to share information about which nursing practices lead to improved outcomes in their patients. This guides future nursing practice.

In addition to the NMDS, several systems have been developed to classify nursing practice. Some of these **nursing classification systems** are the North American Nursing Diagnosis Association (NANDA), the Omaha System, the Home Healthcare Classification, the Nursing Interventions Classifications System (NIC) (Hyun & Park, 2002), and the Nursing Outcomes Classification (NOC). Use of these classification systems allows nurses to communicate and research which interventions produce the best outcome for their patients.

Nursing Report Card In 1995, the ANA developed a *Nursing Report Card for Acute Care Settings*, which lists indicators for patient-focused outcomes, structures of care, and care processes. These patient-focused outcome indicators are listed in Table 2-2.

Monitoring these outcome indicators allows nurses to begin to research which practices lead to the best outcomes.

HEALTH CARE VARIATION

Methods for review and summarization of evidence have undergone dramatic advances. A. Cochrane of the Cochrane Library group was a pioneer in the movement and preparation of high-quality reviews. In 1978, Cochrane suggested that only 15% to 20% of patient care interventions were supported by objective evidence. This finding highlighted the variation in health care delivery and supports the need for EBP.

Nurses today are concerned with this health care variation. Research on variation in medical care practice first began to be reported in the 1970s (Wennberg & Gittelsohn, 1973). Depending on what part of the country you lived in, patient outcomes and costs varied significantly for the same health care condition. Studies on unnecessary surgery (Leape, 1987) and the occurrence of preventable complications in patients (Adams, Fraser, & Abrams, 1973) led to more research into variations in physician practice patterns. Nursing and physician clinicians, as well as patients, began to consider what health care practices led to the best health care outcomes.

Best Practice Guidelines

In 1989, the Agency for Healthcare Research and Quality (AHRQ), an agency of the United States Public Health Service, was formed. The AHRQ began to develop clinical practice guidelines using the best available evidence as a basis. National committees of clinical nurses, physicians, and other health care experts worked on these evidence-based clinical practice guidelines for various topics. The AHRQ also supported research into the effectiveness of medical practice (McCormick, Cummings, & Kovner, 1997).

TABLE 2-2
ANA NURSING REPORT CARD, PATIENT-FOCUSED OUTCOME INDICATORS

Indicator	Definition
Mortality rate	A measure of the number of patients who die following admission to a hospital for care (can be examined over a number of different time periods)
Length of stay	Duration of the inpatient hospital component of a defined episode of illness
Adverse incident rate (total)	Measures the rate at which patients admitted to a hospital for care experience adverse incidents during the course of their stay that are not directly related to the reason for their admission
Medication error rate	Rate at which errors in the administration of medications occur within a given institution
Patient injury rate	Rate at which patients fall or incur physical injuries (unrelated to a surgical or diagnostic procedure) during the course of their hospital stay
Total complication rate	Rate at which additional diseases or conditions that are related to the patient's original diagnosis are developed in patients receiving care at a hospital
Decubitus ulcer rate	Rate at which patients receiving care at a hospital experience skin breakdown
Nosocomial infection rate (total)	Rate at which patients experience infections (all sites) originating in the hospital
Nosocomial urinary tract infection rate	Rate at which catheterized patients experience urinary tract infection originating in the hospital
Nosocomial pneumonia rate	Rate at which inflammation of the lungs with exudation and consolidation develops in patients during the course of their hospitalization
Nosocomial surgical wound infection rate	Rate at which patients experience surgical wound infections
Patient or family satisfaction with nursing care	A patient's or family's opinion of care received from nursing staff

(continues)

Table 2-2 *(continued)*

Indicator	Definition
Patient/family willingness to recommend hospital to others or to use hospital again	Rate at which patients or family would recommend the hospital providing their care to others or agree to return to the hospital for care in the future
Patient adherence to discharge plan	Rate at which patients fully and correctly execute the therapeutic regimen established for the period immediately following discharge
Readmission rate	Rate at which patients return to the hospital within a defined period of time following a hospital stay for unplanned or emergent care related to the same diagnosis addressed during the prior admission
Postdischarge emergency room visits	Number of patient visits to the emergency room, for preventable complaints related to a previous hospital stay, during a defined time period following discharge
Post discharge unscheduled physician visits	Number of unplanned physician visits, for preventable physician complications related to a previous hospital stay, during a defined period following discharge
Patient knowledge	The extent to which patients possess the knowledge and skills necessary to care for themselves following discharge, or if the patient is unable to do so, an appropriate member of the patient's social support network is able to provide that care

From *Nursing Care Report Card for Acute Care Settings*. Copyright 1995 by American Nurses Publishing, American Nurses Foundation/American Nurses Association, Washington, DC. Reprinted with permission.

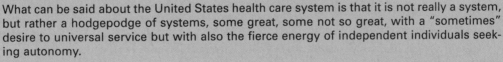

REAL WORLD INTERVIEW

What can be said about the United States health care system is that it is not really a system, but rather a hodgepodge of systems, some great, some not so great, with a "sometimes" desire to universal service but with also the fierce energy of independent individuals seeking autonomy.

Ellyn Stecker, MD

Today, clinical practice guidelines are being developed by more than 60 organizations in at least 10 countries (Rogers, 1995). Most of these organizations are emphasizing the use of the best evidence-based clinical information in developing these guidelines (Titler, Mentes, Rakel, Abbott, & Baumler, 1999; Lang, 1999; Lohr & Carey, 1999; Sackett et al., 1996).

Health Care Ratings

Solucient, a health care information company based in Evanston, Illinois, has reviewed the clinical and financial performance of some 6,000 acute care hospitals of all types and sizes. It annually publishes a listing of the 100 top hospitals nationally, both generally and in selected specialties ("100 Top Hospitals," 2001). *U.S. News and World Report* annually publishes a list of the top hospitals nationally ("America's Best Hospitals," 2001). Look at the health care ratings at http://www.healthgrades.com.

Malcolm Baldridge National Quality Award

In 1999, health care organizations were eligible to consider a framework for health care quality and to apply for the Malcolm Baldridge National Quality Award. In 1995, 46 health care organizations and 19 educational institutions participated in a pilot program for health care and education. The Baldridge Award highlights the importance of leadership; strategic planning; and a focus on patients, other customers, and markets in building a quality health care system. Baldridge also stresses the importance of focusing on staff and monitoring organizational performance results (Baldridge National Quality Program, 2000). The importance of collecting good data and analyzing information using tools is also emphasized.

Other Outcome Measurements

Outcome measurements are used by nurses today to indicate an individual's clinical state, such as their severity of illness, course of illness, and the effect of interventions on their clinical state. Outcome measures involving a patient's functional status evaluate a patient's ability to perform activities of daily living (ADLs). These can include measures of physical health in terms of function, mental and social health, cost of care, health care access, and general health perceptions. The measures can distinguish the concepts of physical and mental health and identify the five indicator categories of clinical status, functioning, physical symptoms, emotional status, and patient/family evaluation and perceptions about quality of life. Selected quality-of-life measures include quality-adjusted life years (QALY), quality-adjusted life expectancy (QALE), and quality-adjusted healthy life years (QUALY) (Drummond, Stoddart, & Torrance, 1994).

The Medical Outcomes Study (MOS) "Short Form 36" Health Survey is one of the many health indices that have been developed since 1950. The SF-36, as it is commonly known (Ware & Sherbourne, 1992), measures physical functioning, role limitations due to physical health, bodily pain, social functioning, general mental health, role limitations due to emotional problems, vitality, and general health perceptions.

Other Health Assessment Tools

Other health status assessment surveys in use by nurses today include the Quality of Life Index (Spitzer, 1998), developed to measure the general health and well-being of terminally ill individuals; the COOP Charts for primary care practice patients; the functional status questionnaire (Jette & Cleary, 1987), a self-administered general health and social well-being survey for ambulatory patients; the Duke Health Profile (Parkerson, Broadhead, & Tse, 1990), which evaluates health status in primary care patients; the Sickness Impact Profile (Bergner, Bobbit, Carter, & Gilson, 1981), which was developed to measure changes in an individual's behavior as a result of illness; and the Nottingham Health Profile (Hunt, McKenna, McEwen, Williams, & Papp, 1981), developed as a measure of perceived general health status for primary care patients and general population health surveys.

STAKEHOLDERS IN HEALTH CARE

Public and private stakeholders, both voluntary and involuntary, affect the delivery of health care services in a variety of settings in the United States. Figure 2-2 shows some of the stakeholders in a large U.S. hospital that nurses today may work with.

Subcultures of Health Professionals

Several subcultures of individual disciplines work in the various health care settings of health care—nursing, medicine, physical therapy, social work, hospital administration, dietary, pharmacy, to name a few. These subcultures affect patient care delivered in the various settings. Table 2-3 lists generalized characteristics of

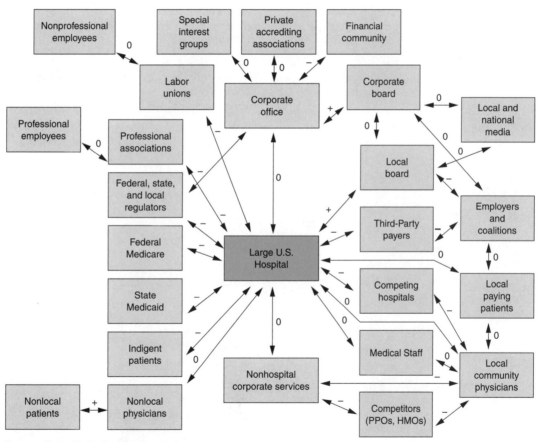

Key: + = Generally Positive Relationship
0 = Generally Neutral Relationship
− = Generally Negative Relationship

Figure 2-2 Stakeholders in a Large U.S. Hospital (From Fottler, M. D., Blair, J. D., Whitehead, C. J., Laus, M. D., & Savage, G. T. Assessing key stakeholders: Who matters to hospitals and why? *Hospital and Health Services Administration*. Winter 1989; 34: 530. Copyright 1989. Foundation of the American College of Healthcare Executives.)

TABLE 2-3
GENERALIZED CHARACTERISTICS OF THREE
SUBCULTURES OF HEALTH PROFESSIONALS TODAY

Characteristics	Nursing	Medicine	Health Care Administration
Major task	Patient care	Diagnosis and treatment of disease	Organizational continuity, managing change and stability
Membership	Historically female, white, middle class; humanistic	Historically male, white, middle and upper class; scientific	Historically male-dominant,* rational
Leading role strength	Comforter, nurturer, health educator	Life-saver and problem-solver; miracle-worker	Keeper of the house, protector
Role centrality	Coordinator of health services	Gatekeeper of health services	Proprietor of health services; holder of the purse strings
Relationships with other professional groups	Collaborative ethic	Autonomy; directing the team	Negotiating, seeks cooperation
Model of authority within profession	Hierarchy	Collegiality, equality	Hierarchy
Perspective	Patient-centered, clinical unit/area	Patient- and practice-centered	Hospital's business and market relations
Conflict management	Interpersonal approach	Use leverage available, e.g., resources and authority, to maintain control	Structural and rational approach
Core dilemmas in era of health care reform	Degree of proactivity within context of high uncertainty; traditional vs. new role initiatives	Choice of organizational and network affiliations, and the conditions and extent of affiliation; the future destiny of medical specialists	Where to invest strategic resources in an era of high future uncertainty

(continues)

Table 2-3 *(continued)*

Characteristics	Nursing	Medicine	Health Care Administration
Major threats (current)	Decrease in job security; constraints on staffing levels and other resources; (undesirable) changes in role	Health economics; changes in role; losses in authority, income; malpractice	Organization survival, job security

*The management of Catholic hospitals, typically run by orders of Catholic sisters, is a notable exception to the generalizations about health care administrators.

three of these subcultures of health professionals identified by Byers (1997). These characteristics are dynamic and constantly changing the culture of the health care organization and the groups that nurses today work with to provide quality health care.

POPULATION-BASED HEALTH CARE

Nurses today are working increasingly in population-based health care practices. **Population-based health care** encompasses three levels: the community; systems within the community; and individuals, families, and groups. Population-based, community-focused practice changes community norms, attitudes, practices, and behaviors. Population-based, system-focused practice changes laws, power structures, policies, and organizations. Population-based, individual-focused practice changes the knowledge, attitudes, beliefs, practices, and behaviors of individuals, families, and groups (Keller, Strohschein, Lia-Hoagberg, & Schaffer, 1998). Figure 2-3 depicts the Minnesota Department of Health Public Health Intervention II Wheel.

Population-based health care addresses the health care needs of a population of people

and patients rather than focusing only on care delivery to individual patients. Research into health and illness has now recognized the contribution of social, economic, and environmental factors to health, and a critical body of evidence is beginning to document the influence of these factors on morbidity and mortality (Gruman & Chesney, 1995). Table 2-4 summarizes what selected evidence-based studies have found.

Population-based health care encourages society to direct resources toward strengthening the determinants of health: health care system influences (e.g., access to medical care, cost, etc.); individual influences (lifestyle, genetics, etc.); interpersonal, social, and work influences (job satisfaction, social support, etc.); community influences (services, programs, etc.); and environmental influences (air, water, etc.) (Donatelle & Davis, 1998). A society that spends so much on medical care that it cannot or will not spend adequately on other health-enhancing activities may actually be reducing the health of its population (Evans & Stoddard, 1990).

Nursing today has begun to direct some of its efforts to population-based interventions designed to improve the health of populations by reducing smoking, substance abuse, violence, risky sexual behaviors, and obesity. See Table 2-5.

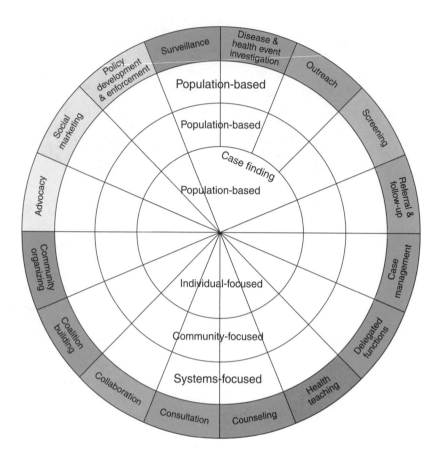

Population-based
Population-based
Case finding
Population-based
Individual-focused
Community-focused
Systems-focused

Surveillance
Disease & health event investigation
Policy development & enforcement
Outreach
Social marketing
Screening
Advocacy
Referral & follow-up
Community organizing
Case management
Coalition building
Delegated functions
Collaboration
Health teaching
Consultation
Counseling

Figure 2-3 The Minnesota Department of Health Public Health Interventions II Wheel. Used with permission of the Section of Public Health Nursing, Minnesota Department of Health. Retrieved from http://www.health.state.mn.us/ on July 13, 2001.

ACCREDITATION

Nurses today work in accredited health care organizations. The Joint Commission on Accreditation of Healthcare Organizations (JCAHO) is the current national organization that develops standards and accredits health care organizations. This accreditation is important to hospitals because it is one of the ways hospitals can be certified to receive federal government Medicare and Medicaid reimbursement for delivery of patient care services.

As many as 50% of the JCAHO's hospital accreditation standards were written to correspond with Medicare's conditions of participation, a comprehensive set of criteria that hospitals and other care providers must meet to qualify for reimbursement. The JCAHO's adherence to the conditions stems from its "deemed" status with Medicare, which means that JCAHO-accredited hospitals are assumed to have met the Medicare participation standards. Hospitals pay an average of $20,000 for a JCAHO survey (Lovern, 2001). See Table 2-6

TABLE 2-4
EVIDENCE-BASED STUDIES: WHAT THEY SHOW

- A 7-year follow-up of women diagnosed with breast cancer showed that those who confided in at least one person in the 3 months after surgery had a 7-year survival rate of 72.4%, as compared to 56.3% for those who did not have a confidant (Maunsell, Brisson, & Deschenes, 1995).

- In a study examining the correlation of social ties to susceptibility to common cold viruses, increased diversity in types of ties to friends, family, work, and community was significantly associated with increased host resistance to infection (Cohen, Doyle, Skoner, Rabin, & Gwaltney, 1997).

- In studies examining the effect of nursing care on patient outcomes, there were fewer complications, fewer adverse events, shorter lengths of stay, and lower incidence of nurse-sensitive negative patient outcomes when nursing staffing was appropriate (Aiken, 2002; Dimick, Swoboda, Provonost, et al., 2001; Needleman, Buerhaus, et al., 2001; Provonost, Dang, Dorman, et al., 2001).

TABLE 2-5
POPULATION-BASED HEALTH CARE INITIATIVES

Global Group	Initiatives
World Health Organization	Health for All by the Year 2000. Principles delineated in the Health for All by the Year 2000 plan include (1) the right to health, (2) equity in health, (3) community participation, (4) intersectoral collaboration, (5) health promotion, (6) primary health care, and (7) international cooperation (Bastian, 1989, p. 15).
United Nations	Cairo Action Plan for Women's Health. This plan illustrates the clear link between education, poverty, gender equality, culture, national politics and economies, population growth, and the health status of women (Nelson, Proctor, Regev, Barnes, Sawyer, Messias, Yoder, & Meleis, 1996).

(continues)

Table 2-5 *(continued)*

National and Regional Group	Initiatives
Great Britain	Saving Lives: Our Healthier Nation. This initiative focused on the prevention of 300,000 deaths in a 10-year period (Mitchell, 1999).
United States	Healthy People 2010. This initiative highlights health indicators related to the leading causes of death, including health behaviors, physical and social and environmental factors, and health systems factors. (Healthy People, n. d.).
American Public Health Association (APHA)	Recommends the development of a universal health care system to provide for the uninsured and disenfranchised of the country. Commentary on the State of the Public's Health (American Public Health Association, 2001).

State	Initiatives
Arizona	Tobacco Education and Prevention Program (TEPP). Centers for Disease Control and Prevention. (2001). Tobacco use among adults—Arizona, 1996 and 1999. *Morbidity and Mortality Weekly Report May 25, 2001, 50:20; 402-406.* Retrieved from http://www.cdc.gov/mmwr on 3/27/03.
Arkansas	Community-oriented primary care (COPC) model utilizing family nurse practitioners (Hartwig & Landis, 1999).
New Hampshire	The New Hampshire Coalition Against Domestic and Sexual Violence (Hastings, 2001).
New Mexico	"Roll Up Your Sleeves" campaign to combat the high incidence of hepatitis B in the state's population. (Harris, Kerr, & Steffen, 1997).
Tennessee	Tenncare, a program to extend health care benefits to the uninsured and to slow down the rapid growth of Medicaid spending (Lyons & Scheb, 1998).

for the list of chapters in the accreditation manual. Each chapter highlights a hospital function and how quality is reviewed for that function. All hospitals and long-term care organizations seeking JCAHO accreditation monitor patient outcomes and use a performance measurement system to provide data about these patient outcomes and other indicators of care. Nurses today monitor accreditation standards and the other forces influencing health care (Shortell & Kaluzny, 2000). See Table 2-7.

HEALTH INSURANCE PORTABILITY AND ACCOUNTABILITY ACT

The Health Insurance Portability and Accountability Act of 1996 (HIPAA) includes measures to standardize and computerize the business transactions of health care billing, claims processing, and reimbursement. The law dictates

TABLE 2-6
HOSPITAL ACCREDITATION STANDARDS OVERVIEW

Patient-focused functions

- Patients rights and organization ethics
- Assessment of patients
- Care of patients
- Education
- Continuum of care

Organization-focused functions

- Improving organization performance
- Leadership
- Management of the environment of care

- Management of human resources
- Management of information
- Surveillance, prevention, and control of infection

Structures with functions

- Governance
- Management
- Medical staff
- Nursing

© Joint Commission Resources: *CAMH: 2003 Comprehensive Accreditation Manual for Hospitals.* Oakbrook Terrace, IL: Joint Commission on Accreditation of Healthcare Organizations, 2003. Reprinted with permission.

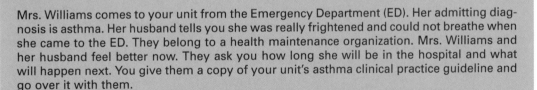

CASE STUDY 2-1

Mrs. Williams comes to your unit from the Emergency Department (ED). Her admitting diagnosis is asthma. Her husband tells you she was really frightened and could not breathe when she came to the ED. They belong to a health maintenance organization. Mrs. Williams and her husband feel better now. They ask you how long she will be in the hospital and what will happen next. You give them a copy of your unit's asthma clinical practice guideline and go over it with them.

How can you use the University of Colorado's Model for Evidence-Based practice to improve Mrs. Williams care?

How will you work with your health care system and the community you serve to ensure that Mrs. Williams and other asthma patients in the community are not admitted with asthma again soon? What kind of teaching will Mrs. Williams need to prevent future attacks?

that patients' data be transmitted securely and handled confidentially, all of which will require fundamental changes in administrative operations and information services for most providers (Morrissey, 2001). Table 2-8 includes HIPAA privacy regulations.

TABLE 2-7
NINE FORCES INFLUENCING HEALTH CARE DELIVERY TODAY

External Force	Management Implication
1. Capitated payment, expenditure targets, or global budgets for providing care to defined populations	• Need for increased efficiency and productivity • Redesign of patient care delivery • Development of strategic alliances that add value • Increased growth of networks, systems, and physician groups
2. Increased accountability for performance	• Information systems that link financial and clinical data across episodes of illness and "pathways of wellness" • Effective implementation of clinical practice guidelines • Ability to demonstrate continuous improvements of all functions and processes
3. Technological advances in the biological and clinical sciences	• Expansion of the continuum of care, need for new treatment sites to accommodate new treatment modalities • Increased capacity to manage care across organizational boundaries • Need to confront new ethical dilemmas
4. Aging of the population	• Increased demand for primary care, wellness, and health promotion services among the age 65 to 75 group • Increased demand for chronic care management among the 75 plus group • Challenge of managing ethical issues associated with prolongation of life
5. Increased ethnic or cultural diversity of the population	• Greater difficulty in understanding and meeting patient expectations • Challenge of managing an increasingly diverse health services workforce
6. Changes in the supply and education of health professionals	• Need for creative approaches in meeting the population's need for disease prevention, health promotion, and chronic care management services • Need to compensate for shortages in some categories of health professionals (i.e., physical therapy, pharmacy, and some areas of nursing) • Need to develop effective teams of caregivers across multiple treatment sites

(continues)

Table 2-7 *(continued)*

External Force	Management Implication
7. Social morbidity (AIDS, drugs, violence, "new surprises")	• Ability to deal with unpredictable increases in demand • Need for increased social support systems and chronic care management • Need to work effectively with community agencies
8. Information technology	• Training the health care workforce in new information technologies • Increased ability to coordinate care across sites • Challenge of managing an increased pace of change due to more rapid information transfer • Challenge of dealing with confidentiality issues associated with new information technologies and HIPAA legislation
9. Globalization and expansion of the world economy	• Need to manage cross-national and cross-cultural tertiary and quaternary patient care referrals • Increasing the competitiveness and productivity of the American labor force • Managing global strategic alliances, particularly in the areas of biotechnology and new technology development

Shortell & Kaluzny, 2000.

TABLE 2-8
HIPAA PRIVACY REGULATIONS

- Allows patient to review and request amendments to their medical records

- Gives consumers control over how their personal health information is used and limits the release of information without a patient's consent

- Restricts the amount of patient information shared between physicians and other care-givers to the "minimum necessary"

- Requires privacy-conscious business practices, such as hiring a privacy officer and training employees about patient confidentiality

- Requires that paper records and oral communications be protected from privacy breaches

KEY CONCEPTS

- The JCAHO is the national organization that accredits health care organizations. This accreditation is one of the ways hospitals can be certified to receive federal government reimbursement for health care delivery to Medicare patients.
- Research in 1970 revealed much variation in health care, and clinical practice guidelines based on the best available evidence were developed by AHRQ to guide and improve care.
- The Pew Health Professions Commission identified 21 competencies for the 21st century for health care providers. Nursing and other health care professions will have to adapt to a fast-changing environment in the future.
- Caring, transdisciplinary nursing practice promises to be an important part of nursing's future role in health care.
- The focus on EBC can be expected to remain a driving force in the health care arena in the foreseeable future.
- Nursing can make significant contributions to the advancement of evidence-based care.
- The focus of population-based health care is to reduce health disparities that exist among diverse population groups.
- The goals of population-based health care are access, quality, cost containment, and equity.
- Nurses play key roles in the successful development and implementation of population-based health care services.

KEY TERMS

evidence-based practice

Medicare's conditional participation

nursing classification systems

nursing minimum data set

nursing report card for acute care settings

population-based health care practice

REVIEW QUESTIONS

1. What is the major purpose of evidence-based care (EBC)?
   A. To increase variability of care
   B. To cause a link to be missing in clinical care
   C. To determine what medical models can be applied by nursing
   D. To provide evidence-based care that supports clinical competency
2. Population-based nursing interventions are directed at
   A. all individuals who need health services.
   B. people without health care insurance.
   C. the health needs of the total community.
   D. only vulnerable groups within the community.
3. The four goals of population-based nursing practice are
   A. access, cost, empowerment, equity.
   B. access, cost, equity, resilience.
   C. access, cost, equity, quality.
   D. cost, equity, resilience, quality.
4. The national organization that accredits health care organizations is known as which of the following?
   A. American Nurses Association
   B. Pew Health Professions Commission
   C. Agency for Healthcare Research and Quality
   D. Joint Commission on Accreditation of Healthcare Organizations

REVIEW ACTIVITIES

1. Compare and contrast individual-focused nursing practice with population-based nursing practice. What nursing knowledge and skills do you need to practice population-based nursing care?

2. Hilfinger (2001) believes that nurses should adopt a global framework for the empowerment of women to reduce health disparities. Discuss what you think this framework should include. How could you become a nursing advocate for this at the local, national, and international levels?

3. Review the Pew Health Professions Commission competencies. Consider how you can improve your own knowledge level in any of the competency areas in which you do not feel comfortable.

EXPLORING THE WEB

- Where could you find information to help serve the health care needs of immigrants? National Institutes of Health:
  http://www.nih.gov

  Office of U.S. Surgeon General:
  http://www.surgeongeneral.gov

- Go to the site for the Joanna Briggs Institute for Evidence Base Nursing and Midwifery.
  http://www.joannabriggs.edu.au

- Go to the Health Care Information Resources—Nurses Links:
  http://www-hsl.mcmaster.ca

- Go to the site for the *Online Journal of Knowledge Synthesis for Nursing,* sponsored by Sigma Theta Tau International.
  http://www.stti.iupui.edu

- Go to the Core List for Evidence-based Practice at the University of Sheffield in England and note the references you see there.
  http://www.shef.ac.uk

- Go to *http://www.google.com* and type in evidence-based care

- Visit the site of the Oncology Nursing Society Evidence-Based Practice Online Resource Center.
  http://www.ons.org

- What sites could you recommend to patients and families seeking information about self-help, hospital accreditation, research, and clinical practice guidelines, for example, the JCAHO and the Agency for Healthcare Research and Quality?
  http://www.selfhelpweb.org
  http://www.jcaho.org
  http://www.ahrq.gov
  http://www.centerwatch.com
  http://www.guideline.gov
  http://www.cdc.gov
  http://www.netdoctor.co.uk
  http://www.health.gov

- Go to the sites for the Malcolm Baldridge National Quality Award and the IOM Report. What information did you find there?
  http://www.quality.nist.gov

- Search the Web, checking these sites: Medicare, National Institute of Health, American Nurses Association, National League for Nursing, American Cancer Society, American Heart Association, diabetes, Ellis Island records, Delmar Learning. What did you find?
  www.medicare.gov
  www.nih.gov
  www.ana.org
  www.nln.org
  www.cancer.org
  www.americanheart.org
  www.diabetes.org
  www.delmarhealthcare.com
  www.ellisislandrecords.org

- Go to Pubmed. What did you find there? Can you access nursing and medical journals? Would you recommend this site to patients? *http://www.ncbi.nlm.nih.gov*

- What are some helpful sites for nurses?
  http://www.allnurses.com

http://www.nursingworld.org
http://www.continuingeducation.com
http://www.hotnursejobs.com
http://www.freelawyer.co.uk
http://www.nln.org
http://www.hospitalsoup.com

- Where could you go for information on the eHealth Internet Code of Ethics? *http://www.ihealthcoalition.org*

REFERENCES

Adams, D. F., Fraser, D. B., & Abrams, H. L. (1973). The complications of coronary arteriography. *Circulation, 48*(3), 609–618.

Aiken, L. (2001). Superior outcomes for magnet hospitals: The evidence base. In M. L. McClure & A. S. Hinshaw (Eds.), *Magnet hospitals visited: Attraction and retention of professional nurses* (pp. 61–81). Washington, DC: American Nurses Publishing.

American Nurses Association. (1995), *Nursing care report card for acute care settings.* Washington, DC: American Nurses Publishing.

American Public Health Association. (2001). *The fourteen points for the campaign for universal health care—the nation's health.* Retrieved July 9, 2001, from http://www.apha.org/legislative/issues/reform.htm

America's best hospitals. (2001, July 23). *U.S. News and World Report,* 44–105.

Aroskar, M. (1998). Ethical working relationships in patient care. *Nursing Clinics of North America, 33*(2), 313–323.

Baldridge National Quality Program. (2000). *Health care criteria for performance excellence.* Gaithersburg, MD: Baldridge National Quality Program.

Bastian, H. (1989). A guide to WHO and "WHO speak." *Consumer Health Forum,* 9, 15.

Bellack, J. P., & O'Neil, E. H. (2000). Recreating nursing practice for a new century: Recommendations and implications of the Pew Health Professions Commission's final report. *Nursing and Health Care Perspectives, 21*(1), 14–21.

Bergner, M., Bobbit, R. A., Carter, W. B., & Gilson, B. S. (1981). The Sickness Impact Profile: Development and final revision of a health status measure. *Medical Care, 19*(8), 787–805.

Byers, S. A. (1997). *The executive nurse—leadership for new health care transitions.* Clifton Park, NY: Delmar Learning.

Carroll-Johnson, R. (2001). Redefining interdisciplinary practice. *Oncology Nursing Forum, 28*(4), 619.

Centers for Disease Control and Prevention. (2001). Tobacco use among adults—Arizona, 1996 and 1999. *Morbidity and Mortality Weekly Report May 25, 2001, 50:20*; 402–406.

Cochrane Library at McMaster University. (2000, March). *Using Medline to search for evidence.* Retrieved from http://www.londonlinks.ac.uk/evidence_strategies/coch_search.htm

Cohen, S., Doyle, W. J., Skoner, D. P., Rabin, B. S., & Gwaltney, J. M., Jr. (1997). Social ties and susceptibility to the common cold. *Journal of the American Medical Association, 277*, 1940–1944.

Dimick, J., Swoboda, S., Pronovost, P. Lipsett, P. A. (2001). Effect of nurse-to-patient in the intensive care unit on pulmonary complications and resource use after hepatectomy. *American Journal of Critical Care.*

Donatelle, R., & Davis, L. G. (1998). *Access to health* (8th ed.). Needham Heights, MA: Allyn & Bacon.

Drummond, M. F., Stoddart, F. L., & Torrance, G. W. (1994). *Methods for the economic evaluation of health care programmes.* Oxford, England: Oxford University Press.

Evans, R., & Stoddard, G. (1990). Consuming health care, producing health. *Social Science and Medicine, 31*(12), 1347–1363.

Fottler, M. D., Blair, J. D., Whitehead, C. U., Laus, M. D., & Savage, G. T. (1989). Assessing key stakeholders: Who matters to hospitals and why? *Hospital and Health Services Administration, 34*(530).

Gordon, M. (2000). *Manual of Nursing Diagnosis* (9th ed.). St. Louis, MO: Mosby.

Gruman, J., & Chesney, M. (1995). Introduction for superhighways for disease. *Psychosomatic Medicine, 57,* 207.

Harris, P. A., Kerr, J., & Steffen, D. (1997). A state-based immunization campaign: the New Mexico experience. *Journal of School Health, 67*(7) 273–276.

Hartwig, M. S., & Landis, B. J. (1999). The Arkansas AHEC model of community-oriented primary care. *Holistic Nurse Practitioner, 13*(4), 28–37.

Hastings, D. P. (2001). The New Hampshire health initiative on domestic violence. *Nursing Forum, 36*(1), 31–35.

Healthy People. (n. d.). *What are the leading health indicators?* Retrieved January 20, 2002, from http://www.health.gov

Hilfinger, D. K. (2001). Globalization, nursing, and health for all. *Journal of Nursing Scholarship, 33*(1), 9–11.

Huber, D., Schumacher, L., & Delaney, C. (1997). Nursing management minimum data set (NMMDS). *Journal of Nursing Administration, 27*(4), 42–48.

Hunt, S. M., McKenna, P., McEwen, J., Williams, J., & Papp, E., (1981). The Nottingham Health Profile: Subjective health status and medical consultations. *Social Science and Medicine, 15*(3, Pt. 1), 221–229.

Hyun, S., & Park, H. A. (2002, June). Cross-mapping the ICNP with NANDA, HHCC, Omaha System and NIC for unified nursing language system development. *International Nursing Revue, 49*(2), 99–110.

Jette, A. M., & Cleary, P. D. (1987). Functional disability assessment. *Physical Therapy, 67,* 1854–1859.

Joint Commission on Accreditation of Healthcare Organizations. (2001). *Manual for hospitals.* Chicago: Author.

Keller, L. O., Schaffer, M., Lia-Hoagberg, B., & Strohschein, S. (in press). Assessment, program planning, and evaluation in population-based public health practice. *Journal of Public Health Management and Practice.*

Keller, L. O., Strohschein, S., Lia-Hoagberg, B., & Schaffer, M. (1998). Population-based public health nursing interventions: A model from practice. *Public Health Nursing, 15*(3), 207–215.

Lang, N. M. (1999). Discipline approaches to evidence-based practice: A view from nursing. *Joint Commission Journal on Quality Improvement, 25*(10), 539–544.

Leape, L. (1987). Unnecessary surgery. *Health Services Research, 24*(3), 351–407.

Lohr, K. N., & Carey, T. S. (1999). Assessing "best evidence": Issues in grading the quality of studies for systematic reviews. *Joint Commission Journal on Quality Improvement, 25*(9), 470–479.

Lovern, E. (2001, May 28). Oh no, not that type of review. JCAHO singling out more hospitals for noncompliance with standards. *Modern Healthcare, 31*(22), 4–5.

Lyons, W., & Scheb, J. M., II. (1998). Managed care and Medicaid reform in Tennessee: The impact of Tenncare on access and health-seeking behavior. *Journal of Health Care for the Poor and Underserved, 10*(3), 328–337.

Maddox, P. (2001). Update on national quality of care initiatives. *Nursing Economic$, 19*(3), 121–124.

Maunsell, E., Brisson, J., & Deschenes, L. (1995). Social support and survival among women with breast cancer. *Cancer, 76,* 631–637.

McCormick, K. A., Cummings, M. A., & Kovner, C. (1997). The role of the Agency for Health Care Policy and Research in improving outcomes of care. *Nursing Clinics of North America, 32*(3), 5.

Minnesota Department of Health, Section of Public Health Nursing. (2001). *Public health interventions—applications for public health nursing practice.* St. Paul, MN: Minnesota Department of Health. Retrieved April 20, 2002, from http://www.health.state.mn.us/

Minnesota Department of Health, Section of Public Health Nursing. (2001). Getting behind the wheel. *Public Health Nursing Newsletter.* Retrieved January 30, 2002, from http://health.state.mn.us/divs/chs/phn/index.html

Mitchell, P. (1999). UK government aims to prevent 300,000 deaths over ten years. *Lancet, 354,* 139.

Morrissey, J. (2001, January 1). Slow down: HIPAA ahead. *Modern Healthcare,* 30.

Needleman, J., Buerhaus, P., Mattke, S., Stewart, M., Zelerinsky, K. (2001) *Nurse staffing and patient outcomes in hospitals (Final report).* Washington, DC: U.S. Dept. of Health and Human Services.

Nelson, M., Proctor, S., Regev, H., Barnes, D., Sawyer, L., Messias, D., Yoder, L., & Meleis, A. I. (1966). International population and development: The United Nations' Cairo action plan for women's health. *Image: Journal of Nursing Scholarship,* 28(1), 75–80.

Nightingale, F. (1914). Florence Nightingale to her nurses: A selection from Miss Nightingale's addresses to probationers and nurses of the Nightingale School at St. Thomas's Hospital [p. 1; Address in May 1872]. London: Macmillan.

100 top hospitals. (2001, February). *Modern Healthcare,* 6–29.

O'Neil, E. H., & The Pew Professions Commission. (1998). *Recreating health professional practice for a new century.* San Francisco, CA: Pew Health Professions Commission.

Parkerson, G. R., Jr., Broadhead, W. E., & Tse, C.-K. J. (1990). The Duke health profile: A 17 item measure of health and dysfunction. *Medical Care, 28,* 1056–1072.

Pronovost, P., Dang, D., Dorman, T., Lipsett, P. A., Garrett, E., Jenckes, M., Bass, E. B. (2001). Intensive care unit nurse staffing and the risks for complications after abdominal aortic surgery. *Effective clinical practice.*

Rogers, E. M. (1995). Lessons for guidelines from the diffusion of innovations. *Joint Commission Journal on Quality Improvement, 21*(7), 324–328.

Sackett, D. L., Rosenberg, W. M. C., Gray, J. A. M., Haynes, R. B., & Richardson, W. S. (1996). Evidence-based medicine: What it is and what it isn't. *British Medical Journal, 312*(7023), 71–72.

Schoon, P. (2003). Population-Based Health Care Practice. In P. Kelly-Heidenthal (Ed.), *Nursing leadership & management.* Clifton Park, NY: Delmar Learning.

Shortell, S. M., & Kaluzny, A. D. (2000). *Health care management* (4th ed.). Clifton Park, NY: Delmar Learning.

Soukup, M. (2000). The Center for Advanced Nursing Practice evidence-based practice model: Promoting the scholarship of practice. *Nursing Clinics of North America, 35*(2), 301–309.

Soukup, M. (2002). Evidence-based nursing practice [Preface]. *Nursing Clinics of North America, 35,* xvii–xviii.

Spitzer, W. O. (1998). Quality of life. In D. Burley & W. H. W. Inman (Eds.), *Therapeutic risk: Perception, measurement, and management.* New York: Wiley.

Strasen, L. (1999). The silent health care revolution: The rising demand for complementary medicine. *Nursing Economic$, 17*(5), 246–256.

Titler, M. G., Mentes, J. C., Rakel, B. A., Abbott, L., & Baumler, S. (1999). From book to bedside: Putting evidence to use in the care of the elderly. *Joint Commission Journal on Quality Improvement, 25*(10), 545–546.

Ware, J. E., & Sherbourne, C. D. (1992). The MOS 36-item short form health survey I: Conceptual framework and item selection. *Medical Care, 30,* 473–478.

Wennberg, J. E., & Gittelsohn, A. M. (1973). Small area variations in health care delivery. *Science, 182*(117), 1102–1108.

SUGGESTED READINGS

Bakken, S., & McArthur, J. (2001). Evidence-based nursing practice: A call to action for nursing informatics. *Journal of the American Medical Informatics Association, 8,* 289–290.

Benner, P. (2000). The wisdom of our practice. *American Journal of Nursing, 100*(10), 99–103.

Boggs, P. B., Hayati, F., Washburne, W. F., & Wheeler, D. A. (1999). Using statistical process control charts for the continual improvement of asthma care. *Joint Commission Journal on Quality Improvement, 25*(4), 163–170.

Bradham, D., Mangan, M., Warrick, A., Geiger-Brown, J., Reiner, J. I., & Saunders, H. J. (2000). Linking innovative nursing practice to health services research. *Nursing Clinics of North America, 35,* 557–568.

Carroll-Johnson, R. M. (2002, May). Nursing diagnosis in the 21st century. *Oncology Nursing Forum, 29*(4), 621.

Closs, S., & Cheater, F. (1999). Evidence for nursing practice: A clarification of the issues. *Journal of Advanced Nursing, 30*(1), 10–17.

Codman, E. (1914). The product of a hospital. *Surgical Gynecology and Obstetrics, 18,* 491–494.

Coile, R. C., Jr. (1999, October). Managed care in the millennium. New forecast for the "five stages of managed care." *Russ Coile's Health Trends, 11*(12), 1, 3–7.

Crow, K., Matheson, L., & Steed, A. (2000). Informed consent and truth-telling: Cultural directions for healthcare providers. *Journal of Nursing Administration, 30*(3), 148–152.

Cullum, N. (2000). Users' guides to the nursing literature: An introduction. *Evidence Based Nursing, 3,* 71–72.

Deaton, C. (2001). Outcomes measurement and evidence-based nursing practice. *Journal of Cardiovascular Nursing, 15*(2), 83–86.

Doenges, M. E., Moorhouse, M. F., & Geissler-Murr, A. C. (2002). *Nursing pocket guide: Diagnoses, interventions, and rationales* (8th ed.).

Donabedian, A. (1966). Evaluating the quality of medical care. *Milbank Memorial Fund Quarterly, 44,* 194–196.

Ferguson, S. L. (1999). Institute for Nursing Leadership: A new program to enhance the leadership capacity of all nurses. *Nursing Outlook,* 91–92.

Fos, P. J., & Fine, D. J. (2000). *Designing health care for populations.* San Francisco: Jossey-Bass.

Ginsberg, E. (1996). *Tomorrow's hospital: A look to the twenty-first century.* New Haven, CT: Yale University Press.

Goode, C. J. (2000). What constitutes the "evidence" in evidence-based practice? *Applied Nursing Research, 13,* 222–225.

Graves, J. R. (1998). The Sigma Theta Tau International nursing research classification system. In J. J. Fitzpatrick (Ed.), *Encyclopedia of nursing research.* New York: Springer.

Guadagnoli, E., Epstein, A. M., Zaslavsky, A., Shaul, J. A., Veroff, D., Fowler, F. J., Jr., & Cleary, P. D. (2000). Providing consumers with information about the quality of health plans: The consumer assessment of health plans demonstration in Washington State. *Joint Commission Journal on Quality Improvement, 26*(7), 410–420.

Guyatt, G. H., Haynes, R. B., Jaeschke, R. Z., Cook, D. J., Green, L., Naylor, C. D., Wilson, M. C., & Richardson, W. S. (2000). Users' guides to the medical literature: XXV, Evidence-based medicine: Principles for applying the users guides to patient care. *Journal of the American Medical Association, 284,* 1290–1296.

Heller, B. R., Oros, M. T., & Durney-Crowley, J. (2000). The future of nursing education: Ten trends to watch. *Nursing and Health Care Perspectives, 21*(1), 9–13.

Hewison, A. (1997). Evidence-based medicine: What about evidence-based management? *Journal of Nursing Management, 5,* 195–198.

Ingersoll, G. L. (2000). Evidence-based nursing: What it is and what it isn't. *Nursing Outlook, 48,* 151–152.

Kindig, D. A. (1999). Purchasing population health: Aligning financial incentives to improve health outcomes. *Nursing Outlook, 47,* 15–22.

Kitson, A. (2000). Towards evidence-based quality improvement: Perspectives from nursing practice. *International Journal for Quality in Health Care, 12,* 459–464.

Kizer, K. (2000). Promoting innovative nursing practice during radical health system change. *Nursing Clinics of North America, 35,* 430–449.

Kohn, L., Corrigan, J., & Donaldson, M. (Eds.). (1999). *To err is human: Building a safer health system.* Washington, DC: Committee on Quality of Care in America, Institute of Medicine, National Academy Press.

Kohn, L., Corrigan, J., & Donaldson, M. (Eds.). (2001). *Crossing the quality chasm: A new health system for the 21st century.* Washington, DC: Committee on Quality of Care in America, Institute of Medicine, National Academy Press.

Lindeman, C. A. (2000). The future of nursing education. *Journal of Nursing Education, 39*(1), 5–12.

McBride, A. B. (1999). Breakthroughs in nursing education: Looking back, looking forward. *Nursing Outlook, 47*(30), 114–119.

McGinnis, J. M., & Foege, W. H. (1993). Actual causes of death in the United States. *Journal of the American Medical Association, 270*(18), 2207–2212.

McLaughlin, C. P., & Kaluzny, A. D. (1999). *Continuous quality improvement in health care* (2nd ed.). Gaithersburg, MD: Aspen.

McPheeters, M., & Lohr, K. N. (1999). Evidence-based practice and nursing: Commentary. *Outcomes Management for Nursing Practice.* 3, 99–101.

Mehta, N., & Jain, A. (2001). Finding evidence-based answers to clinical questions online. *Cleveland Clinic Journal of Medicine, 68,* 307–317.

Moorhead, S., Head, B., Johnson, M., & Maas, M. (1998, August). The nursing outcomes taxonomy: Development and coding. *Journal of Nursing Care Quality, 12*(6), 56–63.

Norton, D., & Kaplan, R. (2001). *The strategy-focused organization: How balanced scorecard companies thrive in the new business environment.* Boston: Harvard Business School Press.

O'Grady, E. (2000). Access to health care: An issue central to nursing. *Nursing Economic$, 18*(2), 88–90.

Pesut, D. J., & Rezmerski, C. J. (2000). *Future think. Nursing Outlook, 48*(1), 9.

Rosen, W., & Donald, A. (1995). Evidence based medicine: An approach to clinical problem solving. *British Medical Journal, 310,* 1122–1125.

Rosenfeld, P., Duthie, E., Bier, J., Bowar-Ferres, S., Fulmer, T., Iervolino, L., McClure, M. L., McGivern, D. O., & Roncoli, M. (2000). Engaging staff nurses in evidence-based research to identify nursing practice problems and solutions. *Applied Nursing Research, 13*(4), 197–203.

Rosswurm, M. A., & Larrabee, J. H. (1999). A model for change to evidence-based practice. *Image: Journal of Nursing Scholarship, 31,* 317–322.

Shortell, S. M. (1996). *Remaking health care in America: Building organized delivery systems.* San Francisco: Jossey-Bass.

Shorten, A., Wallace, M. C., & Crookes, P. A. (2001). Developing information literacy: A key to evidence-based nursing. *International Nursing Review, 48,* 86–92.

Simms, L. M., Price, S. A., & Ervin, N. E. (2000). *Professional practice of nursing administration* (3rd ed.). Clifton Park, NY: Delmar Learning.

Simpson, K. R., & Knox, G. E. (1999). Strategies for developing an evidence-based approach to perinatal care. *MCN American Journal of Maternal Child Nursing, 24,* 122–131.

Stetler, C. B., Brunell, M., Giuliano, K., Morsi, D., Prince, L., & Newell-Stokes, V. (1998a). Evidence-based practice and the role of nursing leadership. *Journal of Nursing Administration, 28*(7/8), 45–53.

Stetler, C. B., Morsi, D., Rucki, S., Broughton, S., Corrigan, B., Fitzgerald, J., Giuliano, K., Havener, P., & Sheridan, E. A. (1998b). Utilization-focused integrative reviews in a nursing service. *Applied Nursing Research, 11*(4), 195–206.

Stetler, C. B., Corrigan, B., Sander-Buscemi, K., & Burns, M. (1999). Integration of evidence into practice and the change process: Fall prevention program as a model. *Outcomes Management for Nursing Practice, 3,* 102–111.

Stevens, K. R., & Cassidy, V. R. (1999). *Evidence-based teaching.* NLN Press. Boston: Jones and Bartlett.

Sullivan, E. J. (1999). *Creating nursing's future: Issues, opportunities, and challenges.* St. Louis, MO: Mosby.

Urbshott, G. B., Kennedy, G., & Rutherford, G. (2001). The Cochrane HIV/AIDS review group and evidence-based practice in nursing. *Journal of the Association of Nurses in AIDS Care, 12*(6), 94–101.

U.S. Department of Health and Human Services. (2000). *Healthy people 2010: Understanding and improving health* (2nd ed.). Washington, DC: U.S. Government Printing Office.

Uys, L. R. (2001). Universal access to health care: If not now, when? *Reflections on Nursing Leadership, 27*(2), 21–23.

Weeks, W. B., Hamby, L., Stein, A., & Batalden, P. B. (2000). Using the Baldridge Management System framework in health care: The Veterans Health Administration experience. *Joint Commission Journal on Quality Improvement, 26*(7), 379–387.

Wells, M. I. (2000). Beyond cultural competence: A model for individual and institutional cultural development. *Journal of Community Health Nursing, 17*(4), 189–199.

Williams, C. A. (2000). Community-oriented population-focused practice: The foundation of specialization in public health nursing. In M. Stanhope & J. Lancaster (Eds.), *Community and public health nursing* (5th ed., pp. 2–19). St. Louis, MO: Mosby.

Willis, E. M., Biggins, A. L., & Donovan, J. E. (1999). Population-focused practice. In J. E. Hitchcock, P. E. Schubert, & S. A. Thomas, *Community health nursing* (pp. 209–223). Clifton Park, NY: Delmar Learning.

World Health Organization. (2000). *A massive effort for better health among the poor.* Retrieved July 7, 2001, from http://www.who.int/inf-new/conclu.htm

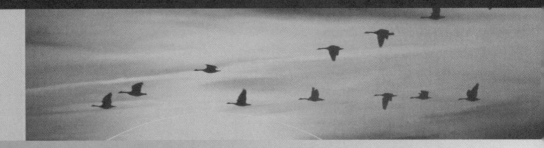

CHAPTER 3

Fundamentally who we are and how we work together is what our patients receive. (Nancy Moore, 2000)

Team Building and Organizational Communication

OBJECTIVES

Upon completion of this chapter, the reader should be able to:

1. Discuss the concept and purpose of a health care team.
2. Review the process of communication.
3. Discuss the stages of group process.
4. Identify elements of the Myers-Briggs Type Indicator.
5. Explore teamwork on a patient care unit.
6. Explore elements of communication with members on a health care team.
7. Discuss organizational communication.
8. Discuss how to overcome communication barriers.

As a new nurse, you are making the day's assignments for a 34-bed medical-surgical unit. Working with you today will be another two registered nurses, two licensed practical nurses, and one nursing assistant. You graduated only a year ago but you were recently promoted to the role of charge nurse. Today, one of the licensed practical nurses and the nursing assistant are challenging your patient care assignments, saying you do not have enough experience to make a fair assignment, and they are trying to get the two registered nurses to side with them. It appears that the two registered nurses often work together, as do the two licensed practical nurses. You know you made the best assignment given the staff available, yet you are wondering if there is a better solution.

What are your thoughts on how to proceed?

What would be the best way to address their concerns?

How can you work with your team to ensure fair patient assignments?

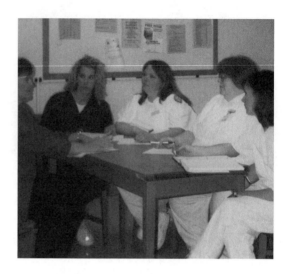

Leadership and management skills in nursing often include some element of effective teamwork. Nurses generally do not work in isolation but provide care with a team that is interdependent and provides expertise to help the patient achieve optimal wellness. This chapter discusses the key factors that build a successful nursing team. It also discusses the group process and ways in which a nurse can communicate on effective teams. Finally, it discusses organizational communication.

DEFINITION OF A TEAM

Katzenbach and Smith (1993) define a **team** as "a small number of people with complementary skills who are committed to a common purpose, performance goals, and approach for which they hold themselves accountable (p. 45)." Senge, Roberts, Ross, Smith, and Kleiner (1994) further elaborate that a team is a group that has a purpose and needs each member's contributions to succeed. On health care teams, the purpose is to meet patient care needs. On some teams all members may have similar backgrounds and abilities, such as a nursing policy and procedure team. Other teams may be developed with interdisciplinary members who have a variety of skills and talents, to provide different perspectives and ideas on how to solve problems.

Everyone on an interdisciplinary team is trained in his or her specialty and looks at care delivery with a different focus: nurses, physicians, social workers, dieticians, case managers. Sometimes having so many viewpoints can be difficult, though, especially if a single decision is needed and everyone has varying opinions.

To get the work of an organization completed, multiple formal and informal teams or groups may develop. Formal teams or groups may be a temporary ad hoc group that meets to accomplish a specific purpose, such as preparing for accreditation by the Joint Commission on Accreditation of Healthcare Organizations (JCAHO). Another formal team may be a permanent standing group or committee that meets regularly to accomplish organizational objectives, such as the Intensive Care Committee.

Informal groups may also evolve in organizations because of staff needs for social interaction. These informal groups and their leaders may not be part of the formal organization. It is very important to identify these informal leaders and groups to enlist their assistance in meeting the organization's goals.

A team may be advisory, such as a committee that meets to discuss concerns of the professional nursing staff and then reports back to the chief nurse executive for decision making, or the team may be self-directed and make decisions on its own. Whatever the type, all teams must communicate to achieve their objectives.

Communication Process

Communication is the exchange of information or opinions (Ruthman, 2003). See Figure 3-1. The message begins with the sender, who communicates it to the receiver. When the receiver reacts by changing his or her behavior or sending a feedback message back to the sender, communication has occurred. Unfortunately, the communication may be altered by the emotions, needs, perceptions, values, education, culture, and goals of both the sender and the receiver.

This fact makes it imperative that both the sender and receiver communicate with each other regularly to ensure clear understanding.

Note that communication is affected by following the rules of civility (Forni, P., 2003). Some of these rules are highlighted in Table 3-1.

Electronic Communication

Communication is shifting to an electronic mode, with computer technology playing an increasingly dominant role. Health care providers are using a variety of technologies, including telephones, voice mail, personal data assistants, fax, e-mail, and video conferencing. These methods require careful communication. For example, e-mail now allows almost instantaneous communication around the world, but it also accommodates individual preferences with respect to the timing of the response. This allows a person to send a message early in the day and allows the team members the opportunity to respond as their schedules permit. The speed with which exchanges can now be made using computers has reduced the acceptable response time. Therefore,

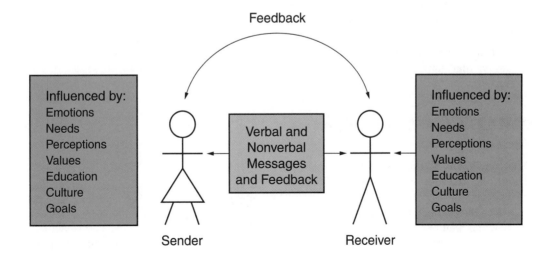

Figure 3-1 Process of Communication

TABLE 3-1
SELECTED TIPS ON CIVILITY

- Smile.
- Give praise.
- Admit you are wrong.
- Let others be kind to you.

- Keep your voice low in public places.
- Do not ridicule, humiliate, or demean others.
- Show consideration.

the first tip when communicating using e-mail is to respond in a timely manner. Answer personal e-mail within 48 hours and business e-mail within 24 hours. Respect the recipient's time and refrain from sending trivial messages (Forni, P., 2003). Next, keep in mind that accurate spelling, correct grammar, and organization of thought assume greater importance in the absence of verbal and nonverbal cues that are given in face-to-face encounters. E-mail can be informal but should not be abusive. Always proofread messages prior to sending them. Imagine yourself the recipient of the message. Look for complete sentences, logical development of thought and reasoning, accuracy, and appropriate use of grammar such as punctuation and capitalization. Finally, don't forward e-mails without the owner's permission, and always remember that your e-mail may be forwarded without your permission.

Building a Successful Team

Davis, Hellervik, Sheard, Skube, and Gebelein (1996) offer the following suggestions for building a successful team:

- Value the contributions of all team members: all members are critical to the success of the team regardless of their position on the team.
- Encourage interaction among group members: know when verbal and nonverbal behavior is appropriate and inappropriate and keep the flow of communication going.
- Discourage "we versus they" thinking: build teamwork that encourages inter-team participation and relationships.
- Involve others in shaping plans and decisions: involving the total team in the problem solving and decision making will strengthen any suggested changes made by the team because the entire team is able to support the decisions.
- Acknowledge and celebrate team accomplishments: publicly and frequently acknowledge positive contributions by team members, and keep the team members abreast of the positive changes they are actively involved in making.
- Evaluate your effectiveness as a team member: being an effective team leader includes being an effective team member. Are you carrying your weight, or are you expecting others to carry out your directives?

STAGES OF GROUP PROCESS

All teams go through predictable phases of group development as they evolve from an immature stage to a mature stage. It is critical to note that not all teams reach maturity, for a vari-

STOP AND THINK

You are the nurse who is working with Mr. Ward, a 76-year-old male who is admitted for congestive heart failure and chronic kidney disease. Mr. Ward is well known to the staff at Memorial Hospital for his multiple admissions. During this admission, his blood pressure is unusually high and he appears sluggish. His wife is visiting her relatives out of town, and he is by himself. When you attend the daily care management conference, you note most of the interdisciplinary team is present: the nurse case manager, the social worker, the nurse caring for him, the hospital chaplain, the dietician, the pharmacist, and his primary care physician.

What perspective does each of the team members bring to the discussion on the care of Mr. Ward? How would the team proceed to develop Mr. Ward's plan of care? Is this a formal team or an informal team?

ety of reasons: perhaps there is ineffective leadership, problematic members, unclear goals and communication, or lack of focus or energy. Some teams may become fully functional and mature quickly, bypassing a stage or two along the way. It is usual for high-functioning teams whose members are familiar with one another to be able to make decisions quickly and accurately; it may take longer for other teams, whose members need to get to know and trust one another before the actual work can take place.

Tuckman and Jensen (1977) and Lacoursier (1980) identified five stages that a group normally progresses through as it reaches maturity. These stages are known as **group process** and consist of: forming, storming, norming, performing, and adjourning (Figure 3-2).

The first stage is the forming stage, in which several critical phases begin: the expectation phase, the interaction phase, and the boundary formation phase. The expectation phase starts when the first meeting begins. Everyone is curious what the group is all about—how will it meet their needs, what they will need to do to fit in, and what they can gain from group membership. During the interaction phase, opinions are beginning to be formed as the group takes shape, and expectations and boundaries are more clearly defined. The group is establishing its

identity, with the help of the group leader. The group leader needs to provide the team with information on the purpose of the group meeting and the vision and boundaries of what the group is expected to accomplish.

The second stage of the group process is the storming phase. As everyone begins to feel more comfortable in the group setting, certain feelings and statements are made that may result in members finding a position within the group to which they can contribute. The storming phase is generally difficult because of conflict that may, at times, be quite apparent. Differences among group members—including even the group leader, perhaps—become obvious, with people often taking sides on certain concerns or issues. Although this phase is tension filled and confrontational, it is often necessary for a group to journey through the storming phase to encourage resolution of the emerging problems and to actively solve the issues at hand.

Stage three is the norming phase, which follows the conflict and confrontation of the storming stage. While the problems are not yet solved and decisions may not be made, there is a general understanding at least of what the issues are and who will be progressing toward solving them. Positions within the group are now established, with members having a sense of

Forming	Storming	Norming	Performing	Adjourning
• Expectations	• Tension	• Positioning	• Actual work	• Closure
• Interactions	• Conflict	• Goal setting	• Relationships	• Evaluation
• Boundary formation	• Confrontation	• Cohesiveness	• Group maturity	• Outcomes review

Figure 3-2 Stages of Group Process (Drawing on Tuckman & Jensen, 1977, and Lacoursier, 1980)

belonging and of setting goals to meet the expectations outlined in the forming stage. Conflict has converted into cohesiveness.

Performing is the fourth stage in the maturity of a group and is probably the most enjoyable phase. Agreement is a foremost activity—everyone knows what their role is and what they are supposed to do, and obvious progress is made toward the plan to achieve the overall group goal. The group is considered mature at this stage, and the individual members are now ready to focus on the actual work that will meet the group's objectives. Another strength of the performing stage is the emphasis placed on maintaining effective relationships with group members, as the individual members function as a whole (Tappen, 2001).

The final stage of the group process is adjourning. The group has met its stated and some unstated objectives, with closure activities the primary focus. Closure is the process by which the team members review the team's progress. Were the goals and objectives of the team met? Was there anything that would be done differently if the team were to start all over? During the final stage, the group should evaluate whether the stated purpose was accomplished. What were the outcomes of both the group process and the individuals' participation? So many times groups are disbanded without this closing review, leaving some members feeling empty and without a feeling of accomplishment.

COMMON MEMBER ROLES

In any team, there are bound to be both participants who are helpful and those who are not helpful in their behaviors. Sometimes the behaviors are unconsciously acted out. At other times, a team member is quite clear and focused about the role he or she is playing, such as the aggressor. In any case, it is imperative that the astute team leader be aware of everyone's roles and use excellent communication skills to facilitate the group process.

Common member roles in groups fit into three categories: group task roles, group maintenance roles, and self-oriented roles. Note that successful teams include both group leader roles and group follower roles.

Group task roles help a group develop and accomplish its goals. Among these roles are the following:

- Initiator-contributor: Proposes goals, suggests ways of approaching tasks, and recommends procedures for approaching a problem or task
- Information seeker: Asks for information, viewpoints, and suggestions about the problem or task
- Information giver: Offers information, viewpoints, and suggestions about the problem or task
- Coordinator: Clarifies and synthesizes various ideas in an effort to tie together the work of the members

- Orienter: Summarizes, points to departures from goals, and raises questions about discussion direction
- Energizer: Stimulates the group to higher levels and better quality of work

Group maintenance roles do not directly address a task itself but instead help foster group unity, positive interpersonal relations among group members, and development of the ability of members to work effectively together. Group maintenance roles include the following:

- Encourager: Expresses warmth and friendliness toward group members, encourages them, and acknowledges their contributions
- Harmonizer: Mediates disagreements between members and attempts to help reconcile differences
- Gatekeeper: Tries to keep lines of communication open and promotes the participation of all members
- Standard setter: Suggests standards for ways in which the group will operate and checks whether members are satisfied with the functioning of the group
- Group observer: Watches the internal operations of the group and provides feedback about how participants are doing and how they might be able to function better
- Follower: Goes along with the group and is friendly but relatively passive

Self-oriented roles are related to the personal needs of group members and often negatively influence the effectiveness of a group. These roles include the following:

- Aggressor: Deflates the contributions of others by attacking their ideas, ridiculing their feelings, and displaying excessive competitiveness
- Blocker: Tends to be negative, stubborn, and resistive of new ideas—sometimes in order to force the group to readdress a viewpoint that it has already dealt with
- Recognition seeker: Seeks attention, boasts about accomplishments and capabilities, and works to prevent being placed in an inferior position in the group
- Dominator: Tries to assert control and manipulate the group or certain group members by using methods such as flatter-

ing, giving orders, or interrupting others (Bartol & Martin, 1998)

Myers-Briggs Type Indicator

If a team is to succeed, it is critical to get the right blend of personalities, experience, and temperaments in the group to work toward a common goal.

Personality theories emphasize how personality differences affect communication. Traits such as introversion or extroversion, preference for rational objectivity or instinctive "gut feeling" affect the individual's communication. An example is a theory based on the Myers-Briggs Personality Dichotomies (Table 3-2), which in turn are based on personality theories of Carl Jung (Briggs Myers, & Myers, 1995).

This theory suggests that personality is made up of four complementary sets of traits: extroversion-introversion, sensing-intuition, thinking-feeling, and judging-perceiving. Within each of these sets, there is a sliding scale, so to speak. For example, on the extroversion-introversion scale, 1 might be completely extroverted, 10 completely introverted, and 5 equally both. See Figure 3-3. In most cases, one or the other usually dominates. Through testing, an individual can be identified as one of 16 possible types, based on the person's score in each of the four areas. The personality type is identified by a four-letter indicator. For example, an INTJ would be an introvert-intuitive-thinking-judging personality. An ESFP would be an extrovert-sensory-feeling-perceiving personality. In the theories of Jung and Myers-Briggs, each personality type has specific characteristics that affect the individual's approach to life experiences, including learning. Extroverts prefer to interact with people; introverts prefer to be alone. Thinking personalities prefer an objective, unwavering approach; feeling personalities are more likely to bend the rules if they think it makes people happy.

Such personality differences can affect the way individuals approach and engage in communication. Note that there are many personality instruments in current use (Pervin, 1993).

TABLE 3-2
MYERS-BRIGGS PERSONALITY DICHOTOMIES

Extroversion	Prefer interaction with people, conversation; learn when explaining to others or selves	vs.	Introversion	Reflective, focus on inner thoughts; think more than talk; need to establish frameworks for information they learn; see global view
Sensing	Rely on senses; detail oriented, prefer facts; prefer linear, structured presentation	vs.	Intuition	Seek patterns and relationships in information; rely on hunches; learn by discovery, prefer big picture or framework
Thinking	Prefer analysis and logic when making decisions; stress objectivity and fairness; want clear goals and objectives; want their learning expectations stated in clear, precise, and concrete terms	vs.	Feeling	Oriented toward human values and needs when making decisions; stress empathy and harmony; enjoy group exercises
Judging	Decisive, goal-oriented; value action and planning	vs.	Perceiving	Curious, adaptable, spontaneous; process-oriented rather than goal-oriented; continually gather information; may be pursuing many goals simultaneously; may learn better when given small and frequent tasks and deadlines

Compiled from *Gifts Differing*, by I. Briggs Myers and P. B. Myers, 1995, Palo Alto, CA: Davies-Black.

GREAT TEAM GUIDELINES

Great teams don't just happen; there is behind-the-scenes planning, preparation, and forward thinking before anyone works together. Theories of effective teams have been discussed in the literature for several decades by Lewin (1951), McGregor (1960), Argyris (1964), Burns (1978), Bennis (1989), and Senge (1990). What are the guidelines for encouraging great teams? A great team accomplishes what it sets out to do, with everyone on the team participating to achieve the desired outcomes. See Figure 3-4 for great team guidelines.

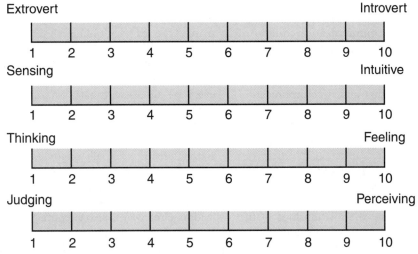

Figure 3-3 MBTI Scale

First and foremost, the team must have a clearly stated purpose: what are the goals? What are the objectives? What does the leader see the team accomplishing? An effective team keeps the larger organization's goals in mind as it progresses; otherwise, its goals will be inconsistent with those of the parent organization. Second is an assessment of the team's composition: what are the team members' personal strengths and weaknesses? How do the team members see themselves as individuals? Do they see themselves as part of a cohesive team? Are any

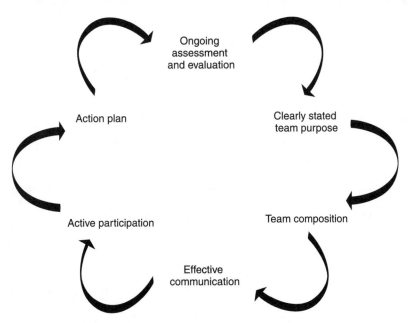

Figure 3-4 Great Team Guidelines

additional members with special expertise needed? What are the roles of each team member?

Third is the communication link. Are effective communication patterns in place? Is there a need to improve communication, either in written format or verbal format? Does the team work well together and is communication open, with minimal hidden agendas by the members? Can the truth be told in order to reach a difficult decision, in a compassionate and sympathetic manner?

Active participation by all team members is a critical fourth item. Does everyone have a designated responsibility? Do people listen to one another? What are the relationships of the team members? Is there mutual trust and respect for members and their decisions, however unpopular? Are there turf issues that must be resolved before proceeding? *Turf*, according to Husting (1996), is the primary reason that early team-building efforts may not work. Therefore,

it is important for the team leader to work on resolving turf-related problems early. The climate of the team should be relaxed but supportive.

Is there a clear plan as to how to proceed? This fifth element leads to an action plan that everyone agrees with early on, and one that is revisited at certain designated times. Feedback by team members and others affected by the team's decisions is necessary to keep focus. The sixth guideline is actually ongoing, in that assessment and evaluation are continuous throughout the team's history. Outcomes have to be consistent and related to the expectations of the organization. Creativity is also encouraged at the team level; perhaps a member has an idea to solve a problem that no one has ever tried. In a supportive environment, pros and cons of all reasonable ideas should be freely discussed. A team needs to periodically evaluate its progress. See Table 3-3.

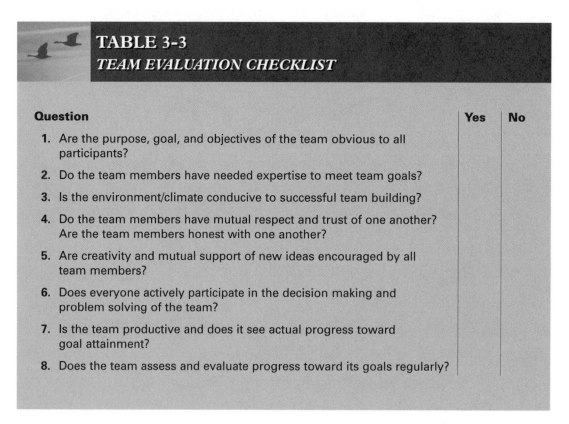

TABLE 3-3
TEAM EVALUATION CHECKLIST

Question	Yes	No
1. Are the purpose, goal, and objectives of the team obvious to all participants?		
2. Do the team members have needed expertise to meet team goals?		
3. Is the environment/climate conducive to successful team building?		
4. Do the team members have mutual respect and trust of one another? Are the team members honest with one another?		
5. Are creativity and mutual support of new ideas encouraged by all team members?		
6. Does everyone actively participate in the decision making and problem solving of the team?		
7. Is the team productive and does it see actual progress toward goal attainment?		
8. Does the team assess and evaluate progress toward its goals regularly?		

REAL WORLD INTERVIEW

An elderly nonverbal patient with a history of schizophrenia was admitted to our surgical unit for dehydration. She was in need of total care, especially with respect to hygiene, which had been neglected. She was dependent on staff to turn and position her. Her level of awareness suggested she was unable to use a call light for help.

This patient challenged staff for a variety of reasons. First, due to multiple other health problems, she was not a candidate for surgery. This placed her among the patients who don't really "fit" the surgical unit where she was admitted. Nonetheless, my goal was to advocate for comfort care with her physician while also encouraging subordinates to provide quality care even though the goal was not for cure with this particular patient. The patient's inability to communicate verbally added to the challenge. It was unclear how aware the patient was of the care she was receiving. Her nonverbal status blocked her ability to dialogue. This caused us to rely on nonverbal cues. Respect for patients with or without their verbal feedback is essential. The CNA and I tackled the needed bed bath together. Teamwork kept the focus on the goal for the patient, which was to optimize comfort and maintain skin integrity. It allowed me to complete a thorough assessment and to model desired communication with the patient, whom I addressed by name. I inquired whether she was in pain, to which she responded with twisting motions. I continued the one-way conversation, attempting to clarify what her nonverbal responses meant. She pointed to her shoulder, so we repositioned her and she settled down, resting quietly. As is often the case, the CNA willingly returned to reposition the patient with confidence the remainder of the shift. The patient's inability to verbalize needs was perceived as less of a barrier once we were successful in overcoming it together.

I find that CNAs will often volunteer to complete entire tasks they feel capable of performing independently. They also need to be assured that they will not be expected to handle clinical situations for which they do not feel qualified. This mutual respect for each other is essential to an ongoing working relationship. They honor my standard of care and will often complete tasks, going above and beyond what I ask. For example, later in the afternoon, the CNA returned to the patient and washed and braided her hair. Since this same patient would not likely use the call light, I also explained our goal to the high school student volunteer and I asked her to check the patient's position whenever she went by the room. I instructed her to let me know if the patient appeared uncomfortable, assuring her that I would reposition the patient as needed. The student expressed that she thought it was cool how nurses communicate with patients who can't talk. I believe through effective communication our team achieved the goal of optimizing this patient's comfort in spite of many potential barriers.

Lari Summa, RN, BSN

Team Leader

TEAMWORK ON A PATIENT CARE UNIT

The role of the nurse is multifaceted. Depending on the scenario, a nurse may work directly or indirectly with a wide variety of staff on the health care team. A registered nurse (RN) is directly responsible for the care of the patient, but that care encompasses ensuring that the physician and nursing orders are carried out and that unlicensed assistive personnel document the intakes and outputs accurately for the shift. The RN ensures that the licensed practical nurse completes the ordered treatments; that discharge planning is coordinated with the social worker, the case manager, the pharmacist, and the administration; that the family understands how to dress the patient's wound; and finally, that the patient understands the discharge instructions. The role of the RN team leader incorporates the entire spectrum of care provided to the family by a wide variety of people. The effective nurse will possess excellent communication skills, both written and verbal; be sensitive of others' cultural and value differences; be aware of others' abilities; and show genuine interest in the team members.

Communicating with Superiors

Communicating with a superior about team problems can be intimidating, especially for a new nurse. It is important to communicate with your superiors in order to develop a good working relationship (Gabarro & Kotter, 1993). See Table 3-4. Note that observing professional courtesy is an important first step. Alert your supervisor to any problems immediately, follow the policy and procedure of your agency, and, if it is not an emergency, request an appointment to discuss a problem further. This demonstrates respect and allows for the conversation to occur at an appropriate time and place. Be prepared to state the concern

TABLE 3-4
MANAGING YOUR BOSS

Know your boss's

1. Goals and objectives
2. Pressures
3. Strengths, weaknesses, blind spots
4. Preferred work style

Know your

1. Strengths and weaknesses
2. Personal style
3. Predisposition toward dependence on authority figures

Develop a relationship that

1. Fits both your needs and styles
2. Is characterized by mutual expectations
3. Keeps your boss informed
4. Is based on dependability and honesty
5. Selectively uses your boss's time and resources

clearly and accurately. Provide supporting evidence. State a willingness to cooperate in finding a solution and then match behaviors to words. Persist in the pursuit of a solution.

Communicating with Coworkers

Nurses depend on their coworkers in many ways to collectively provide quality patient care. Nowhere is this more important than in the acute care setting where nursing services are nonstop around the clock. Transfer of patient care from nurse to nurse is one of the most important and frequent communications between coworkers. It depends on fluid communication to achieve quality nursing care.

The Golden Rule

An excellent guide for communicating with coworkers is the golden rule: "Do unto others as you would have them do unto you." As a nurse who will be responsible for overseeing others' work, a valuable perspective for you to maintain is that all members of the team are important to successfully realize quality patient care. Offering positive feedback such as, "I appreciate the way you interacted with Mr. T. to get him to ambulate twice this shift," goes a long way toward team building, and it improves coworkers' sense of worth. Nurses also have an opportunity to act as teachers to coworkers. Often in a hospital setting, nurses teach by example. Demonstrating the desired behavior allows the coworker to copy the behavior. It is important to allow time for return demonstrations to evaluate that the coworker has learned the intended skill. For example, as the nurse, you may demonstrate how to position a patient with special needs, encouraging the coworker to assist and ask questions. The next time repositioning is indicated, accompany the coworkers and observe his or her ability to successfully complete the task. Offer constructive feedback. Be patient. Remember your own learning curve when mastering new skills and behaviors and allow those you supervise the opportunity to grow. Be open to the possibility that coworkers, particularly those with experience, may have a few pearls of wisdom to share with you as well.

Communicating with Other Practitioners and Physicians

Sometimes new graduates are intimidated by other practitioners and physicians they work with. Cardillo (2001) gives several tips on working with other practitioners. She suggests that it is useful to establish rapport and introduce yourself to the other practitioners you work with. Do not be intimidated. You and the other practitioners are all on the health care team to meet the patient's goals. At least one study has indicated that when nurses and physicians work together, patient death rates or readmission rates decrease (Baggs & Ryan, 1990). Both you and the other practitioners are important to your patient's welfare.

Cardillo (2001) also suggests that nurses be assertive. Do not call another practitioner or doctor and say, "I'm sorry to bother you." You are not bothering her. That is her job and you are doing your job by calling her. If you do not understand something, ask questions. Many practitioners and physicians love to teach. Be honest and up front. Tell the practitioner if something is new to you.

Show respect and consideration for the practitioner you work with but do not be a doormat. Give due respect and expect the same from them. Present information in a straightforward manner, clearly delineating the problem, supported by pertinent evidence. This is especially important when reporting changes in patient conditions. Nurses are responsible for knowing classic symptoms of conditions, orally apprising the physician of changes, and recording all observations in the chart (Sanchez-Sweatman, 1996). See Table 3-5. If the other practitioner is out of line, you might say, "I don't appreciate being spoken to in that way," or "I would appreciate being spoken to in a civil tone of voice and I promise to do the same with you," or something similar.

TABLE 3-5

TOOL TO ORGANIZE INFORMATION FOR CALLING ANOTHER PRACTITIONER OR PHYSICIAN FOR ASSISTANCE

Patient name and room	
All diagnoses	
Allergies	
Current medications and IV fluids	
Current and baseline vitals, level of consciousness, urine output	
Current problem	
Potential outcome of problem for patient	
Action needed from practitioner or physician	
Urgency of call	

Calfee (1998) offers suggestions for handling telephone miscommunications. For example, if a physician hangs up, document that the call was terminated and fill out an incident report. If the physician gives an inappropriate answer or gives no orders, for example, for a patient complaint of pain, document the call, the information relayed, and the fact that no orders were given. In addition, document any other steps, such as notifying the supervisor, that were taken to resolve the problem.

Cardillo (2001) suggests that nurses seek clarification from the practitioner if an order is unclear. If an order is inappropriate or incorrect, rather than saying, "This order does not seem appropriate for this patient," which would likely put the practitioner on the defensive, try, "Teach me something, Dr. Jones; I've never seen a dose of Lopressor that high. Can you explain the therapeutic dynamics to me?" or "Dr. Smith, I can't figure out why you ordered a brain scan on this patient. Can you help me out here?" This approach often results in the practitioner either reevaluating an order or changing it. If the practitioner does not change an order that you think is inappropriate or you can't reach the practioner, let your supervisor know and follow the chain of command guidelines of the agency where you work.

Communicating with Patients and Families

Communication with patients and families is optimized by many skills, including touch. Nurses routinely use touch as a way to communicate caring and concern. Occasionally, lan-

REAL WORLD INTERVIEW

A nurse working in a factory setting was presented with a patient who entered the nursing office complaining that he didn't feel good. The nurse's initial assessment, including vital signs, revealed that the only abnormality was an elevated blood pressure. In this situation, like in any clinical situation, it is important to distinguish the urgent from the nonurgent. With hypertensive patients, it is important to realize that an urgent situation is suggested by evidence of acute end organ damage. Specifically, in this situation, it was important to know whether the patient was experiencing altered sensorium, headache, visual disturbance, chest pain, or dyspnea. The presence of any of these findings should be communicated to the physician and would dictate urgent transport to the hospital. In their absence, the patient can be referred for more elective blood pressure control.

In any clinical situation, such as the one above, the nurse can facilitate communications by being organized and objective. Be prepared to discuss the basics such as the patient's chief complaint, his vital signs, his medications, and any changes from baseline. Know why you are worried about observed changes and communicate this to the physician.

John C. Ruthman, MD

guage barriers will limit communication to the nonverbal mode. For instance, a stroke patient who cannot process words can still interpret a gentle hand on his shoulder.

Communication requires an openness and honesty with concurrent respect for patients and families. In addition, it is important to honor and protect patients' privacy with the nurse's actions and words. Recent HIPAA legislation guarantees this to patients. See Chapter 2.

ORGANIZATIONAL COMMUNICATION

Avenues of communication are often defined by an organization's formal structure. The formal structure establishes who is in charge and identifies how different levels of personnel and various departments relate within the organization. When the chief executive officer of an organization announces that the company will adopt a new policy that all employees will follow, that is

downward communication. The message starts at the top and is usually disseminated by levels through the chain of communication. Upward communication is the opposite of downward communication. The idea originates at some level below the top of the structure and moves upward. For example, when a nurse recommends a more efficient approach to organizing care to his nurse manager, who takes the recommendation to her superior, who uses the recommendation to develop a new policy, that is upward communication. Lateral communication often occurs among people with similar status. Two nurses discussing how to best change a patient's dressing are engaged in lateral communication. Diagonal communication occurs when members of the team who may be on different levels of the organizational chart discuss a patient care concern such as discharge planning. The organizational structure within nursing also determines who is responsible for representing nursing concerns in this type of interaction. For example, if the department

LITERATURE APPLICATION

Citation: DiBartola, L. (2001, June). Listening to patients and responding with care. *Joint Commission Journal on Quality Improvement*, 27(6), 315–323.

Discussion: Clinicians who want to improve their listening skills benefit from identifying the way in which patients are most comfortable interacting. A tool for assessing this is demonstrated. Once the patient's interaction style is identified, the clinician uses this information to move closer to where the patient is comfortable communicating. This article discusses a communication model for improving patient communication. Figure 3-5 describes behavioral characteristics of the four communication modes.

The framework for this model is the continuum of two intersecting axes. The horizontal axis poles are inquisitive and assertive. The vertical axis poles are objective and subjective. People who are most comfortable communicating in an inquisitive way and tend to be objective are called investigators. Those who are most comfortable communicating in an inquisitive way but are subjective in nature are called unifiers. People who are most comfortable communicating in an assertive way and favor subjectivity are called energizers. Those who are most comfortable communicating in an assertive way and tend to be objective are called enterprisers. Behavioral markers can be used to identify someone's preferred communication mode (Figure 3-6).

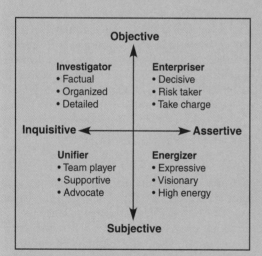

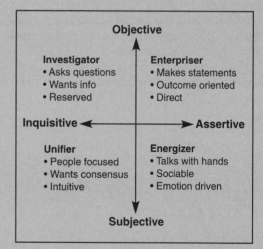

Figure 3-5 Behavioral Characteristics of the Four Communication Modes (From "Listening to Patients and Responding with Care," by L. DiBartola, 2001, *Joint Commission Journal on Quality Improvement*, 27(6), 319. Reprinted with permission.)

Figure 3-6 Behavioral Markers for the Four Communication Modes (From "Listening to Patients and Responding with Care," by L. DiBartola, 2001, *Joint Commission Journal on Quality Improvement*, 27(6), 322. Reprinted with permission.)

(continues)

Literature Application *(continued)*

Using your observation skills, determine where your patient is on the inquisitive-assertive scale. Typical markers that would identify someone who is close to the inquisitive side are asking questions, attending carefully to detail, listening carefully to what the other person is saying, showing caution in making a decision without having adequate time to think about it, and preferring facts over intuition. On the other side of the scale, markers for someone who prefers to communicate in an assertive way are showing concern about wasting time, being quick to make a decision, being more interested in outcomes than in process, being willing to take risks, and making strong statements rather than asking questions.

In addition, you will want to make observations about the patient's preference for objectivity or subjectivity. Whereas people with an objective preference are more interested in facts than intuition and in the project outcome than the process, people who are more subjective show more interest in the people who are working on the project than the project itself, are more willing to trust intuition than the facts, and show greater interest in being satisfied than in being right.

Nonverbal cues include the use of gestures or hands while talking for those on the assertive side, and reserve and control for those on the inquisitive side. To apply this model, think of an interaction that did not go well. Notice where both parties fit on the scale. The closer both parties are on the scale, the easier it will be for them to communicate.

Implications for Practice: Once you understand the way in which both you and another person are most comfortable communicating, you can decide to communicate in a way that may be more comfortable. You are not expected to change who you are; the goal of this approach is to know yourself, understand the other person, and then move closer to him or her. This will build trust and respect, and result in both parties feeling satisfied in the interaction. An important understanding for a nurse is that not all people feel and communicate in the same way as the nurse.

practices within a primary nursing model, the primary nurse is responsible for representing nursing concerns. In team nursing, the team leader rather than the nurse delivering care is responsible. A final avenue worth mentioning, which is not a formal avenue, is the grapevine. The grapevine is an informal avenue in which rumors circulate. It ignores the formal chain of command. The major benefit of the grapevine is the speed with which information is spread, but its major drawback is that it often lacks accuracy. For example, nurses who inform an oncoming shift about a rumor that layoffs or mandatory overtime is imminent in the absence of any information from the hospital's adminis-

tration are participating in grapevine communication. Skilled nurses participate in both formal and informal communication.

OVERCOMING COMMUNICATION BARRIERS

DuBrin (2000) has identified nine strategies and tactics for overcoming communication barriers. See Table 3-6.

In addition to these strategies, it is helpful to use stress management techniques to avoid communication barriers.

TABLE 3-6
OVERCOMING COMMUNICATION BARRIERS

Concept	Application
Understand the receiver	Ask yourself, What's in it for the other person?
	Work to develop understanding of the other person's needs.
Communicate assertively	Be direct. Use "I" statements; e.g., "I want you to . . ."
	Explain ideas clearly and with feeling.
	Repeat important messages.
	Use various communication channels; e.g., written, e-mail, verbal, and so on.
Use two-way communication	Ask questions.
	Communicate face to face.
Unite with a common vocabulary	Define the meaning of important terms, such as high quality.
Elicit verbal and nonverbal feedback	Request and offer verbal feedback often.
	Document important agreements.
	Observe nonverbal feedback.
Enhance listening skills	Pay attention to what is said, what is not said, and nonverbal signals.
	Continue listening carefully even when you don't like the message.
	Give summary reflections to ensure understanding; e.g., "You say you are late giving medication because the pharmacy did not deliver meds on time."
	Engage in concluding discussions; e.g., "Has your unit been late with medications due to problems with pharmacy deliveries before?"
	Ask questions to explore problems.
	Paraphrase the speaker's words to decrease miscommunication rather than blurting out questions as soon as the other person finishes speaking.

(continues)

Table 3-6 *(continued)*

Concept	Application
Be sensitive to cultural differences	Know that cultural communication barriers exist.
	Show respect for all workers.
	Minimize use of jargon specific to your culture.
	Be sensitive to cultural etiquette; e.g., use of first names, eye contact, hand gestures, personal appearance.
Be sensitive to gender differences	Be aware that men and women may have some differences in communication style; e.g., men may call attention to their accomplishments and women tend to be more conciliatory when facing differences.
	Know that male-female stereotypes often don't fit the person you are working with.
	Avoid barriers by knowing differences exist, and don't take things personally.
	Males can improve communication by showing more empathy, and, females, by becoming more direct.
Engage in metacommunication	Communicate about your communication to resolve a problem; e.g., "I'm trying to get through to you, but either you don't react to me or you get angry. What can I do to improve our communication?"

Compiled with information from DuBrin, 2000.

KEY CONCEPTS

- Teams are essential to the effective functioning of any health care organization.
- Teams may be formed for a variety of reasons, including the need for professional affiliation, the need for socialization, and the need for psychological fulfillment.
- Teams consist of people who come together for a common purpose and who need each other's contributions to achieve the overall goal.
- Each group goes through defined stages of increasing maturity.
- Team members can perform various roles, which may ultimately enhance or hinder the team's progress toward goal attainment.
- The MBTI helps identify personality types.
- Great teams have clearly stated purposes, effective communication, an action plan, and continuously evaluate their progress.
- Clear communication is essential to achieving goals.

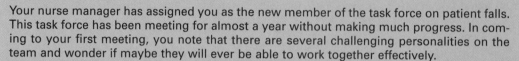

CASE STUDY 3-1

Your nurse manager has assigned you as the new member of the task force on patient falls. This task force has been meeting for almost a year without making much progress. In coming to your first meeting, you note that there are several challenging personalities on the team and wonder if maybe they will ever be able to work together effectively.

Jamie is a new graduate nurse and volunteers for everything. Angela likes details, often asking everyone to repeat what they said so that she can get more information on the topic. Samantha is the passive one and just looks annoyed at having to be there. You noticed she was doing some of her patient charting while in the meeting. Anabelle attempts to keep the team on track, but with her soft-spoken voice, she is not well heard. Finally, no matter what anyone says, Beth is critical and comes up with a reason why something will not work.

Would the Myers-Briggs Type Indicator give you any more information about the members of this team?

It would be interesting to use the MBTI and have every member of the team identify their personal MBTI type. Then they can see how other members of the team identify the MBTI type of each of the other members and compare the two views. See the online test in the Web Exercises.

KEY TERMS

communication   team
group process

REVIEW QUESTIONS

1. In forming a team, the leader should keep in mind that
   A. the team should decide the goals and objectives.
   B. the team is responsible for developing its vision.
   C. the team should be constructed of similar personality types.
   D. the team should encourage active participation by all members.

2. Which is the normal sequencing of group process?

   A. Forming, norming, storming, performing, adjourning
   B. Norming, forming, storming, performing, adjourning
   C. Forming, storming, norming, performing, adjourning
   D. Forming, storming, conforming, norming, adjourning

3. One of the primary duties of effective team leaders on their team is to
   A. ensure that all the details are taken care of all the time.
   B. enable the team to envision their goals and objectives.
   C. take effective minutes of the meetings.
   D. allow everyone a chance to participate, even if the work takes longer than expected.

4. In maintaining an environment conducive to team building, it is important to
   A. have an autocratic management style by leaders.
   B. encourage creativity within the organization.

C. reward employees who consistently revise the team's objectives.

D. hold an evaluation session at the completion of the team's work.

REVIEW ACTIVITIES

1. You are a nurse on a 38-bed medical surgical unit. In light of some vacancies, the nurse manager has hired a licensed practical nurse to fill a position in which only registered nurses had worked before.
   - What are some things you can do to assist the new person in becoming a member of your team?
   - Would nursing assignments change with the addition of the new practical nurse?

2. Because of the increase in patient complaints about the quality of care, you have been asked to work on a team to address patient care issues.
   - What are your expectations of the five stages of group process?
   - How will you work with the team members to progress though each stage?

3. On the unit on which you work as a registered nurse, the team is quite interdisciplinary in nature: you directly work with licensed practical nurses, unlicensed assistive personnel, a secretary, one housekeeper, one respiratory therapist, one case manager, and one clinical nurse specialist.
   - What are some of the advantages of working with interdisciplinary teams?
   - What are some of the challenges of working with interdisciplinary teams?
   - How does one best communicate with an interdisciplinary team?

EXPLORING THE WEB

- Where would you find additional information on effective team building on the Internet?
  http://www.accel-team.com
- What type of leadership style do you have in a team situation?
  http://www.onlinewbc.gov
- Check the type descriptions and online test based on Jung Myers-Briggs typology or updated version of the Jung Typology Test
  http://www.humanmetrics.com

REFERENCES

Argyris, C. (1964). *Integrating the individual and the organization.* New York: Wiley.

Baggs, I. G., & Ryan, S. A. (1990). ICU nurse physician collaboration and nursing satisfaction. *Nursing Economic, 8*(6), 386–392.

Bartol, K. M., & Martin, D. C. (1998). *Management* (3rd ed.). Boston: McGraw-Hill.

Bennis, W. (1989). *Why leaders can't lead.* San Francisco: Jossey-Bass.

Briggs Myers, I. & Myers, P. B. (1995). *Gifts differing.* Palo Alto, CA: Davies-Black.

Burns, J. M. (1978). *Leadership.* New York: Harper & Row.

Cardillo, D. W. (2001). *Your first year as a nurse.* Roseville, CA: Prima.

Davis, B. L., Hellervik, L. W., Sheard, J. L., Skube, C. J., & Gebelein, S. H. (1996). *Successful manager's handbook*, N. p.: Personnel Decisions International.

DiBartola, L. (2001, June). Listening to patients and responding with care. *Joint Commission Journal on Quality Improvement, 27*(6), 315–323.

DuBrin, A. J. (2000). *The active manager.* London: South-Western College Publishing.

Forni, P. (2003). *Choosing civility*. Parade Magazine. New York: St. Martin's Press.

Gabarro, J. J., & Kotter, J. P. (1993). Managing your boss. *Harvard Business Review*, May–June, 150–157.

Husting, P. M. (1996). Leading teams and improving performance [Electronic version]. *Nursing, 27*(9), 35.

Katzenbach, J. R., & Smith, D. K. (1993). *The wisdom of teams: Creating the high-performance organization*. New York: Harper Business.

Lacoursier, R. B. (1980). *The life cycle of groups: Group development stage theory*. New York: Human Sciences Press.

Lewin, K. (1951). *Field theory in social sciences*. New York: Harper & Row.

McGregor, D. (1960). *The human side of enterprise*. New York: McGraw-Hill.

Pervin, L. A. (1993). *Personality: Theory and research* (6th ed.). New York: Wiley.

Ruthman, J. L. (2003). Personal and interdisciplinary communication. In P. L. Kelly-Heidenthal, *Nursing management and leadership*. Clifton Park, NY: Delmar Learning.

Sanchez-Sweatman, L. (1996, September). Communicationg with physicians. *The Canadian Nurse, 92*(8), 49–50.

Senge, P. M. (1990). *The fifth discipline*. New York: Doubleday Books.

Senge, P. M., Roberts, C., Ross, R. B., Smith, B. J., & Kleiner, A. (1994). *The fifth discipline fieldbook: Strategies and tools for building a learning organization*. New York: Doubleday/Currency.

Tappen, R. M. (2001). *Nursing leadership and management: Concepts and practice* (4th ed.). Philadelphia: F. A. Davis.

Tuckman, B. W., & Jensen, M. A. C. (1977). Stages of small group development revisited. *Group and Organizational Studies, 2*(4), 419.

SUGGESTED READINGS

Farrell, M. P., Schmitt, M. H., & Heinemann, G. D. (2001). Informal roles and the stages of interdisciplinary team development. *Journal of Interprofessional Care, 15*(3), 281–295.

Jain, V. K., & Lall, R. (1996). Nurses' personality types based on the Myers-Briggs Type Indicator. *Psychology Reporter, 78*(3 pt. I), 938.

Keirsey, D., & Bates, M. (1978). *Please understand me: Character and temperament types*. Del Mar, CA: Prometheus Nemesis Books.

Kennedy, M. M. (2001). What do you owe your team? Survival tips for people who dread teamwork. *Physician Executive, 27*(4), 58–60.

Opt, S. K., & Loffredo, D. A. (2000). Rethinking communication apprehension: A Myers-Briggs perspective. *Journal of Psychology, 134*(5), 556–570.

Shope, T. C., Frohna, J. G., & Frohna, A. Z. (2000). Using the Myers-Briggs Type Indicator (MBTI) in the teaching of leadership skills. *Medical Education, 34*(11), 956.

Wilson, R. D., Mateo, M. A., & Brumm, S. K. (1999). Revitalizing a departmental committee. *Journal of Nursing Administration, 29*(3), 45–48.

CHAPTER 4

Planning Care in Organizations

The greater thing in this world is not so much where we stand as in what direction we are going. (Oliver Wendell Holmes)

OBJECTIVES

Upon completion of this chapter, the reader should be able to:

1. Discuss assessment of the external and internal environment of health care.
2. Review SWOT analysis.
3. Be able to articulate the importance of aligning the organization's strategic vision both with the organization's own mission, philosophy, and goals and also with the goals and values of the communities served by the organization.
4. Review common organizational structures.
5. Discuss shared governance.

Mary has been assigned the nursing care of several patients on her unit. She has been working as an RN on the unit for two months. What elements in the organization should Mary consider? What elements on the unit should Mary consider? How can Mary work within the care delivery structure and processes of the unit to achieve optimal patient care outcomes?

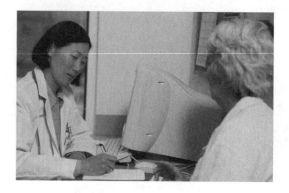

Planning nursing care in organizations utilizes the nursing process to plan, implement, and evaluate the outcomes of care for groups of patients rather than individual patients.

Successful patient care management requires governance structures, patient care delivery, goals and processes, and measures of the outcome of care delivery. These must be consistent with the needs of the patients, the community, and the mission and vision of the organization. It is built on a philosophy of professional nursing practice.

This chapter discusses assessment of a health care organization's external and internal environment, identifies the importance of the mission and vision to achieving goals, and then reviews common organizational structures. Finally, this chapter discusses shared governance in a nursing care organization.

ASSESSMENT OF EXTERNAL AND INTERNAL ENVIRONMENT

As outlined in Figure 4-1, planning patient care involves clarifying the organization's philosoph-

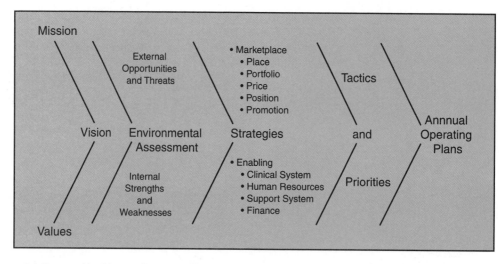

Figure 4-1 Bassett Healthcare Strategic Planning Framework (Framework developed by Gennaro J. Vasile, PhD, FACHE)

ical values; identifying the mission of why the organization exists; articulating a vision statement; and then conducting an environmental assessment, or SWOT analysis, which examines the Strengths, Weaknesses, Opportunities, and Threats of the organization. See Figure 4-2.

Surveys and questionnaires, focus groups and interviews, advisory boards, and a review of the literature can also contribute information useful to the planning stage and add to the data that drive the development of 3- to 5-year strategies for the organization. Tactics are then created and prioritized. Finally, goals and objectives are concretized into annual operating work plans for the organization. This same process is used for unit or departmental planning.

DEVELOPMENT OF A PHILOSOPHY VISION, MISSION, AND GOALS

A **philosophy** is a statement of beliefs based on core values—inner forces that give us purpose (Yoder-Wise, 2002). A unit's mission and vision are most authentic if they are developed based on the philosophy or core beliefs of the work team (Wesorick, Shiparski, Troseth, & Wyngarden, 1997). Core beliefs may be complex as those expressed in Table 4-1. Or they can be short statements developed from a staff brainstorming session, such as "patient centered," "partnering," "healing environment," and the like. A unit's core

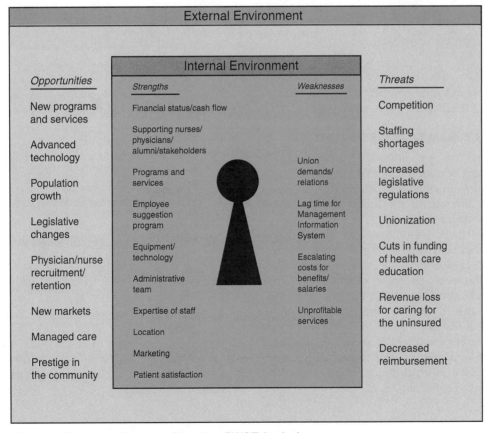

Figure 4-2 Key to Success in Strategic Planning: SWOT Analysis

TABLE 4-1
CORE BELIEFS

- Quality exists where shared purpose, vision, values, and partnerships are lived.

- Each person has the right to health care, which promotes wholeness in body, mind, and spirit.

- Each person is accountable to communicate and integrate his/her contribution to health care.

- Partnerships are essential to plan, coordinate, integrate, and deliver health care across the continuum.

- Continuing to learn and think in different ways is essential to improve health.

- A healthy culture begins with each person and is enhanced through self-work, partnerships, and systems supports.

From "Mission and Core Beliefs," by B. Wesorick, *CPMRC Connections . . . for Continuous Learning*, December 2000, 3, p. 3.

beliefs or values are then incorporated into the unit's mission and vision statements.

Mission Statement

A mission is a call to live out something that matters or is meaningful (Wesorick et al., 1997). An organization's mission reflects the purpose and direction of the health care agency or a department within it.

Covey (1990) states, "An organizational mission statement—one that truly reflects the shared vision and values of everyone within that organization—creates a unity and tremendous commitment" (p. 139). For the unit mission statement to have the greatest effect, all members of the unit work team should participate in its development and it should be written and easily available to all staff to encourage the development of an organization or unit that is focused on meeting its mission.

Questions to be answered by the group charged with development of the unit mission include the following:

- What do we stand for?
- What principles or values are we willing to defend?
- Who are we here to help?

There are three elements to a unit mission statement:

1. A mission statement is no longer than a couple of sentences.

2. It states the unit's purpose using action words.

3. It should be simple and from the heart. (Jones, 1996)

Mission statements are so broad that, often, patient care units adopt the organization's mission statement.

STOP AND THINK

Examine these two mission statements and then respond to the questions that follow.

Hospital A: "Our mission is to ensure the highest quality of care for the patients in our community. We believe that each patient has the right to the most innovative care that current science and technology can provide. To that end, we have assembled a world-renowned medical staff who will strive to ensure that the latest developments in medical science are used to combat disease."

Hospital B: "Our mission is to provide excellence in care to all. Our health care staff, nurses, physicians, and other professionals believe that care can best be provided in an atmosphere of collaboration and partnership with our patients and community. We believe in education—for our patients, for our staff, and for future health care providers. At all times we strive for optimal health promotion and the prevention of disease and disability."

Which of these institutions do you think would be more likely to have a patient lecture series on living with diabetes? Value the contributions of nursing? Provide experimental therapy for cancer? Be open to scheduling routine patient care visits for uninsured patients?

Vision Statement

The unit vision statement reflects the organization's vision of the future. A unit vision statement then exemplifies how the mission and vision of the unit will be actualized within the organization's mission and vision.

Following are four elements of a vision for the future:

1. It is written down.

2. It is written in present tense, using action words, as though it were already accomplished.

3. It covers a variety of activities and spans broad time frames.

4. It balances the needs of providers, patients, and the environment. This balance anchors the vision to reality. (Wesorick et al., 1997)

The surgical unit vision statement in Table 4-2 exemplifies the core values of the unit: patient centered, partnering, healing environment, and knowledge. The written statement tells the reader the work of the unit, why it is done, how, and for what reasons. In short, it delineates how the unit will continue to fulfill its mission in the future.

Goals and Quality Measures

The next step in the planning process is for the organization and the work unit to develop goals and quality measures that reflect the mission. A goal is a specific aim or target that the unit wishes to attain within the time span of 1 year. Measures of the goal may reflect finances, customer satisfaction and services, internal operating efficiency, and learning and growth (Norton & Kaplan, 2001). See Table 4-3.

ORGANIZATIONAL STRUCTURE

Organizations are structured or organized to facilitate the execution of their mission, goals, reporting lines, and communication within the

TABLE 4-2
SURGICAL UNIT VISION STATEMENT

The work we do: Affects the outcomes that patients desire in their pursuit of wellness.

Why we do it: To provide a healing environment in which an individual's physical, mental, emotional, and spiritual well-being will be nurtured.

Who we are: Practicing within partnering relationships that communicate respect while recognizing and valuing diversity.

How we do it: By committing to continued learning. Our knowledge fosters our growth; our mentoring nurtures our practice. (Roesch, 2000)

REAL WORLD INTERVIEW

We plan every year, but I'd say we look at our unit philosophy based on our core values and reevaluate the strategic plan every 2 to 3 years. We had three core values that guided us, and then this year, with all the external pressures, we added a fourth. We keep these core values in the forefront when we do our annual planning. The process we used to develop and reevaluate the core values was really very powerful and staff driven.

SPAN—Staff Planning Action Network—is our unit-based shared governance organization. SPAN met and developed draft mission and vision statements from our philosophy, which is based on our current core values—patient centered, partnering, and healing environment. They then transcribed these draft statements onto three flip charts and for 15 minutes per shift circulated these terms throughout the unit and got staff's reaction and feedback to the statements. Revisions were made from the feedback received. These were then presented at a staff meeting. What was emerging from the feedback was a focus on the need for continuing education and training related to the rapidly changing environment. So we added a fourth value—knowledge.

Our unit philosophy, stemming from our core values, is what we believe in. We've expanded these core values into a vision statement.

Patricia S. Roesch, BSN, RN

Patient Care Manager

TABLE 4-3
MISSION, GOALS, AND QUALITY MEASURES

Mission

The Peoples Choice Healthcare Center provides excellent health care to all patients through partnerships with patients and the community and collaboration with nurses, physicians, and other health care staff. We believe in continuous education for patients, health care staff, and future health care providers. We are committed to optimal health care promotion and prevention of disease and disability.

Goals

1. Collaborate with all health care staff to improve patient care

2. Increase customer satisfaction scores

3. Increase number of emergency room visits

4. Increase patient days

5. Increase use of computers by all staff

6. Increase funding for staff's continued education

7. Encourage all staff to attend one education program yearly

8. Increase number of specialty certifications of staff

9. Monitor nurse sensitive patient outcomes, such as incidence of cardiac arrest, UTI, upper GI bleeding, thrombophlebitis, failure to rescue, and so forth

10. Decrease medication errors

Quality Measures for Emergency Department

Customer/Patient

1. Increase in patient satisfaction

2. Increase in customer return

3. Decrease in patient complaints

4. Increase in market share

5. Decrease in repeat asthma patient visits

6. Develop patient education materials explaining norms for ER stays, well and ill child care, and so on

(continues)

Table 4-3 *(continued)*

Financial

1. Increase use of computers on all units

2. Monitor budget compliance

3. Improve nurse staffing ratios

4. Develop computerized order entry system for medications

Internal Processes

1. Achieve 90% on key Performance Improvement measures

2. Decrease sick time and overtime by 10%

3. Increase number of nursing research projects

4. Achieve Magnet status

5. Increase use of Best Practice Educational Materials for all patients and staff

6. Increase participation of nursing, medicine, unlicensed assistive personnel, and pharmacy staff in quality improvement activities

7. Arrange for all staff to attend one outside conference yearly

8. Set up nursing journal club meetings monthly

9. Set up interdisciplinary committee on medication administration safety

Employee Growth and Learning

1. 50% of the nursing department join a nursing professional association

2. All nurses working in the emergency room are certified in ACLS, PALS, and so forth

3. One-third of nurses are continuing their nursing education

4. 50% of all staff are cross-trained and can work in ICU and ER

5. 90% of employees are very satisfied

6. 90% of staff are retained

7. All nurses are able to use the computer for patient information, to search literature, and so forth

8. 20% of nursing staff present a community program on topics such as stroke and so forth

organization. This is true of entire organizations as well as individual nursing units. There are a number of ways to describe organizational structures.

Types of Organizational Structures

Usually, the existing organizational structures are communicated by means of an organizational chart. Figure 4-3 is an example of an organizational chart for a typical acute care general hospital. This organization has a tall bureaucratic structure with many layers in the hierarchy or chain of command and a centralized formal authority in the board of trustees. It represents a formal, top-down reporting structure.

Matrix Structure

Today, given the greater complexity of the health care system, more organizations are using matrix structures. Note that in this structure, a person may report to two or more managers. Figure 4-4 shows a matrix design (Shortell & Kaluzny, 2000).

Flat Versus Tall Structure

Organizations are considered flat when there are few layers in the reporting structure. A tall organization would have many layers in the chain of command. An example of a flat organizational structure is a department of nursing that has no divisions and has many unit managers reporting to one director of nursing.

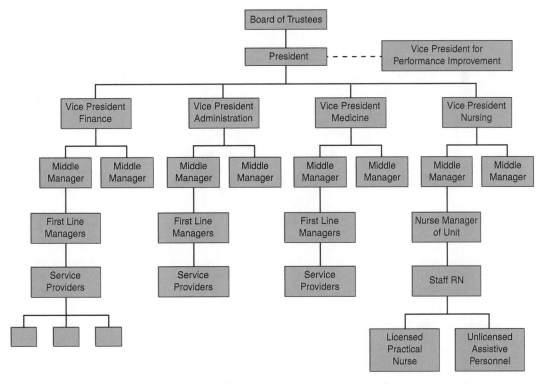

Figure 4-3 Organizational Chart, Formal Authority Structure: Acute Care General Hospital

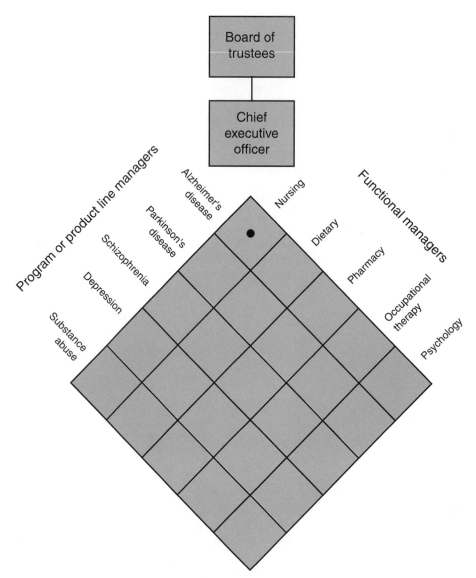

Figure 4-4 Matrix Design: A Psychiatric Center. An individual worker in this example is part of the Alzheimer program as well as a member of the nursing department.

Decentralized Versus Centralized Structure

The terms *centralized* and *decentralized* refer to the degree to which an organization has spread its lines of authority, power, and communication. A tall, bureaucratic design like that in Figure 4-3 would be considered highly centralized. A matrix design like that in Figure 4-4 would be on the decentralized end of the continuum. As can be seen in Figure 4-4, the nursing manager can interface with the Alzheimer's disease program manager without going through a central, hierarchical core, as would happen in a bureaucratic structure like that in Figure 4-3. Note that other characteristics or attributes can also be used to identify organizations (Shortell & Kaluzny, 2000).

Division of Labor

The way the labor force is divided or organized has an effect on how the mission is accomplished. The organizational chart in Figure 4-3 graphically depicts how the formal authority in this organization is functionally structured. At the highest level, the board of trustees delegates authority to the president, who delegates to the vice presidents and so on. At the vice presidential level, there are four department vice presidents. The vice presidents each report to the president. The middle managers report to their vice president. The nurse managers report to the middle managers. The service provider or staff nurses report to the nurse manager. In this design, the division of labor is quite efficient and specialized. A danger with this division of labor is that each individual may be so focused on a specific area that he or she has little perspective about the overall picture. For example, a service provider may focus on one area of a nursing unit and have little information about the total picture.

In the matrix structure shown in Figure 4-4, the structure was less important and the workforce roles and reporting relationships are based on the project or task to be accomplished, rather than on a rigid hierarchy. An example of this is the planning involved in the preparation for a Joint Commission on Accreditation of Healthcare Organizations (JCAHO) review. The JCAHO team could be composed of various individuals at varying levels of responsibility and from programs across the organization, but they could interact with staff at all levels and report as a task force at a high level in the organization.

Division of Labor by Geographic Area.
Care delivery divided according to geography or location can be efficient. It might consist of the hospital and ambulatory care, or at smaller unit levels, the North Team and the West Team. For example, each team may consist of an RN team leader, a licensed practical nurse (LPN), and an unlicensed assistive personnel (UAP).

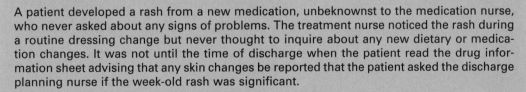

CASE STUDY 4-1

A patient developed a rash from a new medication, unbeknownst to the medication nurse, who never asked about any signs of problems. The treatment nurse noticed the rash during a routine dressing change but never thought to inquire about any new dietary or medication changes. It was not until the time of discharge when the patient read the drug information sheet advising that any skin changes be reported that the patient asked the discharge planning nurse if the week-old rash was significant.

What could have been done differently?

Was anyone at fault? Who?

Why is good communication especially important in a situation in which there is a division of labor by function?

What types of problems could you expect if staff members focused on their own tasks and failed to communicate with each other about the patient's emotional, psychosocial, educational, and discharge needs?

Division of Labor by Product or Service. Sometimes, care delivery is organized around product lines or service lines. This is based on a patient's diagnosis or the specialty care required by a patient. For example, there might be a cardiology service line, a woman's health service line, and an oncology service line. This can lead to improved quality of care and decreased confusion for the patient because the information and protocols used in the outpatient side would be consistent with the information and protocols used in the hospital and across the entire health care system. Figure 4-5 demonstrates a product line design (Shortell & Kaluzny, 2000).

Roles and Responsibilities

Note that exact roles and responsibilities within each level and division are not defined on the organizational charts beyond specifying the given division, for example, nursing. Scope of

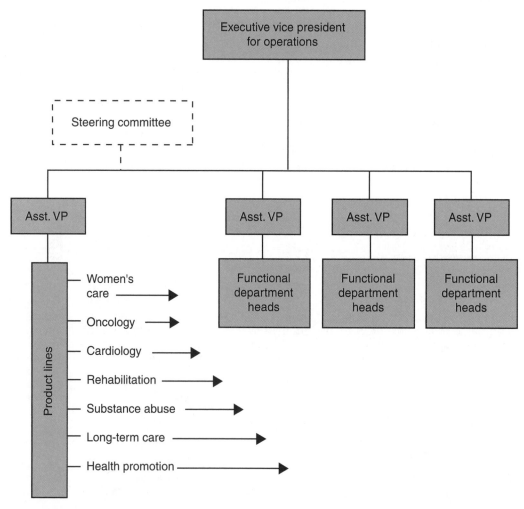

Figure 4-5 Product Line Design

responsibilities, specific duties, and specific job requirements are found in documents such as individual job or position descriptions.

Reporting Relationships

An organizational chart, such as the one that appears in Figure 4-3, allows one to determine the formal reporting relationships. These are shown with a solid line. Sometimes dotted lines are used in an organizational chart to depict dual or secondary reporting relationships. An example of this might be the role of the Vice President for Performance Improvement. This individual might directly report to the President but also have position accountabilities to the board of trustees. The formal reporting relationships may or may not reflect the actual communications that occur within the institution. An example of this occurs when information is communicated outside the formal reporting relationships. This method of information sharing is often referred to as the grapevine. An example of grapevine communication might occur when a nurse had a personal friend who was in a high administrative position who shared information confidentially about pending budget cuts.

SHARED GOVERNANCE

Shared governance is an organizational framework grounded in a philosophy of decentralized leadership that fosters autonomous decision making and professional nursing practice (Porter-O'Grady, 1992). Shared governance, by its name, implies the allocation of control, power, or authority (governance) among mutually (shared) interested vested parties (Stichler, 1992).

In most health care settings, the vested parties in nursing fall into two distinct categories: (1) nurses practicing direct patient care such as staff nurses and (2) nurses managing or

administering the provision of that care such as managers. In shared governance, a nursing organization's management assumes the responsibility for organizational structure and resources. Management relinquishes control over issues related to clinical practice. In return, staff nurses accept the responsibility and accountability for their professional practice.

Unit-based shared governance structures are most successful if there is an organization-wide structure of shared governance in place that unit-based functions can articulate with. Organizational shared governance structures are usually council models that have evolved from preexisting nursing or institutional committees. In a council structure, clearly defined accountabilities for specific elements of professional practice have been delegated to five main arenas: clinical practice, quality, education, research, and management of resources (Porter-O'Grady, 1992). Figure 4-6 illustrates a shared governance model.

Shared Goverance Model

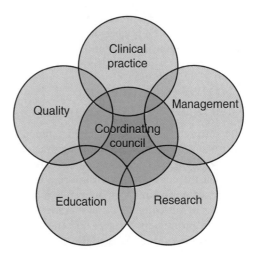

Figure 4-6 A Shared Governance Model

Purpose of the Clinical Practice, Quality, and Education Councils

The purpose of the clinical practice council is to establish nursing practice standards for a unit. The purpose of the quality council is twofold: (1) to make recommendations about hiring, promoting, and credentialing nursing staff and (2) to oversee the unit quality management initiatives.

The purpose of the nursing education council is to assess the learning needs of the unit staff and develop and implement programs to meet these needs.

Purpose of the Research Council

At the unit level, the research council advances research utilization with the intent of incorporating research-based findings into the clinical nursing standards of practice. Research utilization is the process of staff critiquing available research literature and then making recommendations to the practice council so that clinical policies and procedures can be based on evidence-based research findings. The research council may also coordinate research projects if advanced practice nurses practice at the institution.

Purpose of the Management Council

The purpose of the management council is to ensure that the standards of nursing practice and governance agreed upon by unit staff are upheld and that there are adequate resources to deliver patient care. The nurse manager is a standing member of this council. Other members include the assistant nurse managers and the charge or resource nurses from each shift.

Purpose of the Coordinating Council

The purpose of the nursing coordinating council is to facilitate and integrate the activities of the other councils. This council is usually composed of the nurse manager and the chairpeople of the other councils. This council usually facilitates the annual review of the unit mission and vision and develops the annual operational plan (Sellers, 1996).

Unit-based shared governance structures may be less diverse. Often some of the councils are combined into one council, for example, education and research. Or a council may contain subcommittees whose purposes are to perform very specific tasks, for example, credential and promote staff or recruit and retain staff. Unit-based structures are varied, with the primary purpose being to empower staff by fostering professional practice while meeting the needs of the work unit.

 KEY CONCEPTS

- There are increasing opportunities for nurses to become involved in planning for the delivery of health care services in their organizations and communities. To do so effectively, however, they will need a basic understanding of the way in which organizations are structured, how organizational systems function, and how to engage in the planning process.
- Successful orchestration of a patient care unit in today's health care environment is achieved through vision-driven professional practice.
- Shared governance is an organizational framework grounded in a philosophy of decentralized leadership that fosters autonomous

decision making and professional nursing practice.

- The mission statement reflects the organization's values and provides the reader with an indication of the behavior and actions that can be expected from that organization.
- A health care organization needs to have a good idea of where it fits into its environment and what types of programs and services are needed and demanded by its customers or stakeholders.
- The pivotal value of planning is that it requires an organization to focus on its mission and to test how its operations are leading to accomplishment of that mission.
- The purpose of planning is twofold. First, it is important that everyone has the same idea or vision of where the organization is headed; second, a good plan can help to ensure that the needed resources are available to carry out the initiatives that have been identified as important to the unit or agency.
- Organizations are structured or organized in a manner that is designed to facilitate the execution of their mission and their strategic plans.

KEY TERMS

goal
mission

philosophy
shared governance

REVIEW QUESTIONS

1. Shared governance
   A. is an accountability-based care delivery system.
   B. is a tested framework of organizational development.
   C. is a competency-based career promotion system.
   D. implies the allocation of control, power, or authority (governance) among interested parties.

2. A document that describes the institution's purpose and philosophy is
   A. the organizational chain of command.
   B. the organizational chart.
   C. the mission statement.
   D. the strategic plan.

3. Which of the following is the outcome of the processes by which an organization engages in environmental analysis, goal formulation, and strategy development with the purpose of organizational growth and renewal?
   A. Stakeholder assessment
   B. SWOT analysis
   C. Strategic planning
   D. Mission development

4. The most formal and hierarchical organizational structure would be expected to have an organizational chart with
   A. a matrix design.
   B. many layers of command.
   C. a product line design.
   D. a number of dotted lines representing reporting relationships.

5. SWOT means
   A. strengths, weaknesses, opportunities, threats.
   B. strengths, worries, outcomes, threats.
   C. strengths, weaknesses, opportunities, treatment.
   D. structures, worries, outcomes, threats.

REVIEW ACTIVITIES

1. You have been practicing as a new graduate for a little over a year. You are feeling more confident about your clinical practice and think you might want to expand your leadership experience. Your unit governance framework is shared governance. Review the common councils of shared governance. Given your education and experience, which council would you like to join?

2. Having a plan in place can help an organization to make a decision about one alternative over another. For example, an institution whose strategic plan calls for positioning itself as the leading cancer care provider in the area would be well served to advertise for nurses in the *Oncology Nursing Society Journal* rather than in a local newspaper, even if the costs of advertising in the journal were higher. Identify another situation in which a plan could guide an organization in its choices among alternative actions.

3. Write a beginning mission statement for your professional nursing career. Do you plan to care for vulnerable populations in the community, become expert in critical care nursing, or seek advanced education to become a midwife? Once you have identified your mission, outline a plan with objectives to attain your plan. For example, you might want to conduct a SWOT analysis, looking at the external environment; your internal environment (your skills, talents, and preferences); and the strengths, weaknesses, threats, and opportunities that exist in each. Once you have completed this exercise, you will have a better idea of which opportunities to pursue. For example, if you know that you want to work in pediatrics, you might ask for a pediatric journal subscription for your birthday. Additionally, you may be able to select or have input into the selection of your final clinical rotation in school, or you may be able to look for meetings, conferences, or educational sessions in your area of interest.

4. You are asked to help establish the advisory board for your institution's proposed hospice program. What groups of professionals and consumers would you want to see represented on a hospice advisory board? Identify at least 10 candidates and the stake- holder groups that they might represent. Remember to include both professionals and consumer/community representatives. It would be important to assess each individual's sup-

port for hospice concepts and his or her level of interest in becoming involved prior to inviting those individuals to join the advisory board. How might you go about doing this?

5. Examine the organizational structure of an organization or institution with which you are familiar. How would you characterize it using the types of structures that were discussed in this chapter? Is the organization a hierarchy, a matrix, or some other design? Does the way that the institution or organization is structured assist it in meeting its goals? Why or why not?

 EXPLORING THE WEB

- You have been asked by your nurse manager and members of the credentialing committee to revamp the current clinical promotion ladder so that it more clearly differentiates and rewards nurses for their education level as well as expertise. Go to *http://www.uchsc.edu*. Note the University of Colorado's nursing differentiated practice model that can be accessed there.

- Upon completion of your nursing degree, you plan to interview for a position at an area hospital. In preparation for your interview, you want to understand the mission as well as other information about that institution. Today that information is readily available on the Web. For example, if you were planning to apply at Loyola University Chicago (*http://www.luc.edu*) you would go to *http://www.luhs.org*. By clicking the About Us tab (on the home page) and then the Mission Statement tab, you can view the mission statement.

- What impressions do you form about these organizations and their missions? Does the stated mission seem to fit with the general "feel" that you get from the Web site? Could you easily find information about positions available? About the institution?

Try this exercise with your local hospital or medical center.

- Go to the magnet hospitals site at *http://www.nursingworld.org.* Type in Magnet, and then click Magnet. What information do you find here?
- Go to *http://www.nursingsociety.org.* This site provides weekly literature updates from Sigma Theta Tau International, the nursing profession's honor society. What new books and periodicals are available that may be helpful to you in your practice?

Stichler, J. F. (1992). A conceptual basis for shared governance. In N. D. Como & B. Pocta (Eds.), *Implementing shared governance: Creating a professional organization* (pp. 1–24). St. Louis, MO: Mosby.

Wesorick, B., Shiparski, L., Troseth, M., & Wyngarden, K. (1997). *Partnership council field book: Strategies and tools for co-creating a healthy work place.* Grand Rapids, MI: Practice Field.

Yoder-Wise, P. S. (2002). *Leading and managing in nursing* (2nd ed.). St. Louis, MO: Mosby.

REFERENCES

Covey, S. R. (1990). *The seven habits of highly effective people.* New York: Hay House.

Jones, L. B. (1998). *The path: Creating your mission statement for work and for life.* New York: Hyperion.

Jones, R., & Beck, S. (1996). *Decision making in nursing.* Clifton Park, NY: Delmar Learning.

Norton, D. P., & Kaplan, R. S. (2000). *The strategy focused organization.* Boston, MA: Harvard Business School.

O'Malley, A. A., & Androwich, I. M. (2003). Strategic Planning and Organizing Patient Care. In P. L. Kelly-Heidenthal (Ed.), *Nursing Management and Leadership.* Clifton Park, NY: Delmar Learning.

Porter-O'Grady, T. (1992). *Implementing shared governance: Creating a professional organization.* St. Louis, MO: Mosby-Year Book.

Roesch, P. (2000, October). Surgical unit practice. *Nursing Matters, 7*(3), 1. Bassett Healthcare, Cooperstown, NY.

Sellers, K. F. (1996). *The meaning of autonomous nursing practice to staff nurses in a shared governance organization: A hermeneutical analysis.* Unpublished doctoral dissertation, Adelphi University, Garden City, New York.

Shortell, S., & Kaluzny, A. (2000). *Health care management: Organization design and behavior* (4th ed.). Clifton Park, NY: Delmar Learning.

SUGGESTED READINGS

Aiken, L. H., Havens, D. S., & Sloane, D. M. (2000, March). The magnet nursing services recognition program. *American Journal of Nursing, 100*(3), 26–35.

Alspach, J. (1984). Designing a competency-based orientation for critical care nurses. *Heart and Lung, 13,* 655–662.

Benner, P. (1984). *From novice to expert.* Menlo Park, CA: Addison-Wesley.

Bennis, W. (1999, Summer): The end of leadership: Exemplary leadership is impossible without full inclusion, initiatives, and cooperation of followers. *Organizational Dynamics,* 71–80.

Bridges, W. (2000). *Managing transitions: Making the most of change.* New York: Perseus Books Group.

Dreyfus, S. E., & Dreyfus, H. L. (1980). *A five stage model of the mental activities involved in directed skill acquisition.* Unpublished report supported by the Air Force Office of Scientific Research, USAF (Contract F49620-79-C-0063), University of California at Berkeley.

Havens, D. S., & Aiken, L. H. (1999). Shaping systems to promote desired outcomes: The magnet hospital model. *Journal of Nursing Administration, 29*(2), 14–20.

Kaplan, R. S., & Norton, D. P. (2001). *The strategy focused organization.* Boston, MA: Harvard Business School.

Sellers, K. F., Hargrove, B., & Jenkins, P. (2000). Asthma disease management programs improve clinical and economic outcomes. *MEDSURG Nursing, 9*(4), 201–203, 207.

Senge, P. (1990). *The fifth discipline.* New York: Doubleday.

Silvetti, C., Rudan, V., Frederickson, K., & Sulivan, B. (2000, April). Where will tomorrow's nurse managers come from? *Journal of Nursing Administration, 30*(4), 157–159.

Zemke, R., Raines, C., & Filipczak, B. (2000). *Generations at work: Managing the clash of veterans, boomers, xers and nexters in your workplace.* New York: AMACOM.

CHAPTER 5

Delegation

> The authority was delegated to me to care for this patient and, by assuming this responsibility for the patient, I will then be accountable for this patient's care. (Phyllis Franck and Marjorie Price, 1980)

OBJECTIVES

Upon completion of this chapter, the reader should be able to:

1. Discuss concepts of delegation, authority, responsibility, accountability, supervision, and assignment.
2. Utilize the National Council of State Boards of Nursing Delegation Decision–Making Grid.
3. Discuss the role of state boards of nursing in delegation.
4. Describe the five rights of delegation.
5. Identify responsibilities of health team members.

Magda Golbrida was admitted to the hospital for a ventricular shunt placement to divert her excess cerebrospinal fluid. Magda had a failed shunt insertion recently and had returned to the hospital for repeat surgery. She is now 2 days post-op and needs neurological assessments to be performed at the onset of every shift and whenever necessary, as indicated by changes in her condition. The night nurse assessed the patient at the beginning of her shift and noted that the patient's neurological status was intact. During the night, the nurse checked on the patient every 2 hours but did not awaken her. A sitter was in the room with the patient. The sitter had assured the nurse that the patient was "doing fine." When the sitter had assisted the patient to the bathroom at the start of the shift, the patient had no difficulty. Then, upon assisting the patient the second time, the sitter noted that the patient was leaning to one side so badly that she could not stand and required help from two additional aides. This change in the

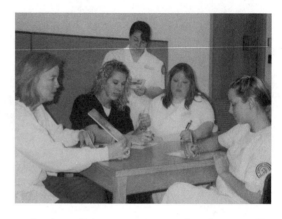

patient's condition was not reported to the nurse. The patient ended up with fluid retention in the shunt and permanent paralysis.

- *Could this have been prevented?*
- *Who is accountable?*
- *What are the responsibilities of the nurse, the sitter, and the two aides?*

According to the American Nurses Association (ANA) Code for Nurses With Interpretive Statement, 2001, "The nurse is responsible and accountable for individual nursing practice and determines the appropriate delegation of tasks consistent with the nurse's obligation to provide optimum patient care."

A priority responsibility for nurses is to deliver safe patient care. To ensure that this responsibility is met, nurses are accountable under the law for patient care delivered by them and other personnel under their supervision. These personnel may include other registered nurses (RN), licensed practical/vocational nurses (LPN/LVN), and unlicensed assistive personnel (UAP). UAP is an umbrella term applied to many categories of unlicensed workers such as nurse aides, nurse technicians, patient care technicians, nurse support personnel, nurse extenders, personal care attendants, unit assistants, nursing assistants, and other non-licensed personnel. UAP are trained to

function in an assistive role to the licensed RN in the provision of patient care activities as delegated by the nurse (ANA, 1992). Note that in some states, assistive personnel are licensed (National Council of State Boards of Nursing [NCSBN], 1997).

This chapter discusses the concepts of delegation, authority, responsibility, accountability, supervision, and assignment of nurses. It also describes the National Council of State Boards of Nursing Delegation Decision–Making Grid, the role of state boards of nursing in delegation, the responsibilities of health team members, the five rights of delegation, and using the chain of command.

PERSPECTIVES ON DELEGATION

Florence Nightingale is quoted as saying, "But then again to look to all these things yourself does not mean to do them yourself. . . . But can you not insure that it is done when not done by yourself?" (1859, p. 17). Nursing delegation was discussed by Nightingale in the 1800s and has continued to evolve since then. Delegation is particularly needed because of the advent of cost containment, the shortage of nurses, increases in patient acuity levels, an elderly chronic population, and advances in health care technology. It is a must for the new nurse as well as for the experienced nurse. Delegating to personnel with different educational levels from a variety of nursing educational programs requires nurses to be vigilant and ensure that safety is maintained for the patient. RNs are accountable for using the nursing process to achieve good outcomes of patient care. When delegating to UAP who are not trained in the nursing process, the RN is additionally accountable for monitoring all aspects of the nursing process, including the evaluation of patient outcomes. For example, when an RN delegates the process of ambulating a patient to UAP, the RN remains accountable for the safe implementation of the process of ambulation as well as for monitoring the patient's safe outcome; that is, the patient is protected from falls. The RN must monitor both the competency, education, and skill of UAP and the stability of the patient needing a delegated task initially and in an ongoing fashion. Thus, efficient delegation protects the patient.

DELEGATION

Delegation is defined as "the transfer of responsibility for the performance of an activity from one individual to another while retaining accountability for the outcome. Example: the nurse, in delegating an activity to an unlicensed individual, transfers the responsibility for the performance of the activity but retains professional accountability for the overall care" (ANA, 1992). There are two types of patient care activities that may be delegated: direct and indirect.

Direct Patient Care Activities

Direct patient care activities include activities such as assisting the patient with feeding, drinking, ambulating, grooming, toileting, dressing, and socializing. Direct patient care activity may also involve collecting, reporting, and documenting data related to these activities. These data are reported to the RN, who uses the information to make a clinical judgment about patient care. Activities delegated to UAP do not include health counseling or teaching, or require independent, specialized nursing knowledge, skill, or judgment. **Nursing judgment** is defined as the process by which nurses come to understand the problems, issues, or concerns of patients, to attend to salient information, and to respond to patient problems in concerned and involved ways. This includes both conscious decision-making and intuitive response (ANA, 1992).

Indirect Patient Care Activities

Indirect patient care activities are necessary to support patients and their environment and only incidentally involve direct patient contact. These activities assist in providing a clean, efficient, and safe patient care milieu. They typically encompass chore services, companion care, housekeeping, transporting, clerical, stocking, and maintenance tasks (ANA, 1992).

Underdelegation

Personnel in a new job role such as new nurse managers or new nursing graduates often underdelegate. Believing that older, more experienced staff may resent having someone new delegate to them, new nurses may simply avoid delegation. Or they may seek approval from other staff members by demonstrating their capability to complete all assigned duties without assistance. New nurses can become frustrated and overwhelmed if they fail to delegate properly. They may fail to delegate the appropriate authority to go with certain responsibilities. Perfectionism and refusal to allow mistakes also can overwhelm new nurses.

Overdelegation

Overdelegation of duties can also be a problem. Delegating duties that are inappropriate for personnel to perform because they have been inadequately educated is dangerous and against the state nurse practice act. The reasons for overdelegation are numerous. Personnel may feel uncomfortable performing duties that are unfamiliar to them, and they may depend too much on others. They may be unorganized or inclined to either avoid responsibility or immerse themselves in trivia. Overdelegating duties can overwork some personnel and underwork others. See Table 5-1 for other obstacles to delegation.

AUTHORITY

Authority is the right to act or to command the action of others. Authority comes with the job and is required for a nurse to take action. The person to whom a task and authority has been delegated must be free to make decisions regarding the activities involved in performing those tasks. Without authority the nurse cannot function to meet the needs of patients. Authority is commonly delegated to the nurse in the nurse's job description and it is based on each individual state's nurse practice act. For example, if a nurse is in charge of a group of patients, he or she must have the authority or the right to act or command the action of others. Note that there are four possible levels of authority to be used by the RN when delegating a task to another nurse (Cox, 1997). See Table 5-2.

TABLE 5-1
OBSTACLES TO DELEGATION

1. Fear of being disliked

2. Inability to give up any control of the situation

3. Inability to prioritize using Maslow's Hierarchy of Needs

4. Lack of confidence to move beyond being a novice nurse

5. Tendency to isolate oneself and choosing to complete all tasks alone

6. Lack of confidence to delegate to staff who were previously one's peers

7. Inability to communicate effectively and develop working relationships with other team members

8. Thinking of oneself as the only one who can complete a task the way "it is supposed" to be done

9. Lack of knowledge of the capabilities of staff, including their competency, experience, and level of education

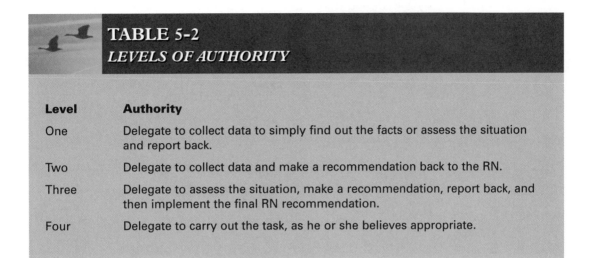

TABLE 5-2
LEVELS OF AUTHORITY

Level	Authority
One	Delegate to collect data to simply find out the facts or assess the situation and report back.
Two	Delegate to collect data and make a recommendation back to the RN.
Three	Delegate to assess the situation, make a recommendation, report back, and then implement the final RN recommendation.
Four	Delegate to carry out the task, as he or she believes appropriate.

An understanding of the level of authority at the time the task is delegated and the level of authority that is mandated by the state nurse practice act prevents each party from making inaccurate assumptions about authority for delegated assignments.

THE NATIONAL COUNCIL OF STATE BOARDS OF NURSING (NCSBN) DELEGATION DECISION-MAKING GRID

The NCSBN has developed a Delegation Decision-Making Grid with seven elements. Rating the seven elements on the grid assists the nurse in delivering care based on such elements as the level of client stability and the competency of the UAP and licensed nurse. A lower rating on the grid indicates that the activity can be safely delegated. A higher rating on the grid cautions against delegation. For example, if the level of client stability is ranked a 3 (client condition is unstable or acute or has a strong potential for change) and the level of UAP competence is also rated a 3 (novice in performing nursing care activities in the defined client population), that activity should probably not be delegated. Each one of the seven grid elements is scored to assist in making the delegation decision. See Figure 5-1.

STATE BOARDS OF NURSING

Many states specify nursing tasks that may be delegated in their rules and regulations. For excerpts from the Board of Nurse Examiners for the State of Texas January 2003, see Table 5-3. Although the excerpts in this example are similar to those of some other states, there is some variation in these rules and regulations from state to state. Check your state requirements with your state board of nursing at http://www.ncsbn.org.

THE FIVE RIGHTS OF DELEGATION

The NCSBN has spelled out Five Rights of Delegation (NCSBN, 1997) that nurses may apply to practice. These five rights are the right task, the

STOP AND THINK

Following are some examples of appropriate delegation of authority:

• An RN asks the UAP to take a stable patient in a wheelchair for a chest x-ray.

• The charge nurse asks another experienced RN to be in charge while the charge nurse goes to dinner.

Why are these delegations appropriate?

Why must the nurse evaluate staff qualifications and competency as well as patient needs prior to delegation?

right circumstance, the right person, the right direction and communication, and the right supervision. See the Web site for more information at http://www. ncsbn.org. See Table 5-4.

KNOWLEDGE AND SKILL OF DELEGATION

Note that delegation is not a skill that is simply learned in a classroom. Delegation requires discussion of knowledge and concerns related to delegation and clinical mentorship or practice in responsibilities related to that delegation. The process also includes discussion of how to handle situations where tasks were not accomplished when delegated (Salmond, 1994). See Table 5-5.

RESPONSIBILITY

Responsibility is the obligation involved when one accepts an assignment. The delegation process is not complete until the person who receives the assignment accepts it. Without this acceptance of obligation or responsibility, authority cannot be delegated. Further, if a person does not have the knowledge, skill, expe-

rience, or willingness needed to complete an assignment, it is inappropriate to accept responsibility for an assignment. There must be documented evidence of the competency of all assigned personnel.

Responsibility cannot be delegated if the assumption of the responsibility is not taken by the receiver of the assignment. Once a person accepts responsibility for an assignment, this responsibility is retained. For example, after the UAP's assigned duty is performed, he or she is responsible to give feedback to the nurse about the performance and outcome of the duty. This feedback information is given in a specified time frame. Note that feedback works two ways. It is the UAP's responsibility to give feedback as well as the registered nurse's responsibility to follow up with ongoing supervision and evaluation of the UAP's activities. The nurse transfers authority for the completion of a delegated task but retains responsibility for monitoring the delegated task's outcome.

RESPONSIBILITIES OF HEALTH TEAM MEMBERS

New graduate nurses may feel overwhelmed in their first nursing position by the responsibility of

Delegation Decision-Making Grid

Elements for Review		client A	client B	client C	client D
Activity/task	**Describe activity/task:**				
Level of Client Stability	**Score the client's level of stability:** 0. client condition is chronic/stable/predictable 1. client condition has minimal potential for change 2. client condition has moderate potential for change 3. client condition is unstable/acute/strong potential for change				
Level of UAP Competence	**Score the UAP competence in completing delegated nursing care activities in the defined client population:** 0. UAP – expert in activities to be delegated, in defined population 1. UAP – experienced in activities to be delegated, in defined population 2. UAP – experienced in activities but not in defined population 3. UAP – novice in performing activities and in defined population				
Level of Licensed Nurse Competence	**Score the licensed nurse's competence in relation to both knowledge of providing nursing care to a defined population and competence in implementation of the delegation process:** 0. Expert in the knowledge of nursing needs/activities of defined client population *and* expert in the delegation process 1. Either expert in knowledge of needs/activities of defined client population and competent in delegation or experienced in the needs/activities of defined client population and expert in the delegation process 2. Experienced in the knowledge of needs/activities of defined client population *and* competent in the delegation process 3. Either experienced in the knowledge of needs/activities of defined client population *or* competent in the delegation process 4. Novice in knowledge of defined population *and* novice in delegation				
Potential for Harm	**Score the potential level of risk the nursing care activity has for the client (*risk is probability of suffering harm*):** 0. None 1. Low 2. Medium 3. High				
Frequency	**Score based on how often the UAP has performed the specific nursing care activity:** 0. Performed at least daily 1. Performed at least weekly 2. Performed at least monthly 3. Performed less than monthly 4. Never performed				
Level of Decision-Making	**Score the decision-making needed, related to the specific nursing care activity, client (both cognitive and physical status) and client situation:** 0. Does not require decision making 1. Minimal level of decision making 2. Moderate level of decision making 3. High level of decision making				
Ability for Self Care	**Score the client's level of assistance needed for self-care activities:** 0. No assistance 1. Limited assistance 2. Extensive assistance 3. Total care or constant attendance				
	TOTAL SCORE				

Figure 5-1 NCSBN Delegation Decision-Making Grid (Reprinted and used by permission of the National Council of State Boards of Nursing Inc. [NCSBN]. Copyright 1997 National Council of State Boards of Nursing [NCSBN]). This information can be found on the NCSBN Web site at http://www.ncsbn.org.

TABLE 5-3
EXCERPTS FROM THE BOARD OF NURSE EXAMINERS FOR THE STATE OF TEXAS, RULES AND REGULATIONS RELATING TO PROFESSIONAL NURSE EDUCATION, LICENSURE, AND PRACTICE JANUARY, 2003

Nursing tasks that may not be delegated

- Assessment (physical, psychological, and social assessment that requires professional nursing judgment, intervention, referral, or follow-up). Note that data collection without interpretation is not assessment
- Planning of nursing care and evaluation of the client's response to the care rendered
- Implementation that requires judgment
- Health teaching and health counseling other than reinforcement of what the RN has already taught
- Medications

Tasks that are most commonly delegated

- Noninvasive and nonsterile treatments
- Collecting, reporting, and documentation of data such as
  - Vital signs, height, weight, intake and output, capillary blood and urine test for sugar, and hematest results
  - Ambulation, positioning, and turning
  - Transportation of the client within the facility
  - Personal hygiene and elimination, including cleansing enemas
  - Feeding, cutting up of food, or placing of meal trays
  - Socialization activities
  - Activities of daily living
  - Reinforcement of health teaching planned or provided by the RN

Nursing tasks that may not be routinely delegated

(Note that these may sometimes be delegated if the UAP has received special credentialing; e.g., education and competency testing.)

- Sterile procedures
- Invasive procedures, such as inserting tubes in a body cavity or instilling or inserting substances into an indwelling tube
- Care of broken skin other than minor abrasions or cuts generally classified as requiring only first aid treatment

Excerpts January 2003 from http://www.bne.state.tx.us/rr218.htm#218.5. Accessed January 2, 2003.

CASE STUDY 5-1

Applying the NCSBN Delegation Decision-Making Grid

The staff for 2 East on the night shift included three registered nurses, Mary, Colleen, and Steve; a nursing assistant, Jill; and a sitter, Jane. Mary is a new graduate who has just completed orientation. Steve, the charge nurse for the night shift, made the following assignment:

2501–2504	RN, Mary
2505–2508	RN, Steve
2509–2512	RN, Colleen
2501–2512	Nursing assistant, Jill
2504	Sitter, Jane

It is just about 11:30 P.M. when Steve finishes listening to the shift report from the 3–11 nurse. He prepares to give the report to Jill, the nursing assistant, who has worked with Steve on 2 East for the past 7 years. Steve tells Jill, "the patient in 2505 just received a pain shot and probably will not be needing anything for pain for the next few hours. If he does complain of pain, let me know."

In the shift report, Steve was told that the patient's blood pressure (BP) in 2506 was coming down although he was still hypertensive with a BP of 180/102. The patient had just been given one dose of Lopressor. The dose was to be repeated every 6 hours as needed for a systolic blood pressure greater than 170 mm Hg or a diastolic blood pressure greater than 100 mm Hg. Steve told Jill to check this patient's blood pressure every half hour for the next 2 hours and to let him know of any changes. Jill is certified by the hospital in taking BPs. Steve also informed Jill that the patient in 2507 was stable, had received a sleeping pill earlier and was sound asleep, and that there would be a new admission in 2508 coming up from the emergency department (ED) any minute. Just then, as Steve was giving the report, the new ED patient with pneumonia was rolled into the room on a cart. The patient was complaining of shortness of breath and needed oxygen.

Fill out the Delegation Decision-Making Grid in Figure 5-2 for the patient in 2506 to determine what tasks Steve can safely delegate to Jill. Then check your answers below.

Was your score any different? If so, why do you think your score was different?

Here is how we scored the patient in 2506. We took into account the fact that Jill is certified and experienced on 2 East in taking and reporting BPs on this unit. With a total score of 13, the patient's BP could be assigned to Jill because this patient was fairly stable with a decreasing BP. Jill was competent in monitoring and reporting BPs. She has been taught signs of an abnormal BP and the importance of reporting abnormalities immediately. The patient's BP has been decreasing daily and Steve is experienced in caring for this type of patient and will continue to assess and monitor the patient and work with Jill. Now fill in the scores for the other 3 patients on the grid. Do your scores agree with ours?

Delegation Decision-Making Grid

Elements for Review		2505	2506	2507	2508
Activity/task	**Describe activity/task:**	Pain assess-ment	Take BP	Monitor sleep	Give O$_2$
Level of Client Stability	**Score the client's level of stability:** 0. client condition is chronic/stable/predictable 1. client condition has minimal potential for change 2. client condition has moderate potential for change 3. client condition is unstable/acute/strong potential for change		3		
Level of UAP Competence	**Score the UAP competence in completing delegated nursing care activities in the defined client population:** 0. UAP – expert in activities to be delegated, in defined population 1. UAP – experienced in activities to be delegated, in defined population 2. UAP – experienced in activities but not in defined population 3. UAP – novice in performing activities and in defined population		1		
Level of Licensed Nurse Competence	**Score the licensed nurse's competence in relation to both knowledge of providing nursing care to a defined population and competence in implementation of the delegation process:** 0. Expert in the knowledge of nursing needs/activities of defined client population *and* expert in the delegation process 1. Either expert in knowledge of needs/activities of defined client population and competent in delegation or experienced in the needs/activities of defined client population and expert in the delegation process 2. Experienced in the knowledge of needs/activities of defined client population *and* competent in the delegation process 3. Either experienced in the knowledge of needs/activities of defined client population *or* competent in the delegation process 4. Novice in knowledge of defined population *and* novice in delegation		0		
Potential for Harm	**Score the potential level of risk the nursing care activity has for the client (*risk is probability of suffering harm*):** 0. None 1. Low 2. Medium 3. High		3		
Frequency	**Score based on how often the UAP has performed the specific nursing care activity:** 0. Performed at least daily 1. Performed at least weekly 2. Performed at least monthly 3. Performed less than monthly 4. Never performed		0		
Level of Decision-Making	**Score the decision-making needed, related to the specific nursing care activity, client (both cognitive and physical status) and client situation:** 0. Does not require decision making 1. Minimal level of decision making 2. Moderate level of decision making 3. High level of decision making		3		
Ability for Self-Care	**Score the client's level of assistance needed for self-care activities:** 0. No assistance 1. Limited assistance 2. Extensive assistance 3. Total care or constant attendance		3		
	TOTAL SCORE		13		

Figure 5-2 Application of the NCSBN Delegation Decision-Making Grid (Reprinted and used by permission of the National Council of State Boards of Nursing Inc. [NCSBN]. Copyright 1997 National Council of State Boards of Nursing [NCSBN]). This information can be found on the NCSBN Web site at http://www.ncsbn.org.

patient care, especially if patient needs are urgent. New nurses may quickly realize that if they do not delegate some of the patient's care, it will not be completed in a timely and effective manner. Other staff can help new graduates begin to develop their role and learn to delegate by making sure that they introduce all the other department staff and explain their roles to the new nurses.

REAL WORLD INTERVIEW

Each agency using the NCSBN Delegation Decision-Making grid may want to adapt the grid to their agency as we have done, defining client stability and the levels of potential for harm to avoid large differences in scores based on intuition or past experience of staff using the grid. See our revised grid in Figure 5-3. Also, the NCSBN grid does not incorporate the availability of the RN as an aspect for consideration, which could make an impact on care and the RN's delegation decisions.

Deloria Armstrong, RN, BSN

Senior Project Coordinator, Nursing Practice,

SETON Medical Center of SETON Healthcare Network of Austin, Texas, Magnet Hospital

Nurse Manager Responsibility

The nurse manager helps develop staff members' ability to delegate. Guidance in this area is necessary because new graduates, wanting to be regarded favorably, often may try to do everything themselves and not ask for assistance. Orientation will cover staff job descriptions, competency, chain of command guidelines, and other organizational resources for the new nurse.

The nurse manager will determine the appropriate mix of personnel on a nursing unit based on the patient's needs, acuity level, and staff competency. From this personnel mix, the nurse manager will identify who can best perform the direct and indirect nursing duties.

New Graduate Registered Nurse Responsibility

The new graduate registered nurse needs to focus on the duties for which they are directly responsible. What duties can they delegate and to what extent? What do UAP do? What do licensed practical/vocational nurses (LPNs/LVNs) do? The state nurse practice act and the job description of each of these staff will help clarify the responsibilities of each staff member.

Registered Nurse Responsibility

The registered nurse is responsible and accountable for the provision of nursing care. Although unlicensed assistive personnel may measure vital signs, intake and output, and other patient status indicators, it is the registered nurse who analyzes these data for comprehensive assessment, nursing diagnosis and development, and evaluation of the plan of care.

Licensed Practical/Vocational Nurses Responsibility

Licensed practical/vocational nursing (LPN/LVN) caregivers who have undergone a standardized training and competency evaluation are able to perform duties and functions that UAPs are not allowed to do. LPN/LVNs are held to a higher standard of care and are responsible for their actions. Common LPN/LVN duties include the duties of the UAP plus instructing patients from a standard care plan and updating initial assessments. In many states, with documented competency, LPN/LVN duties may also include removal of sutures, initiating and/or maintaining intravenous lines, blood transfusion and hyperalimentation lines, giving IV push and

TABLE 5-4
FIVE RIGHTS OF DELEGATION

Right Task	Has the agency established policies, procedures, and standards consistent with the state nurse practice act, federal, state, and legal regulations and guidelines for practice, nursing professional standards, and the ANA Code of Ethics? Can this task be delegated to any staff? Are patient and community needs met?
Right Circumstance	Are the setting and available resources conducive to safe care? Does staff understand how to do the task safely? Do the job description, education, and competency of the RN, LPN/LVN, and UAP match the patient requirements? Do they do it right? Does staff have the resources, equipment, and supervision needed to work safely?
Right Person	Is the right person delegating the right task to the right person to be performed on the right person? Is the patient stable with predictable outcomes? Is it legally acceptable to delegate to this person? Do personnel have documented knowledge, skill, and competency to do the task?
Right Direction/ Communication	Does the RN communicate the task clearly with directions, specific steps of the task, any limits, and expected outcomes? Are times for feedback specified? Is staff understanding of the task clarified? Can staff say, "I don't know how to do this and I need help," without jeopardizing his or her job?
Right Supervision	Are there appropriate monitoring, intervention, evaluation, and feedback as needed? Does the RN answer staff questions and problem solve as needed? Does the staff report task completion and client response to the RN? Does the RN provide follow-up teaching and guidance to staff as appropriate? Are problems, particularly any sentinel events, reported via the chain of command and as needed to the State Board of Nursing?

Compiled with information from www.ncsbn.org. Five Rights of Delegation, 1997.

STOP AND THINK

Identify a group of four patients on the unit where you have your clinical experience. Note the RNs, LPN/LVNs, and UAPs on the unit.

What delegation decisions could you make using the Five Rights of Delegation and the Delegation Decision-Making Grid?

TABLE 5-5
NURSING PROCESS

Ultimately, some professional activities involving the specialized knowledge, judgment, or skill of the nursing process can never be delegated. These include patient assessment, triage, making a nursing diagnosis, establishing nursing plans of care, extensive teaching or counseling, telephone advice, evaluating outcomes, and discharging patients (Zimmermann, 1996). Delegated tasks are typically those that occur frequently, are considered technical by nature, are considered standard and unchanging, have predictable results, and have minimal potential for risks (Westfall, 1998). As a professional standard for all nurses in all states, the assessment, analysis, diagnosis, planning, teaching, and evaluation stages of the nursing process may not be delegated. Delegated activities usually fall within the implementation phase of the nursing process.

piggyback medications, inserting feeding tubes, and so on. The LPN role must be in agreement with the state nurse practice act and should be reflected in policies, job descriptions, methods of assigning, and competency documentation, no matter what the setting. (A sample nurse practice act for LPNs in Louisiana may be found at http://www.lsbpne.com.) The RN must be aware of the job description, skills, and educational background of the LPN prior to delegation of duties. Note that the RN is still primarily responsible for overall patient assessment, planning, and evaluation of the quality of care delegated to the LPN/LVN. See Figure 5-4.

UAP Responsibility

The increased numbers of UAP in acute care settings can pose a degree of risk to patients. UAP may perform duties such as bathing, feeding, toileting, and ambulating patients. UAP also report information related to these activities. The RN delegates to the UAP and is liable for those delegations. If the RN knows or reasonably believes that the assistant has the appropriate training, orientation, and documented competencies, then the RN can reasonably expect that the UAP will function in a safe and effective manner.

Using UAP in acute care settings frees RNs from nonnursing duties and allows them time to complete assessments of patients and their responses to treatments. It is less expensive to have UAP perform nonnursing duties than to have nurses perform them. UAP can deliver supportive care. They cannot practice nursing or provide total patient care. Inappropriate use of UAP in performing functions outside their scope of practice is a violation of the state nursing practice act and is a threat to patient safety. The RN has an increased scope of liability when tasks are delegated to UAP.

ACCOUNTABILITY, SUPERVISION, AND ASSIGNMENT

Accountability, supervision, and assignment are additional important concepts to understand when delegating care. See Table 5-6.

Nursing Accountability

The RN is accountable for the performance of tasks delegated to others, for the tasks the nurse personally performs, and for the act of delegating activities to others. When authority has been delegated and responsibility assumed, the

	TASK/PROCEDURE			PATIENT		UAP		RN
BNE	**Safety of Task**	**Absence of Problem-Solving**	**Interactions of RN to Patient**	**Stability of Patient for Task Per RN Assessment**	**Predictability of Patient's Response to Task**	**Validation of Competency**	**Experience**	**Availability**
C A T E G O R I E S O F B N E T A S K S	High chance of risk; difficult to treat	Potential innovations which are not clearly defined	Requires ongoing RN instruction throughout procedure	Unstable, Probable fluctuation if task is done	Predictable negative response	No Validation of Competency	No experience with task or patient type	Not Available
	0	0	0	0	0	0	0	0
	Moderate chance of risk, treatable over time	Options for innovations are clearly defined, but require a choice	Require intermittent interactions by RN throughout procedure	Currently stable, Possible fluctuation if task is done	Response could be negative or positive	Validation of competency: *Discretionary Deleg.* Org. approved educ. program	Minimal experience with task and/or patient type	Available by phone or in person over time
	1	1	1	1	1	1	1	1
	Low chance of risk; easily treatable, temporary	Problem-solving has clearly defined option identified in procedure/ education	RN interactions completed before and/or after procedure	Stable, Fluctuations unlikely if task is done	Minimal chance for negative response	Validation of competency- *Discretionary Deleg.* Org. approved educ. program	Recent or frequent experience with task and/or patient type	Available; easy to find
	2	2	2	2	2	2	2	2
	Minimal or no chance or risk; no treatment needed	No innovations needed	No RN interactions needed	Consistently stable, No expected fluctuations if task is done	Predictable favorable response	*Most Commonly Deleg. Tasks* Competency validation per delegating RN	Experience with specific task and patient	Immediately available
	3	3	3	3	3	3	3	3

The final decision for delegation is based upon the RN's professional judgment. (BNE 218.10.6)

Guidelines for Decision-Making
If a "O" is selected for any of the criterion in any of the categories (RN, UAP, PATIENT, or TASK), it is recommended that the task not be delegated.
If a "1" is selected in the RN or UAP categories, it is recommended that all criterion in the "PATIENT" and "TASK" categories be a "2" or a "3."
If a "1" is selected for any of the PATIENT or TASK categories, it is recommended that all criterion in the RN and UAP category be a "2" or a "3."
If a "2" or a "3" is selected for each of the criterion in the PATIENT, TASK, RN, or UAP categories, the task may be delegated.
Category "3" represents the ideal criterion for delegation.

SCALE
0 = Not Met
1 = Marginally Met
2 = Adequately Met
3 = Ideally Met

Figure 5-3 Seton Healthcare Network RN Critical-Thinking Grid for Delegation to Unlicensed Assistive Personnel (Used with permission of Joyce Batcheller, Senior Vice President, Chief Nursing Officer, Seton Healthcare Network Austin, TX, Magnet Hospital)

LITERATURE APPLICATION

Citation: Johnson, S. H. (1996). Teaching nursing delegation: Analyzing nurse practice acts. *Journal of Continuing Education in Nursing, 27*(2), 52–58.

Discussion: This author recommends reviewing your state nurse practice act. She notes policies common to many state nurse practice acts. These include:

- Only nursing tasks can be delegated, not nursing practice.
- RN must perform patient assessment to determine what can be delegated.
- LPN and UAP do not practice professional nursing.
- RN can delegate only what is in the scope of nursing practice.
- LPN works under the direction/supervision of RN.
- RN delegates care based on the knowledge and skill of the person selected to perform the task.
- RN determines competency of the person to whom she delegates.
- RN can't delegate activity that requires RN professional skill and knowledge.
- RN is accountable and responsible for delegated tasks.
- RN must evaluate patient outcomes resulting from delegated activity.
- Health care facilities can develop special delegation protocols provided they meet State Board of Nursing delegation guidelines.
- Delegation requires critical thinking by the RN.

The author recommends looking at your own state nurse practice act and looking for the following items to improve your own understanding of delegation:

- Definition of delegation
- Items that cannot be delegated
- Items that cannot be routinely delegated
- Guidelines for RN on what can be delegated
- Description of professional nursing practice
- Description of LPN/LVN and unlicensed nursing assistant roles
- Degree of supervision required
- Guidelines for lowering risk of delegation
- Warning about inappropriate delegation
- Restricted use of the word "nurse" to licensed nurses

continues

Literature Application *(continued)*

Implications for Practice: Reviewing your own state's nurse practice act can increase your knowledge and skill in using delegation appropriately. Note that many State Nursing Board's contact information as well as information about model nurse practice acts are listed at http://www.ncsbn.org.

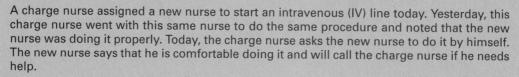

STOP AND THINK

A charge nurse assigned a new nurse to start an intravenous (IV) line today. Yesterday, this charge nurse went with this same nurse to do the same procedure and noted that the new nurse was doing it properly. Today, the charge nurse asks the new nurse to do it by himself. The new nurse says that he is comfortable doing it and will call the charge nurse if he needs help.

Did the charge nurse delegate authority correctly?

Did the new nurse correctly assume responsibility to do the IV?

delegatee is then accountable for the delegated task. The accountability for the performance of the task becomes shared, because the delegator also remains accountable for the completion of the delegated task. The RN is accountable for monitoring changes in the patient's status, noting and implementing treatment for the patient's responses to illness, and assisting in the prevention of complications. Nursing tasks that do not involve direct patient care can be reallocated more freely and carry fewer legal implications for registered nurses than delegation of direct nursing practice activities (American Association of Critical Care Nurses, 1990).

In a hospital, the UAP and LPN/LVN are accountable to the RN. Accountability for the act of delegating involves the appropriate choice of person and activity. For example, an RN might delegate to UAP the authority to perform a certain task. If the RN has not determined in advance that the person understands the assignment and has the skills, knowledge, and judgment to do the task or does not supervise the

task completion, and the UAP does not do it right, the RN would be accountable for this act of improper delegation.

Supervision

A nurse who is supervising care will provide clear direction to his or her staff about what tasks are to be performed for specific patients. The supervisor nurse must identify when and how the task is to be done and what information must be collected as well as any patient-specific information. The nurse must identify what outcomes are expected and the time frame for reporting results. The nurse will monitor staff performance to ensure compliance with established standards of practice, policy, and procedure. The supervisor nurse will obtain feedback from staff and patients and intervene, as necessary, to ensure quality nursing care and appropriate documentation. Hansten and Washburn (1998) identify three levels of supervision, based on the task del-

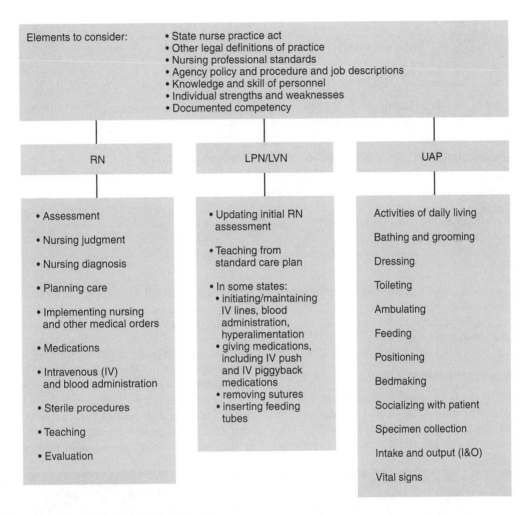

Figure 5-4 Considerations in Delegation

egated and the education, experience, competency, and working relationship of the people involved. The three levels are:

- Unsupervised—occurs when one RN works with another RN. Both are accountable for their own practice.
- Initial direction and periodic inspection—occurs when an RN supervises licensed or unlicensed staff, knows the staff's training and competency level, and has a working relationship with the staff. For example, an RN who has worked with UAP for several weeks is now comfortable giving the UAP initial directions to ambulate two new postoperative patients. The RN follows up with the UAP once during the shift or as needed.
- Continuous supervision—occurs when the RN determines that the delegatee needs frequent-to-continuous support and assis-

LITERATURE APPLICATION

Citation: Sheehan, J. P. (2001). Delegating to UAP—a practical guide. *RN, 64*(11), 65–66.

Discussion: Delegating duties to unlicensed assistive personnel can free up the RN to complete RN level tasks. To do this without endangering patients or increasing the RN's liability, the RN should consider the key questions this article discusses:

What should you do before you delegate? What can you delegate and what can't you delegate? How should you effectively assign tasks? How can you minimize your liability?

Implications for Practice: Specific delegation scenarios are discussed in this article. The National Council of State Boards of Nursing's five rights of delegation are discussed, and the examples are useful for nurses to improve their ability to delegate in various situations.

tance. This level is required when the working relationship is new, the task is complex, or the delegatee is inexperienced or has not demonstrated competency.

Assignment

Assignment is the downward or lateral transfer of both the responsibility and accountability of an activity from one individual to another. The lateral or downward transfer must be made to an individual of skill, knowledge, and judgment. The activity must be within the individual's scope of practice (ANA, 1992). Tasks can properly be assigned to an individual who understands the assignment, has similar skill, knowledge, and judgment, and is within the legal authority or regulatory scope of practice, such as another nurse. An example is a charge nurse assigning the care of four patients to a staff nurse. The person making the assignment is accountable for the decision in making the

TABLE 5-6
DEFINITION OF ACCOUNTABILITY AND SUPERVISION

Accountability	**Accountability** is being responsible and answerable for actions or inactions of self or others in the context of delegation (NCSBN, 1995).
Supervision	**Supervision** is the provision of guidance or direction, evaluation, and follow up by the licensed nurse for accomplishment of a nursing task delegated to UAP. Supervision is generally categorized as on-site (the nurse being physically present or immediately available while the activity is being performed) or off-site (the nurse has the ability to provide direction through various means of written and verbal communications) (NCSBN, 1995).

assignment. For example, it is inappropriate for the charge nurse to assign the care of a very complex patient to a new graduate nurse. However, once the new staff nurse accepts the assignment, he or she will assume responsibility and accountability for the care of that patient. That individual is now practicing on the basis of his or her own credentials. In the true sense of the word, then, assignments can never be made to UAP (Zimmerman, 1996).

Note that there is a significant difference between assigning care to another RN and delegating to an LPN/LVN or UAP. The assignment or delegation must fall within the individual's legal scope of practice. Experienced RNs are expected to work with minimal supervision of their nursing practice. The RN who assigns care to another competent registered nurse does not have the same obligation to closely supervise that person's work as when the care is delegated to an LPN/LVN or UAP.

Assigning full care responsibility to a new graduate or to a nurse working in an unfamiliar specialty may be unsafe. In these instances, the supervising nurse has a greater responsibility to evaluate the abilities and performance of the new nurse (Barter & McLaughlin, 1997). Certain actions may be delegated to an LPN/LVN in keeping with the scope of practice as designated by state regulation. If the LPN is certified in IV therapy, and the policy of the state and the employing institution permits LPNs/LVNs to provide IV treatment, the RN should not have the inordinate duty of supervising the work of the LPN once the LPN/LVN's skills in this area are ensured. Note that prior competency certification may have been done through a skills day or through a competency validation that ensures that, for example, the LPN has been observed inserting an IV successfully three times under direct supervision of an RN in states where this practice by an LPN is allowed. The RN cannot assign responsibility for total nursing care to UAP or LPNs, but can delegate certain tasks to them in keeping with the job description, knowledge base, and demonstrated competency of these individuals. The RN is then responsible for adequate supervision of the person to whom the task is given (Barter & McLaughlin, 1997). See Table 5-7 for delegation suggestions for nurses.

CHAIN OF COMMAND

The RN, including the new graduate nurse, is accountable to the chief nursing executive, for example, the vice president for nursing. The chief nursing executive is accountable to the chief executive officer of the hospital, who is accountable to the board of directors. The board of directors is accountable to the community it serves and often to another larger hospital corporation as well as the state nursing and licensing boards and JCAHO. See Figure 5-6.

Each of these people is accountable for their actions to the patients they serve. Responsibility and accountability cannot be delegated. This contrasts with authority, which can be delegated.

STOP AND THINK

A novice nurse was hired as a staff nurse. The nurse was assigned as spelled out in the job description and nursing Practice Act to give nursing care to patients on the unit. When the nurse accepts this responsibility, he or she is then accountable for the patient's care. Can the nurse's accountability be assigned to UAP?

Is the nurse's accountability shared with the charge nurse?

TABLE 5-7
DELEGATION SUGGESTIONS FOR RNS

- Be clear on the qualifications of the delegate, i.e., education, experience, and competency. Require documentation or demonstration of current competence by the delegatee for each task. Clarify patient care concerns or delegation problems. Consult ANA position papers at http://www.nursingworld.org and your state board of nursing, as necessary.

- Speak to your delegatee as you would like to be spoken to. There is no need to apologize for your delegation. Remember, you are carrying out your professional responsibility. Positively reinforce good attitudes and dependability in your staff.

- Communicate the patient's name, room number, and what you want done and when you want it done. Discuss any changes from the usual procedures that might be needed to meet special patient needs and any potential patient abnormalities that should be reported to you. The expectations for personnel before, during, and after duty performance should be stated in a clear, pleasant, direct, and concise manner.

- Identify realistic, attainable standards that you will use to identify completion of the task. Identify the expected patient outcome.

- Identify the authority necessary to complete the task. Include any limits on the delegatee's authority also.

- Verify the delegatee's understanding of delegated tasks and have him or her repeat instructions, as needed. Be clear, and welcome lots of questions until you are convinced that the delegatee understands what you want done. Verify that the delegatee accepts responsibility for carrying out the task correctly. Require frequent mini reports about patients from staff, and include any specific reporting guidelines, times for interventions, and deadlines for accomplishing any tasks.

- As needed, explain to the delegatee why the task needs to be done, its importance in the overall scheme of things, and any possible complications that may arise during its performance. Invite questions, and don't get defensive if your delegatee pushes you for answers. Seek commitment from your delegatee to complete the task according to standards and in a timely fashion.

- Avoid changing standards or removing duties once performance has begun. Removing duties should be done only when the duty is above the level of the delegatee, such as when the patient's care is in jeopardy because the patient's status has changed.

- Provide support, and monitor the task completion according to standards. Make frequent walking rounds to assess patient outcomes. Be sure your delegatee has the resources, training, and other help to get the task done.

- Accept minor variations in the style in which the duties are performed. Individual styles are acceptable as long as the duty is performed according to standards. Try to provide for continuity of care by the same staff when possible, and consider the geography of the unit and fair, balanced work distribution among staff when assigning care.

continues

Table 5-7 *(continued)*

- If the delegatee doesn't meet the standards, talk with him or her to identify the problem. If this is not successful, inform the delegatee that you will be discussing the problem with your supervisor. Document your concerns, as appropriate. Follow up with your supervisor according to your organization's policy.

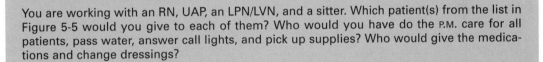

CASE STUDY 5-2

You are working with an RN, UAP, an LPN/LVN, and a sitter. Which patient(s) from the list in Figure 5-5 would you give to each of them? Who would you have do the P.M. care for all patients, pass water, answer call lights, and pick up supplies? Who would give the medications and change dressings?

Room/Name	Patient Description	Special Needs
		Report vitals and outcomes to Mary, RN, at 8:30 P.M. Report anything abnormal STAT
2501/Ms. J. D.	68-year-old female, postop day 1, post shoulder repair Confused; fall risk; side rails up	Up in chair at 6 P.M. Maintain safety Vitals at 4 P.M. and 8 P.M.; check distal pulses Monitor level of consciousness (LOC) Check dressings at 4 P.M. and 8 P.M. Check voiding at 6 P.M. Family at bedside
2502/Mr. D. H.	45-year-old male diabetic, postop day 1, right below the knee amputee Insulin sliding scale Complaining of pain; restless; diaphoretic	Vitals and Accucheck STAT and at 4 P.M. and 9 P.M. Up in chair 6 P.M. Pain medication as needed Monitor dressing No pillow under stump
2503/Mr. H. M.	35-year-old male, history of alcohol abuse Complaining of abdominal pain; new hematemesis of coffee-ground fluid; IV of 0.9% normal saline at 125 cc/hour; alert	Vitals Q 15 minutes Monitor LOC, hematemesis, and possible seizures 16 gauge IV, type and crossmatch Possible transfer to ICU
2504/Mr. J. K.	20-year-old male college student, just admitted; threatening to commit suicide; alert and oriented	Vitals at 4 P.M. and 8 P.M. Do not leave unattended Maintain safety

Figure 5-5 Assignment Delegation Form

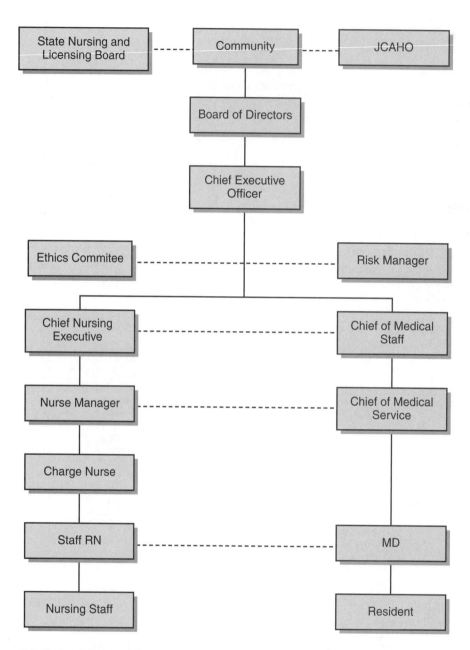

Figure 5-6 Chain of Command

KEY CONCEPTS

- The National Council of State Boards of Nursing defines *delegation* as transferring to a competent individual the authority to perform a selected nursing task in a selected situation. The nurse retains accountability for the delegation.
- Delegation is not a skill that is simply learned in a classroom. It requires discussion of knowledge and concerns related to delegation and clinical mentorship or practice in responsibilities related to that delegation. The process also includes discussion of how to handle situations in which tasks were not accomplished when delegated (Salmond, 1994).
- The NCSBN has identified seven elements of delegation decision making. Rating the seven elements on the grid assists the nurse in evaluating the circumstances, client needs, and available resources, including UAP and licensed nurse competence and potential for client harm to support the delegation decision.
- Certain elements must be in place in an organization in order for efficient delegation to occur.
- Several states specify nursing tasks that may be delegated in their rules and regulations.
- Delegated tasks typically are ones that occur frequently, are considered technical by nature, are considered standard and unchanging, have predictable results, and have minimal potential for risks (Westfall, 1998).
- Authority is the right to act or to command the action of others. There are four possible levels of authority.
- Responsibility is the obligation involved when one accepts an assignment.
- Accountability is being responsible and answerable for actions or inactions of self or others in the context of delegation.
- Note that the assessment, analysis, diagnosis, planning, teaching, and evaluation stages of the nursing process may not be delegated. Delegated activities usually fall within the implementation phase of the nursing process.
- In a hospital, UAP and LPNs/LVNs are accountable to the RN.
- According to the NCSBN, supervision is the provision of guidance or direction, evaluation, and follow-up by the licensed nurse for accomplishment of a nursing task delegated to unlicensed assistive personnel.
- The ANA (1994) defines *assignment* as shifting an activity from one person to another, including the responsibility and the accountability for the task.
- The five rights of delegation are the right task, the right circumstance, the right person, the right direction and communication, and the right supervision.
- Organizations fulfill their responsibility to staff and patients by ensuring that appropriate standards are in place.

KEY TERMS

accountability

assignment

authority

delegation

nursing judgment

responsibility

supervision

UAP

REVIEW QUESTIONS

1. Which of the following statements about RNs and UAP is true?
   A. UAP and RNs have equal responsibilities.
   B. UAP are responsible for all patient care.
   C. RNs are less accountable for patient care when UAP are assisting.
   D. The RN provides patient care, delegating to other RNs or UAP as necessary.

2. Which of the following is an inappropriate task for an LPN/LVN?
   A. Taking vital signs on a new patient
   B. Completing an Accucheck and reporting it to the RN

C. Completing a pain assessment that the UAP identified as being changed from an earlier assessment

D. Discharging the patient after teaching has been completed by the RN

3. If a patient being discharged requires teaching reinforced, the most appropriate caregiver to perform this would be
   A. a unit secretary.
   B. an LPN/LVN.
   C. a CNA.
   D. UAP.

REVIEW ACTIVITIES

1. To determine what your scope of practice is, call your state nurses association for information on your state's laws and regulations.

2. Read the study in the April 14, 1999, *Journal of the American Medical Association*, by Dr. Peter Pronovost and colleagues at Johns Hopkins University. They found that a decreased ICU nurse-patient ratio during the day or evening was associated with increased ICU days and increased hospital length of stay. Could some of this high acuity patient care be safely delegated?

3. Have you had any clinical opportunities to delegate duties? Identify to whom and what you delegated and discuss how it affected the patient and your work. What would you do differently next time?

EXPLORING THE WEB

- Log on to *http://www.aacn.org* and go to Clinical Practice. Click on Public Policy and find the advisory team member of your state. Note what policies, if any, consider delegation of care to UAP and LPNs.

- The state of California is the first state to require all its licensed hospitals to meet fixed nurse-to-patient ratios. Log on to the California Nurses Association Web site at *http://www.calnurse.org* to identify the particulars of this bill.

- Log on to *http://www.nursingworld.org*, the American Nurses Association's (ANA) site, to view safety and quality of care issues.

- Go to *http://nclextestprep.com* as another resource for delegation information as to whom to delegate to and what can be delegated. This site also has review questions for NCLEX covering delegation.

- Logging on to *http://www.nursingsociety. org* and the Sigma Theta Tau International's Web site will access continuing education courses in leadership and management. Read the courses on delegation.

- A paper written by an RN discussing ethical concerns when choosing to delegate can be found at *http://www.e-quipping.com*. The paper is well written and includes a personal opinion summarizing the article. Click on delegation issues to view various views.

- Some of the historical information associated with delegation and how it came to be in individual states are discussed in the site. Go to *http://www.nursingworld.org*. Type in nursing delegation and note what you find there.

- A case study with study questions reviews delegation to unlicensed assistive personnel in oncology at *http://www.nursingspectrum. com*. Click on education and then, self study modules, to access many continuing education courses for a fee.

REFERENCES

American Association of Critical Care Nurses (AACN). (1990). *Delegation of nursing and non-nursing activities in critical care: A framework for decision making*. Irvine, CA: Author.

American Nurses Association (ANA). (1985).

American Nurses Association (ANA). (1995).

American Nurses Association (ANA). (1997). Registered Nurse Utilization of UAP. Washington, DC: American Nurses Publishers.

American Nurses Association (ANA). (2001). Code of ethics for nurses with interpretive statements. Washington, DC: American Nurses Publishing.

Barter, M., & McLaughlin, F. E. (1997). Registered nurse role changes and satisfaction with unlicensed assistive personnel. *Journal of Nursing Administration, 27*(1), 29–38.

Boucher, M. A. (1998). Delegation alert. *American Journal of Nursing, 98*(2), 26–32.

Cox, S. H. (1997, November). Motivation and morale: Coin of the realm. Symposium conducted at Nursing Management Congress, Chicago.

Franck, P., & Price, M. (1980). *Nursing Management.* (2d ed.). New York: Springer.

Hansten, R. & Washburn, M. (1998). Clinical delegation skills: a handbook for professional practice. (2d ed.) Gaithersburg, MD: Aspen Publishers.

Johnson, S. H. (1996). Teaching nursing delegation: Analyzing nurse practice acts. *The Journal of Continuing Education in Nursing, 27*(2), 52–58.

National Council of State Boards of Nursing. (1997). 5 Rights of Delegation. www.ncsbn. org

National Council of State Boards of Nursing. (1995, December). Delegation: Concepts and decision-making process. *Issues,* 1-2.

Nightingale, F. (1859). *Notes on nursing: What it is and what it is not.* London: Harrison & Sons.

Pronovost, P. J., Jenckes, M., Dorman, T., Garrett, E., Breslow, M. J., Rosenfeld, B. J., et al. (1999). Care of the critically ill. *Journal of the American Medical Association, 281,* 1310–1317.

Salmond, S. (1994). *Perceived effectiveness of models of care using clinical nursing assistants.* Pitman, NJ: National Association of Orthopedic Nurses.

Sheehan, J. P. (2001). Delegating to UAP—a practical guide. *RN, 64*(11), 65–66.

Westfall, P. (1998). Nurse attorney organization makes UAP recommendation. *Insight, 7*(2).

Zimmermann, P. G. (1996, June). Delegating to assistive personnel. *Journal of Emergency Nursing, 22*(3), 206–212.

Zimmermann, P. G. (1996). Use of unlicensed assistive personnel: anecdotes and antidotes. *Journal of Emergency Nursing, 22,* 42–48.

 # SUGGESTED READINGS

Ellis, J. R., & Hartley, C. L. (2000). *Managing and coordinating nursing care.* Philadelphia: Lippincott.

Fisher, M. (2000). Do you have delegation savvy? *Nursing2000, 30*(12), 58–59.

Hansten, R., & Washburn, M. (2001, March). Delegating to UAPs: Making it work. *Nurse-Week,* 21–23.

No abuse zone. (2002, March). *Hospitals and Health Networks, 26,* 28.

CHAPTER 6

Staffing

High quality nursing care should be the goal of every nurse, educator, and manager. High quality to me means care that is individualized to a particular patient, administered humanely and competently, comprehensively and with continuity. Primary nursing is one means of accomplishing that quality of care.
(Marie Manthey, 1980)

OBJECTIVES

Upon completion of this chapter, the reader should be able to:

1. Discuss how staffing needs are determined.
2. Identify patient classification systems.
3. Review considerations in developing a staffing pattern.
4. Discuss scheduling on a patient care unit.
5. Discuss the role of nurse staffing in achieving quality nurse-sensitive outcomes.
6. Review models of care delivery.
7. Discuss care delivery management tools, such as clinical pathways, case management, and disease management.

You are a new nurse on a 30-bed medical unit that uses primary nursing as the care delivery model. There are 40 employees who work full and part time on this unit with vacancies for 8 additional full-time staff. The current schedule does not accommodate any 12-hour shifts. There are five long-term staff members who are threatening to leave if they are forced to work 12-hour shifts. You have heard there are several new graduates who will come to work on the unit only if there are 12-hour shifts.

How can the needs of both groups of staff be accommodated?

What effect will the 12-hour shifts have on the care delivery model?

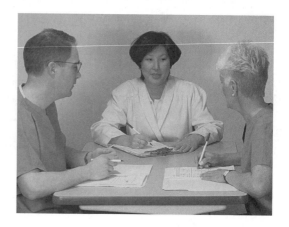

The ability of a nurse to provide safe and effective care to a patient is dependent on many variables. These variables include the knowledge and experience of the staff, the severity of illness of the patients, the amount of nursing time available, the care delivery model, care management tools, and organizational supports in place to facilitate care. This chapter explores factors that affect planning and evaluation of staffing plans. It also discusses classification systems on an inpatient unit.

DETERMINATION OF STAFFING NEEDS

Nurse staffing has varied widely since the inception of nursing as a profession. Nursing staffing ratios have ranged from a ratio of one nurse to many soldiers, as in Florence Nightingale's time, to today when you may see a ratio of one nurse to one patient in a critical care area. Gaining an understanding of the key terms—full-time equivalents (FTEs), productive time, nonproductive time, direct and indirect care, and nurs-

ing hours per patient day (NHPPD)—is helpful to understanding staffing patterns.

FTEs

A **full-time equivalent** (FTE) is a measure of the work commitment of a full-time employee. A full-time employee has traditionally worked 5 days a week or 40 hours per week for 52 weeks a year. This amounts to 2,080 hours of work time (Figure 6-1). Note that the definition of full time as 40 hours per week is changing. See new options in staffing patterns later in this chapter.

A full-time employee who works 40 hours a week is referred to as a 1.0 FTE. A part-time employee who works 5 days in a 2-week period is considered a 0.5 FTE. The FTE calculation is used to mathematically describe how much an employee works (Figure 6-2).

FTE hours are a total of all paid time. This includes worked time as well as nonworked time. Hours worked and available for patient care are designated as **productive hours**. Benefit time such as vacation, sick time, and education time is considered **nonproductive hours**. When

5 days per week	×	8 hours per day	=	40 hours per week
40 hours per week	×	52 weeks per year	=	2,080 hours per year

Figure 6-1 Calculation of Full-Time Equivalent Hours

| 1.0 FTE = 40 hours per week or five 8-hour shifts per week |
| 0.8 FTE = 32 hours per week or four 8-hour shifts per week |
| 0.6 FTE = 24 hours per week or three 8-hour shifts per week |
| 0.4 FTE = 16 hours per week or two 8-hour shifts per week |
| 0.2 FTE = 8 hours per week or one 8-hour shift per week |

Figure 6-2 FTE Calculation for Varying Levels of Work Commitment

considering the number of FTEs you need to staff a unit, you must count only the productive hours available for each staff member. Available productive time can be easily calculated by subtracting benefit time from the time a full-time employee would work (Figure 6-3).

In this case, a full-time registered nurse (RN) would have 1,848 hours per year of productive time available to care for patients.

Employees who work with patients can be classified into two categories: those who provide direct care and those who provide indirect care. **Direct care** is time spent providing hands-on care to patients. **Indirect care** is time spent on activities that are patient related but are not done directly to the patient. Documentation, time consulting with people in other health care disciplines, and time spent following up problems are good examples of indirect care. Even though RNs, licensed practical nurses (LPNs), and unlicensed assistive personnel (UAP) engage in indirect care activities, the majority of their time is spent providing direct care; therefore they are classified as direct care providers. Nurse managers, clinical specialists, unit secretaries, and other support staff are considered indirect care providers because the majority of their work is

indirect in nature and supports the work of the direct care providers.

Nursing Hours per Patient Day

Nursing hours per patient day (NHPPD) is a standard measure that quantifies the nursing time available to each patient by available nursing staff. For example, a nursing unit that has 20 patients at a given point during a 24-hour period, usually the midnight census, and 5 nursing staff each shift would calculate into 6 nursing hours per patient day. NHPPD reflect only productive nursing time available (Figure 6-4). This measure is useful in illustrating nursing care to both nurses and financial staff in an organization.

PATIENT CLASSIFICATION SYSTEMS

To assess cost and how many staff are needed at any given time, it is necessary to determine what

Vacation time	15 days	or	120 hours
Sick time	5 days	or	40 hours
Holiday time	6 days	or	48 hours
Education time	3 days	or	24 hours
Total nonproductive time		=	232 hours

2,080 − 232 = 1,848 hours of productive work time available for each staff member with these benefits.

Figure 6-3 Calculation of Productive and Nonproductive Time

> 20 patients on the unit
>
> 5 staff × 3 shifts = 15 staff
>
> 15 staff each working 8 hours = 120 hours available in a 24-hour period
>
> 120 nursing hours ÷ 20 patients = 6.0 NHPPD
>
> FTE = 8 hours per week or one 8-hour shift per week

Figure 6-4 Calculation of Nursing Hours per Patient Day (NHPPD)

the patients' needs are. A **patient classification system** (PCS) is a measurement tool used to articulate the nursing workload for a specific patient or group of patients over a specific period of time. The measure of nursing workload that is generated for each patient is called the **patient acuity**. PCS data can be used to predict the amount of nursing time needed based on the patient's acuity. As a patient becomes sicker, his acuity level rises, meaning the patient requires more nursing care See Table 6-1. As a patient acuity level decreases, the patient requires less nursing care. In most patient classification systems, each patient is classified using weighted criteria that then predict the nursing care hours needed for the next 24 hours. Criteria reflect care needed in assessment, bathing, mobilizing, supervision, monitoring, evaluation, and so on. In most cases, patients are classified once a day. The ideal PCS produces a valid and reliable rating of individual patient care requirements,

which are matched to the latest clinical technology and caregiver skill variables (Malloch & Conivaloff, 1999). These systems are generally applied to all inpatients in an organization. There are many different classification and acuity systems on the market. Some of these are Medicus, GRASP, OMAHA, NIC, Van Slyk, and RIMS (Diers, Bozzo, and RIMS/Nursing Acuity Project Groups, 1997).

Utilization of Classification System Data

Patient classification data are valuable sources of information for all levels of the organization. On a day-to-day basis, acuity data can be utilized by staff and managers in planning nurse staffing over the next 24 hours. Acuity data and NHPPD are concrete data parameters that are used to

TABLE 6-1
COMPARATIVE VALUES OF ACUITY AND CARE HOURS

PCS Acuity	Care Hours
1	3.00
2	3.60
3	6.00
4	9.99
5	15.00

educate staff on how to adjust staffing levels. For example, for an acuity range of 1.0 to 1.10, the RN staffing may be five RNs on days. For an acuity of 1.10 to 1.15, the RN staffing on days might be six RNs. Experienced staff have the knowledge to manage staffing to acuity levels given the information, boundaries, and authority to do so. In many organizations, a central staffing office monitors the census and acuity on all units and deploys nursing resources to the areas in most need using the classification system data and recommended staffing levels. The manager reviews the results of staffing over the past 24 to 48 hours to adjust staffing to patient requirements. At the unit level, acuity data are also essential in preparing month-end justification for variances in staff utilization. If your average acuity has risen, then there is often a rise in NHPPD to accommodate the increased patient needs.

At an organization level, acuity data have been used to cost out nursing services for specific patient populations and global patient types. This information is also very helpful in negotiating payment rates with third-party payers such as insurance companies to ensure that reimbursement reflects nursing costs. In most organizations, the classification or acuity data are also used in preparation of the nursing staffing budget for the upcoming fiscal year. The data can be benchmarked with other organizations to lend credence to any efforts to change nursing hours. Finally, patient acuity data and NHPPD can be used to develop a staffing pattern. Patient classification and NHPPD data provide an enormous amount of information that serves a multitude of needs.

CONSIDERATIONS IN DEVELOPING A STAFFING PATTERN

Benchmarking is a tool for seeking out the best practices in one's industry so as to improve performance (Swansburg, 1996). In developing a

staffing pattern that leads to a budget, it is important to benchmark your planned NHPPD against other organizations with similar patient populations. Purchased patient classification systems often offer acuity and NHPPD benchmarking data from around the country as part of their system. This kind of data can be helpful in establishing a starting point for a staffing pattern or as part of justification for increasing or reducing nursing hours. Caution must be used, however, because each organization is different.

Regulatory Requirements

Regulatory requirements related to nurse staffing are increasing as the nursing shortage heightens. California has mandated nurse staffing levels in emergency departments and critical care units. Twenty-eight other states have legislation pending (Steefel, 2003). There is considerable controversy within the nursing profession over this issue. There are nurses who are adamant that they need to be protected by law with stipulated staffing levels. There are nurse leaders who are concerned that the mandated staffing levels would soon become the maximum staffing levels rather than the minimum.

The Joint Commission on Accreditation of Healthcare Organizations (JCAHO) surveys hospitals on the quality of care provided. The JCAHO has identified staffing effectiveness screening indicators to assess an organization's ability to provide the right number of competent staff to meet the needs of patients served by the hospital (Zimmermann, 2002). See Table 6-2.

Skill Mix

Skill mix is another critical element in nurse staffing. **Skill mix** is the percentage of RN staff to other direct care staff, LPNs, and unlicensed assistive personnel (UAP). For example, in a unit that has 40 FTEs budgeted, with 20 of them being RNs and 20 FTEs of other skill types, the RN skill mix would be 50%. If the unit had 40

TABLE 6-2
STAFFING EFFECTIVENESS SCREENING INDICATORS

Human Resource

- Overtime
- Staff vacancy rate
- Staff satisfaction
- Staff injuries
- Staff turnover rate
- Sick time
- Nursing care hours per patient day
- On call per diem nurse

Clinical/Service

- Patient falls
- Adverse drug events
- Injuries to patients
- Skin breakdown
- Pneumonia
- Patient complaints
- Family complaints
- Length of stay
- Postoperative infections
- Shock/cardiac arrest
- Gastrointestinal bleeding
- Urinary tract infections

FTEs, with 30 of them being RNs, the RN skill mix would be 75%. The skill mix of a unit should vary according to the care that is required and the care delivery model utilized. For example, in a critical care unit, the RN skill mix will be much higher than in a nursing home where the skills of an RN are required to a much lesser degree.

Staff Support

Another important factor to consider in developing a staffing pattern is the support in place for the operations of the unit or department. For instance, does your organization have a systematic process to deliver medications to the department or do unit personnel have to pick up patient medications and narcotics? Does your organization have staff to transport patients to and from ancillary departments? The less support available to your staff, the more nursing hours have to be built into the staffing pattern to provide care to patients.

ESTABLISHING A STAFFING PATTERN

A **staffing pattern** is a plan that articulates how many and what kind of staff are needed by shift and day to staff a unit or department. There are basically two ways of developing a staffing pattern. It can be generated by determining the required ratio of staff to patients; nursing hours and total FTEs are then calculated. It can also be generated by determining the nursing care hours needed for a specific patient or patients and then generating the FTEs and staff-to-patient ratio needed to provide that care. In most cases, you would use a combination of methods to validate your staffing plan.

Staffing an Inpatient Unit

An **inpatient unit** is a hospital unit that is able to provide care to patients 24 hours a day, 7 days a week. To establish a staffing pattern for this kind of unit, you will utilize a staffing schedule. Plot out the number and type of staff needed during the week and weekend for 24 hours a day for the number of patients you expect to have. Delineate the number and type of staff as well as the additional FTEs for weekend coverage, orientation and education, and benefited time.

For example, on a 24-bed medical unit, you expect to have, on average, 22 patients per day. The ratio of one RN to six patients and one UAP for every twelve patients works well from 7 A.M. to 7 P.M. From 7 P.M. to 7 A.M., the ratio can go to one RN to eight patients. Two UAPs are needed from 7 P.M. to 11 P.M. and then one UAP from 11 P.M. to 7 A.M. This would generate a total of 124 hours per day. The average number of patients on this unit is 22. To calculate the NHPPD see Figure 6-5.

In this example, the number of care hours available would be 5.63 NHPPD.

As you can see, the staffing pattern drives the NHPPD. The more staff available per patient, the higher the NHPPD. Cost is associated with hours of care available and skill mix. There are staffing patterns with many hours of care available, but they may have lower-cost FTEs. The key is to have the right number and

skill level of caregiver available to ensure safe, effective, and appropriate care.

To develop a staffing pattern using NHPPD, you would start with a target NHPPD. If your target NHPPD were 8, for example, and you expected to have 22 patients on your 24-bed unit, you would multiply 8 NHPPD by 22 patients to get 176 productive hours needed every day. Dividing 176 by 8-hour shifts worked by an FTE gives you 22 FTEs needed per day.

You must now calculate the amount of additional staff that will be needed to provide for days off and benefit time. Direct caregivers will need to be replaced, but some other support staff may not need to be replaced for days off or benefited time off. Managers typically are not replaced on days off. Noting that each 8-hour shift for a FTE is equal to 0.2 FTE, to provide coverage for 2 days off a week, add, multiply the number of staff needed per day by a 0.4 FTE. In the example in Figure 6-5, 15.5 FTEs per day multiplied by 0.4 FTE would be an additional 6.2 FTEs to cover 2 days off per week for a total of 21.7 FTEs.

The next step would be to provide additional FTEs for coverage for benefited time away from work. This includes vacations, educational

Skill	Day	Evening	Night	Total
Direct				
ANM				
RN	4	3.5	3	10.5
LPN				
Tech				
UAP	2	2	1	5
Subtotal				

10.5 staff × 8-hour shifts = 84 hours
5 staff × 8-hour shifts = 40 hours
Staff hours available per day = 124 hours

124 hours ÷ 22 patients per day = 5.63 hours of NHPPD
124 hours ÷ 8 hour shifts = 15.5 FTEs to fill the staffing pattern

Figure 6-5 Staffing Plan for a 24-Bed Medical Unit

time, orientation time, and so on. The amount of time away from work varies by organization. If every employee receives 2 weeks of vacation a year and 2 conference days, this would equate to 1,984 hours of productive time per FTE (2,080 possible hours minus 96 hours). Total FTE hours divided by 1,984 hours gives you the total FTEs needed to provide coverage. In the previous example, 21.7 FTEs multiplied by 2,080 hours equals 45,136 hours, and 45,136 hours divided by 1,984 would be 22.75 FTEs or 1.05 additional FTEs to ensure that there are staff available to work when other staff are taking benefited time off. This then means that a total of 22.75 FTEs are needed to staff this 24-bed unit.

SCHEDULING

Scheduling of staff is the responsibility of the nurse manager. The nurse manager must ensure that the schedule places the appropriate staff on each shift for safe, effective patient care. There are many issues to consider as staff are scheduled: the patient needs and acuity, the number of patients, the experience of your staff, and the supports available to the staff. The combination of these factors guides the number of staff scheduled on each shift.

Experience and Scheduling of Staff

Each nurse is different regarding her knowledge base, experience level, and critical thinking skills. A novice nurse takes longer to accomplish the same task than an experienced nurse. An experienced RN can handle more in terms of workload and acuity of patients. If a nursing unit requires special skills or competencies, you would also want to plan for additional nursing hours, so that staff with the special skills are scheduled when the patient care need may arise. The underlying principle of good staffing is that those you serve come first. This may dictate some undesirable shifts but there must be appro-

priate numbers and kinds of staff on hand to care for the patients you serve. Staff are plotted out across a staffing sheet (Figure 6-6).

The scheduled days should be assigned so that there are an even number of staff available across the week. Typically, the spread of FTEs across the 24-hour period falls within the following guidelines: days 33% to 50%, evenings 30% to 40%, and nights 20% to 33%. The spread is based on patient need.

Shift Variations

To attract and retain employees, organizations offer traditional schedules and flexible schedules to meet organizational and employee needs. Traditional staffing patterns are generally 8-hour shifts, 7 A.M. to 3:30 P.M., 3 P.M. to 11:30 P.M., and 11 P.M. to 7:30 A.M. A full-time employee works 10 8-hour shifts in a 2-week period. The start time of 8-hour shifts may vary by organization or by unit and patient need. For example, emergency departments are typically busiest during the evening into the night hours. An 8-hour shift for the ED may be 7 P.M. to 3 A.M. to cover the peak activity times.

New Options in Staffing Patterns

Twelve-hour shifts have become very popular across the country. In many organizations, employees can work less than 40 hours per week and get full-time benefits. In one example, a nurse could work three 12-hour shifts per week and have 4 days off and be full time. Another popular option is weekend programs. Weekend program staff work two 12-hour shifts every weekend and are paid a rate that would make the 24 hours of work equal to 40 hours of work. Some of these programs include full-time benefits as well. These programs are expensive but they can be helpful. See Figure 6-7. Note that any time you implement a scheduling plan, it is critical to assess what the effect will be on the care of patients. For example, workweeks made

REAL WORLD INTERVIEW

Given the need for staffing and financial accountability, I used spreadsheet software to improve the development of staffing patterns in our facility. We had been using a pencil and paper template for managers to use to develop staffing patterns. This manual template concentrated on the weekday staffing needs and applied an overall factor to calculate weekend and benefit time. The FTE number provided did not address orientation and education needs for any of the staff or benefit needs for the weekend staff. Although these staffing patterns were used to project the number of FTEs needed and the distribution of employees to staff the nursing unit, they were not used to drive the budgeted quota for the unit.

Using a computer software program, I developed a spreadsheet template the managers could use to accurately project FTEs needed to meet the staffing pattern. This computerized approach allows for weekday and weekend staffing to be considered independently considering any differences in census or direct NHPPD. A benefit time factor, tailored to our organization's specific benefit package for each skill level, was used to calculate the number of FTEs needed to staff for benefit time. Benefit time was now calculated for weekday and weekend staffing, coverage for a 24/7 operation. Additionally, an orientation and education factor is used to calculate the FTEs needed to provide coverage. For the first time, benefited time off and orientation time were built into each unit's staffing pattern. Additionally, direct and indirect NHPPD are automatically calculated as the staffing pattern is changed, and the calculated FTE needs can be compared to the current budgeted quota for variances. I also worked with Finance to use this template as the basis for a Budgeted Quota Sheet, which is used during the budget process for determining the unit quota for the next year, a quota that now includes benefited time off and orientation time.

One of the biggest assists has been the ability of the nurse managers to use the template for what-if scenarios. When they are planning for a census or patient program change, FTE needs can be quickly calculated and compared to their current budgeted quota. This tool has become part of our business planning process.

Overall, this template has been accepted as a valid management tool, has standardized inclusion of non-productive time into FTE budgets, and has given managers a simple tool to develop new staffing patterns. It has also helped in raising the accountability of managers to develop workable staffing patterns that they can be held accountable to.

Barbara Leafer, RN, BS
Fiscal Administrator for Patient Care

up of three 12-hour shifts have in some units disrupted continuity of care. This is especially true when the 12-hour shifts are not scheduled together. To mediate this impact, 12-hour staff can be paired so that the patient has the same pair of nurses every day for 3 days, and then the patient can be transitioned to a new pair of 12-hour staff. Units that have short patient lengths of stay may have fewer continuity problems than units with longer lengths of stay.

	Monday 04	Tuesday 05	Wednesday 06	Thursday 07	Friday 08	Saturday 09	Sunday 10	Monday 11	Tuesday 12	Wednesday 13	Thursday 14	Friday 15	Saturday 16	Sunday 17
Melinda	D		D	D		D	D	D		D	D	D	D	D
Jason		8.00/1900			N	N	N		8.00/1900		D	D	D	
Eileen	12.00/0900		12.00/0900		D	12.00/0900	12.00/0900	12.00/0900		12.00/0900		N		
Susan	D	8.00/1100		E	E	E		vac		8.00/1100	E	E	E	E
Barbara		14.00/2400	13.00/2400	13.00/2400	D				14.00/2400	13.00/2400	13.00/2400		D	D
Rosemary	D	D	D	D		E			D	N	N		E	E
Robert	N	N	N	N			N	N	N	N	N			N
Jacqueline	E	E	E				E	E	E	E	E	E		
Marcella	E	D		D		D	D	E	D	D		N	N	
Sara				E	8.00/0800		E					8.00/0800		E
Gary		E	E		E	N		D	E	E		12.00/1500		
Cynthia	N	N	N		N			N	N				N	N
Toni	8.00/0730	8.00/0730	8.00/0730	8.00/0730	8.00/0730			8.00/0730	8.00/0730		8.00/0730	8.00/0730	N	

The 1st number in a square is the number of hours scheduled, the second number is the shift start time in military time.

Standard Work Assignments

D 0700–1500
E 1500–2300
N 2300–0700

Figure 6-6 Excerpt from Schedule for an Emergency Department Showing Great Variation in Shift Design

LITERATURE APPLICATION

Citation: Buerhaus, P. I. (2000, May/June). Why are shortages of hospital RNs concentrated in specialty care units? *Nursing Economic$,* 18(3), 111-117.

Discussion: In this study of the nursing shortage in hospital special care units, Dr. Buerhaus utilized data from federal databases to review trends in the nursing workforce and prospects for a future nursing shortage. Significant findings included far fewer young people choosing nursing as a career and the expansion of career opportunities for women. The lack of young people entering the profession will cause the nursing workforce to continue to age at a rapid pace, 3.4 years over the next 10 years. In addition, it can be expected that as the current workforce ages and retires, the number of RNs will remain in 2020 roughly what it was in 2000, causing ongoing nursing shortages, primarily in intensive care units (ICUs) and operating rooms (ORs). ICUs employ younger RNs than other hospital settings. The author notes that it was not until the 1970s that ICUs became prevalent in hospitals and students had rotations in these areas. It is also noted that the challenging and stimulating environment in ICUs attracts younger RNs. On the other hand, operating rooms have a large proportion of older diploma-prepared RNs working in them. Prior to the 1970s, the majority of RNs received their education in hospital-based, 3-year diploma programs, which offered students significantly greater exposure to all hospital clinical areas. The author theorizes that the RN shortage in ICUs is due to the decreasing number of young nurses coming into the profession. The shortage in OR nurses is a reflection of older RNs retiring or reducing work schedules and also the reduction of diploma programs in hospitals.

Implications for Practice: It is clear that there is and will continue to be a nursing shortage for the next decade. In addition to devising global strategies to draw more people into the nursing profession, it is imperative for managers and nurse leaders to create environments that retain staff. This includes planning staff schedules that nurses find compatible with their personal lives. As the nursing workforce ages, we must also take measures to make accommodations for the older worker, including technology to simplify work and physical plant changes to make the work less physically taxing.

CASE STUDY 6-1

You are working on a patient care unit that is planning to begin doing its own scheduling. Using Figure 6-6, make a schedule for your unit. Identify the number of nurses budgeted for each day. Develop a plan to allocate these nurses to cover 24 hours a day, 7 days a week of patient care for 2 weeks.

Weekend staff working at $35 an hour × 24 hours = $840 per weekend

Regular staff working at $20 an hour × 24 hours = $480 per weekend

Difference in cost = $360 per weekend

Six weekend staff members at $360 would cost $2,160 more than regular staff per weekend;

$2,160 × 52 weekends a year would cost $112,320 more than regular staff annually.

Figure 6-7 Annual Cost of a Weekend Program for One Nursing Unit

Self-Scheduling

Self-scheduling is a process in which staff on a unit collectively decide and implement the monthly work schedule (Dearholt & Feathers, 1997). One of the issues that drives nurses from their place of employment is scheduling (Hill-Popper, 2000). Self-scheduling has been implemented to boost staff morale by increasing staff control over their work environment through self-governance activities (Dearholt & Feathers, 1997). This form of scheduling provides maximum flexibility for staff and serves to increase their sense of ownership and shared responsibility in ensuring that their respective work areas are adequately staffed (Shullanberger, 2000). To ensure that patient care needs are met, there must be structure to a self-scheduling program. This is often done by a unit committee, made up of staff that reports to the nurse manager. It is important to spell out the roles and responsibilities of all—the unit-based committee, the chairperson if there is one, the staff, and the manager. Generic boundaries need to be established regarding fairness, fiscal responsibility, evaluation of the self-scheduling process, and the approval process. Table 6-3 spells out specific issues that must be addressed.

NURSE SENSITIVE PATIENT OUTCOMES

Research studies (Lichtig, Knaug, F., Rison-McCoy, & Wozniak, 2000; Needleman, Buerhaus, Mattke, Stewart, Zelinsky, 2002) confirm there is a relationship between nurse staffing and patient outcomes. The studies are finding patient outcomes that show a consistent significant relationship with nurse staffing. Some of the outcomes found to be affected by nurse staffing are length of stay and incidence of pneumonia, postoperative infections, pressure ulcers, urinary tract infections and "failure to rescue" (defined in Needleman et al. study as "death of a patient with one of five life-threatening complications—pneumonia, shock or cardiac arrest, upper gastrointestinal bleeding, sepsis, or deep vein thrombosis" [2002]) for which early identification can influence the risk of death. These nurse sensitive outcomes are negatively affected when nurse staffing or the skill mix is inadequate.

Nurse Staffing and Nurse Outcomes

In addition to patient outcomes, nurse outcomes should also be measured. Staff's perception of the adequacy of staffing should be tracked. There should be the ability for staff to communicate both in written and verbal form regarding staffing concerns. In addition, actual staffing compared to recommended staffing should be tracked. This will give clues to other staffing issues. Medication errors is another measure that has been linked with inadequate NHPPD. When resources are scarce, data are imperative to drive needed changes. The outcomes of ineffective staffing patterns and nursing care can be devastating to patients, staff, and the organization.

REAL WORLD INTERVIEW

As a manager of an intensive care unit, I can say that self-scheduling has greatly increased my staff's satisfaction with their schedules. I think the biggest factor in the success of our process was the initial buy-in from the staff. Before implementing, staff were surveyed to assess their commitment to making the process work. I was looking for 60% to 75% staff buy-in before implementation and found greater than 70%. A second critical factor was having clear guidelines for the process. These included time lines for how and when staff can sign up for time and how time off is prioritized.

During implementation, we learned many things. One key factor was that staff needed to have confrontation and negotiation skills in order for this process to work. Inevitably there were situations when someone had to change their schedule. When confrontation and negotiation didn't take place, there were periods of short staffing and patient care needs not being met. We also learned that this is a time-consuming process. It takes about 16 hours per month for the self-scheduling committee to put the schedule together.

Another key element I found was the manager had to maintain accountability for staffing. I meet with the scheduling committee regularly and oversee the orientation of new staff to the self-scheduling process. I sign off on every schedule to ensure that the schedule maintains appropriate staffing levels at all times. I found that I needed to identify trends that may be affecting staffing and assist the staff in addressing the trends. I also work with the staff on the implementation of any new program that affects the schedule. The weekend program is a good example of this. I worked with the staff to ensure there were appropriate guidelines for staff receiving a reduced weekend commitment. And finally, the most important role I play is to be very clear about the expectations for all—the committee, the staff, and myself. This scheduling process has been one of the most positive quality of worklife efforts for my staff.

Rob Rose, BSN, MSN

Nurse Manager, Cardiopulmonary Surgery Intensive Care Unit

MODELS OF CARE DELIVERY

To ensure that nursing care is provided to patients, the work must be organized. A **nursing care delivery model** organizes the work of caring for patients. The decision of which nursing care delivery model is used is based on the needs of the patients and the availability of competent staff in the different skill levels.

Case Method and Total Patient Care

In the case method, the nurse has one patient whom the nurse cares for exclusively. Total patient care is the modern-day version of the case method. In **total patient care**, the nurse is responsible for the total care for the nurse's patient assignment for the shift the nurse is working. The RN is responsible for several patients. The RN may have some support from

TABLE 6-3
ISSUES TO BE SPELLED OUT IN SELF-SCHEDULING GUIDELINES

1. Scheduling period: Is the scheduling period 2, 4, or 6 week intervals?

2. Schedule time line: What are the time frames for both staff and per diem workers to sign up for regular work, special requests, and overtime?

3. Staffing pattern: Will 8 or 12 hour shifts, or both, be used?

4. Weekends: Are staff expected to work every other weekend? If there are extra weekends available, how are they distributed?

5. Holidays: How are they allocated?

6. Vacation time: Are there restrictions on the amount of vacation during certain periods?

7. Unit vacation practices: How many staff from one shift can be on vacation at any time?

8. Requests for time off: What is the process for requesting time off?

9. Short-staffed shifts: How are shifts that are short staffed handled?

10. On call, if applicable: How do staff get assigned or sign up for on call time?

11. Cancellation guidelines: How and when do staff get canceled for scheduled time if they are not needed?

12. Sick calls: What are the expectations for calling in sick, and how are these shifts covered?

13. Military/National Guard leave: What kind of advance notice is required?

14. Schedule changes: What is the process for changing one's schedule after the schedule has been approved?

15. Shifts defined: What are the beginning and endings of available shifts?

16. Committee time: When does the self-scheduling committee meet and for how long?

17. Seniority: How does it play into staffing and request decisions?

18. Staffing plan for crisis/emergency situations: What is the plan when staffing is inadequate?

LPNs or UAP, but the LPNs and UAP are not assigned to a specific group of patients.

Advantages and Disadvantages

The advantage of total patient care and the case method for the patient is the consistency of one individual caring for patients for an entire shift. This enables the patient, nurse, and family to develop a relationship based on trust. This model provides a higher number of RN hours of care than other models. The nurse has more opportunity to observe and monitor progress of the patient. A disadvantage is that these models utilize a high level of RN nursing hours and are more costly to deliver care, and, in many cases, this level of RN intensity may not be warranted.

STOP AND THINK

Recently, you have been part of a unit committee that is reviewing data on your unit's pressure ulcer rates. In researching further, you discover that your unit's rates are significantly higher than those of other units. Staffing on your unit has been stable and in accordance with the staffing plan. The staff are experienced, and, in fact, they include some of the longest tenured staff in the hospital.

Why is the pressure ulcer rate higher than other units? What could your committee do to investigate this nurse sensitive outcome further?

Functional Nursing Care

Functional nursing divides the nursing work into functional duties. These duties are then assigned to one of the team members. In this model, each care provider has specific duties or tasks they are responsible for. For instance, a typical division of labor for RNs is medication nurse or admission nurse and so on. Decision

making is usually at the level of the head nurse or charge nurse (Figure 6-8).

Advantages and Disadvantages

In this model, care can be delivered to a large number of patients. This system utilizes other types of health care workers when there is a

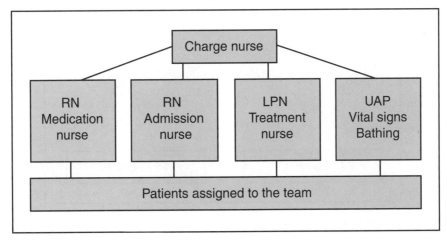

Surgical Unit

Figure 6-8 Functional Nursing Model

shortage of RNs. Patients are likely to have care delivered to them in one shift by several staff members. To a patient, care may feel disjointed. Staff must be aware of this disadvantage and work to eliminate this outcome.

Team Nursing

Team nursing is a care delivery model that assigns staff to teams that then are responsible for a group of patients. A unit may be divided into two teams, and each team is led by a registered nurse. The team leader supervises and coordinates all the care provided by those on his team. The team is most commonly made up of LPNs and UAP, but occasionally there is another RN. Care is divided up into the simplest components and then assigned to the appropriate care provider. In addition to super-

vision duties, the team leader also is responsible for providing professional direction to those on the team regarding the care provided (Figure 6-9).

A modular nursing delivery system is a kind of team nursing that divides a geographic space into modules of patients, with each module cared for by a team of staff led by an RN. The modules may vary in size, but typically there is one RN with an LPN and nursing assistant to make up the team. In this case, the RN is responsible for the overall care of the patients in her module.

Advantages and Disadvantages

In team nursing and modular nursing, the RN is able to get work done through others, but

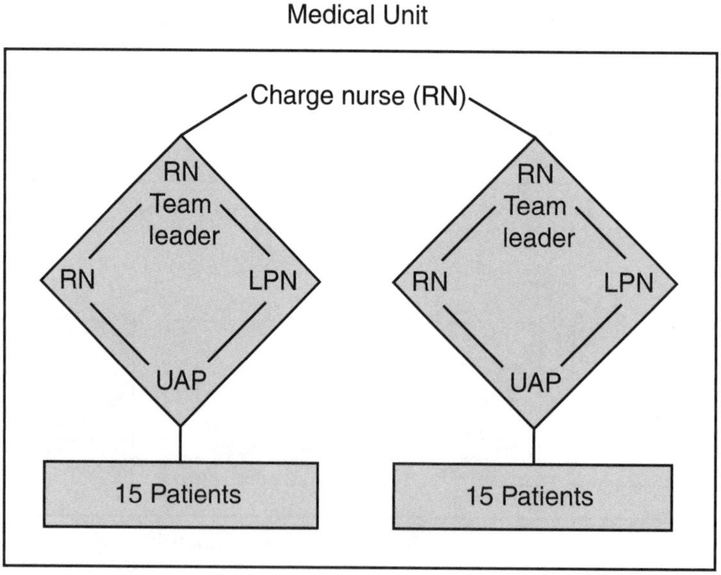

Figure 6-9 Team Nursing Model

patients sometimes receive fragmented, depersonalized care. Communication in these models is complex. There is shared responsibility and accountability, which can cause confusion and lack of accountability. These factors may contribute to RN dissatisfaction with these models. These models require the RN to have very good delegation and supervision skills.

Primary Nursing

Primary nursing is a care delivery model that clearly delineates the responsibility and accountability of the RN and designates the RN as the primary provider of care to patients. Primary nursing is a form of the case model that consists of four elements. These are allocation and acceptance of individual responsibility for the decision making to one individual; assignments of daily care by the case method; direct

person-to-person communication; and one person operationally responsible for the quality of care administered to patients on a unit 24 hours a day, 7 days a week (Manthey, 1980). Patients are assigned a primary nurse, who is responsible for developing with the patient a plan of care that is followed by other nurses caring for the patient. Nurses and patients are matched according to needs and abilities. Patients are assigned to their primary nurse regardless of unit geographic considerations. In the primary nursing model, the role of the head nurse changes to one of leader by empowering the staff RNs to be knowledgeable about their patients and to direct the care of their primary patients. The primary nurse has the authority, accountability, and responsibility to provide care for a group of patients. There are associate nurses who care for the patient when the primary nurse is not working. There will be several associate nurses for each patient (Figure 6-10).

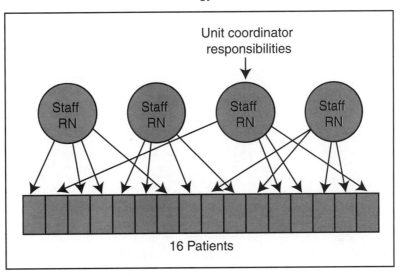

Figure 6-10 Primary Nursing Model

Advantages and Disadvantages

An advantage of this model is that patients and families are able to develop a trusting relationship with one primary nurse. There is defined accountability and responsibility for the nurse to develop a plan of care with the patient and family. There is a holistic approach to care, which facilitates continuity of care rather than a shift-to-shift focus. Nurses, when they have adequate time to provide necessary care, find this model professionally rewarding because it gives the authority for decision making to the nurse at the bedside. Disadvantages include a high cost because there is a higher RN skill mix. With no geographical boundaries within the unit, nursing staff may be required to travel long distances at the unit level to care for their primary patients. Nurses often perform functions that could be completed by other staff. And finally, nurse-to-patient ratios must be realistic to ensure there is enough nursing time available to meet the patient care needs.

Patient-Centered or Patient-Focused Care

Patient-centered care or patient-focused care is designed to focus on patient needs rather than staff needs. In this model, required care and services are brought to the patient. In the highest evolution of this model, all patient services are decentralized to the patient area, including radiology and pharmacy services. Staffing is based on patient needs. In this model, there is an effort to have the right person doing the right thing. Care teams are established for a group of patients. The care teams may include other disciplines such as respiratory or physical therapists. In these teams, disciplines collaborate to ensure that patients receive the care they need. Staff are kept close to the patients in decentralized work stations. For example, on a rehabilitation unit, physical therapists may be members of the care team and work at the unit level rather than in a centralized physical therapy department (Figure 6-11).

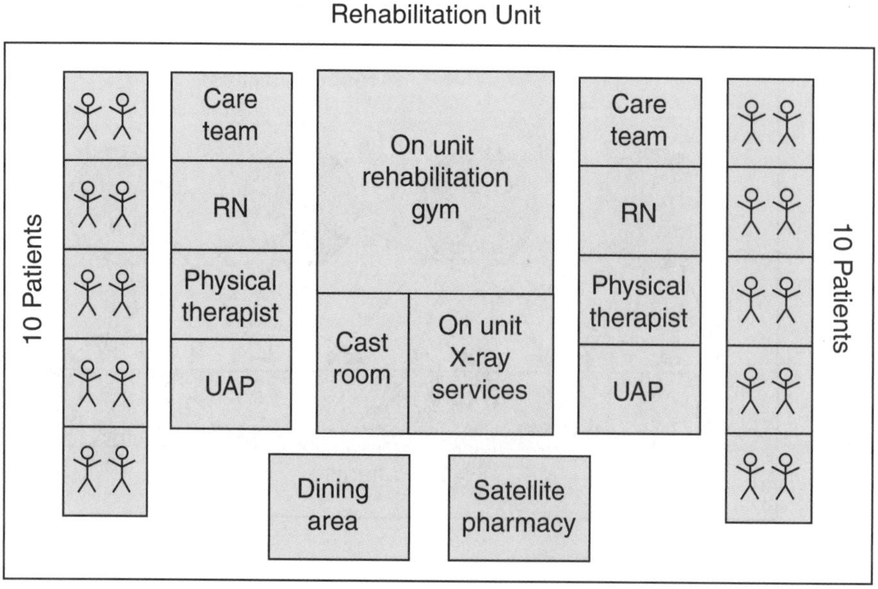

Rehabilitation Unit

Figure 6-11 Patient-Centered Care Model

Advantages and Disadvantages

The pros of the system are that it is most convenient for patients and expedites services to patients. But it can be extremely costly to decentralize major services in an organization. A second disadvantage is that some staff have perceived the model as a way of reducing RNs and cutting costs in hospitals. In fact, this has been true in some organizations, but many other organizations have successfully used the patient-centered model to have the right staff available for the needs of the patient population.

Differentiated Practice

Differentiated nursing practice is a care delivery model that sorts the roles, functions, and work of registered nurses according to some identified criteria, commonly education, clinical experience, and competence (Baker et al., 1997). This model of care delivery emerged in the mid-1980s as a way of articulating the difference in practice of RNs. Educational preparation is grouped into associate degree in nursing (ADN), bachelor of science in nursing (BSN), and master of science in nursing (MSN) as a hierarchy. Nursing competencies are generally measured in three arenas: technical skills, communication skills, and management of care or leadership skills. Pilot implementation projects have shown some positive outcomes from this model. To illustrate how this model works, review the Real World Interview that follows.

Advantages and Disadvantages

Differentiated practice allows nurses to work in specialized roles for which they were educated, leading to greater career satisfaction, and provides appropriate recognition and rewards across the continuum of nurses' care ("Differentiated nursing practice in all care settings," 1995). A disadvantage is that nurses who have gained experience and who have the knowledge and capability to function beyond their original education may not be recognized. These staff may be disenfranchised by a model that does not factor in the learning that takes place outside of the academic setting. In addition, organizations that have established minimal educational requirements for RN positions may have difficulty recruiting staff with the requisite credentials.

CARE DELIVERY MANAGEMENT TOOLS

In the 1980s and 1990s, hospitals looked for opportunities to reduce costs through reduction in the LOS. Clinical pathways, case management, and disease management surfaced as significant strategies.

Clinical Pathways

Clinical pathways are a major initiative to come out of the efforts to reduce LOS and are widely used to enhance outcomes and contain costs within a constrained length of stay (Lagoe, 1998). **Clinical pathways** are care management tools that outline the expected clinical course and outcomes for a specific patient type. Clinical pathways take a different form in each organization that develops them. Typically they are pathways that outline the normal course of care for a patient. Pathways are often done by day, and for each day expected outcomes are articulated. It is the expected outcomes that patient progress is measured against. In some organizations, the pathways include multidisciplinary orders for care, including orders from nursing, medicine, and other allied health professionals such as physical therapy and dietary services. This serves to further expedite care for patients. Figure 6-12 provides an excerpt from a clinical pathway.

REAL WORLD INTERVIEW

In our organization, we have implemented a model of differentiated practice. Our purpose was to match individual competencies with job descriptions to maximize an individual's skills. In our model, there is one staff nurse title, but there are job descriptions and performance expectations based on the nurse's level of education, associate degree, bachelor's degree, or master's degree. Pay is based on level of education and performance. Performance expectations were developed for each education level and organized using the nursing process as a framework. The nursing process statements for each level of education reflect nursing practice from novice to expert. In this model, all nurses may participate in activities like discharge planning, but the performance expectations for a master's-prepared nurse would be different than for a diploma-prepared nurse. Each nurse has an individual performance plan that assists the nurse to meet established performance expectations and to develop and meet individual goals. This performance plan is developed annually by the staff nurse with their nurse manager.

The outcomes of this model have been improved job satisfaction and reduced turnover of the nursing staff. We have noted that more staff have engaged in formal education and are accessing educational opportunities within the organization. Some of the lessons we learned were that we had to look at people as individuals. Staff did not fit into neat categories. We learned that there was fear among the nursing administrative ranks regarding how the staff would react to a differentiated practice model. In reality, the staff accepted the model and the message that everyone has value and brings different skills to the workplace. The goal of the model was to maximize those two things. In communicating to the staff, hierarchy of any sort in the model was minimized.

In retrospect, I would spend more time up front with the managers and other leadership staff. It is key that leadership staff have a complete understanding of the model, how to communicate the key elements of the model, and how to implement the model at the unit level. Even though this was a significant culture change for our organization, the outcomes for the staff have been positive and well worth the efforts put forth.

Kathleen Brodbeck, RN, MSN
Vice President for Patient Care
St. Peter's Health Care Services

These pathways can be used by physicians, nurses, and case managers to care for the patient and measure the patient's progress against expected outcomes. Any variance in outcome can then be noted and acted upon to get the patient back on track. Some organizations have up to 60 pathways implemented.

Case Management

Case management is a second strategy to improve patient care and reduce hospital costs through coordination of care. Typically a case manager is responsible for coordinating care and establishing goals from preadmission through

Clinical Pathway: Lower Extremity Revascularization
EXCERPT

ADDRESSOGRAPH

DAILY ANTICIPATED OUTCOMES							
POD2	Date/Time /Init When met	POD3	Date/Time /Init When met	POD4	Date/Time /Init When met	POD5	Date/Time /Init When met
Patient rates pain 0-2 on pain scale 0-10 using po analgesia.		Graft signal present with doppler		Graft signal present with doppler		Graft signal present with doppler	
Graft signal present with doppler.		Incisional edges will be approximated without drainage.		Able to participate in self-care and adjunct therapies.		Ambulates independently	
Patient will verbalize knowledge of plan of care, testing and treatment.		Site of invasive devices without signs of infection.		Patient viewed diet video.		Patient/significant other will verbalize understanding of activity/diet restrictions, medication use, wound management.	
Ambulate in hall Q I D		Ambulates in hall Q I D.					
Tolerates po solids		Patient/significant other will describe appropriate problem solving skills to decrease anxiety.				Completed nutrition post test	
Voiding without difficulty		Rehab referral started: _yes _no					
		Family support available at discharge, specify _____ _____					

TO BE KEPT IN PROGRESS NOTE SECTION OF CHART AT ALL TIMES.

Figure 6-12 Example of a Clinical Pathway (Excerpt) (Courtesy of Albany Medical Center, Albany, NY)

discharge (Del Togno-Armanasco, Hopkin, & Harter, 1995). In the typical model of case management, a nurse is assigned to a specific high-risk patient population or service, such as cardiac surgery patients. The case manager has the responsibility to work with all disciplines to facilitate care. For example, if a postsurgical hospitalized patient has not met ambulation goals according to the clinical pathway, the case manager would work with the physician and nurse to determine what is preventing the patient from achieving this goal. If it turns out that the patient is elderly and is slow to recover, they may agree that physical therapy would be beneficial to assist this patient in ambulating. In other models, the case management function is provided by the staff nurse at the bedside. This works well if the population requires little case management, but if the patient population requires significant case management services, there needs to be enough RN time allocated for this activity. In addition to facilitating care, the case manager usually has a data function to improve care. In this role, the case manager collects aggregate data on patient variances from the clinical pathway. The data are shared with health care clinicians who participate in the clinical pathway and are then used to explore opportunities for improvement in the pathway or in hospital systems.

Disease Management

Increasingly, health care centers are developing disease management (DM) programs. Disease management is a "systematic, population-based approach to identify persons at risk, intervene with specific programs of care, and measure clinical and other outcomes" (Epstein & Sherwood, 1996). An objective of disease management is cost containment, and research indicates that this is occurring. A study of nurses who managed patients with congestive heart failure in an aged population showed significantly lower numbers of patient readmissions and costs (Rich et al., 1995).

DM can be as simple as a pharmaceutical pamphlet describing how best to use a medication or as complex as nurse managers developing individualized care plans and regularly contacting patients to ensure compliance with the plans.

Disease management strategies use a variety of methods, including telephone, the Internet, and in-person visits, to keep high-risk, high-cost patients out of the hospital. These DM strategies collect data from and send reminders

to patients who need constant monitoring. They also provide information systems that help caregivers develop care plans and gather data for clinical improvement initiatives.

 KEY CONCEPTS

- To plan nurse staffing, you must understand and apply the concepts of full-time equivalents (FTEs) and nursing hours per patient day (NHPPD).
- Patient classification systems predict nursing time required for a specific patient and then whole groups of patients; the data can then be utilized for staffing, budgeting, and benchmarking.
- Determination of the number of FTEs needed to staff a unit requires review of patient classification data, NHPPD, regulatory requirements, skill mix, staff support, historical information, and the physical environment of the unit.
- The number of staff and patients in your staffing pattern drives the amount of nursing time available for patient care.
- In developing a staffing pattern, additional FTEs must be added to a nursing unit budget to provide coverage for days off and benefited time off.
- Scheduling of staff is the responsibility of the nurse manager, who must take into consideration patient need and acuity, volume of patients, and the experience of the staff.
- Whatever staffing variations are chosen, it is critical to assess the effect on patient care and finances.
- Self-scheduling can increase staff morale and professional growth but to be successful requires clear boundaries and guidelines.
- Evaluating the outcomes of your staffing plan on patients, staff, and the organization is a critical activity that should be done regularly.
- Case management and clinical pathways are care management tools that have been developed to improve patient care and reduce hospital costs.

KEY TERMS

benchmarking
case management
clinical pathway
differentiated nursing practice
direct care
disease management
full-time equivalent
functional nursing
indirect care
inpatient unit
modular nursing
nonproductive hours
nursing care delivery model

nursing hours per patient day
patient acuity
patient-centered care
patient classification system
patient-focused care
primary nursing
productive hours
self-scheduling
skill mix
staffing pattern
team nursing
total patient care

REVIEW QUESTIONS

1. Patient classification systems measure nursing workload needed by the patient. The higher the patient's acuity, the more care that is required by the patient. Which of the following statements is a weakness of classification systems?
   A. Patient classification data are useful in predicting the required staffing for the next shift and for justifying nursing hours provided.
   B. Patient classification data can be utilized by the nurse making assignments to determine what level of care a patient requires.
   C. Classification systems typically focus on nursing tasks rather than a holistic view of a patient's needs.
   D. Aggregate patient classification data are useful in costing out nursing services and for developing the nursing budget.

2. To determine the number of FTEs required for a renal transplant unit, you must review all but which of the following?

A. Regulatory requirements from your regional, state, and federal governments
B. The patient population care needs and the impact on your skill mix
C. Organizational structure or supports in place to enable care providers to care for patients
D. The chief financial officer's opinion on the number of staff needed for your unit

3. In calculating the number of FTEs needed to staff your medical-surgical unit, you must provide additional FTEs for all but which of the following?
   A. Benefited time off such as vacation and sick time
   B. Educational time for staff, including orientation of new staff
   C. Indirect patient care staff that support the operation of the direct care staff 24 hours a day
   D. Coverage for other departments that do not staff to cover their own benefited time off

4. If your RN staff members receive 4 weeks of vacation and 10 days of sick time per year, how many productive hours would each RN work in that year if they utilized all of their benefited time?
   A. 2,080 productive hours
   B. 1,840 productive hours
   C. 1,920 productive hours
   D. 1,780 productive hours

5. In building your staffing plan, which of the following would NOT be a major consideration for determining how many staff you need each day and shift?
   A. The need for your staff to have more weekends off
   B. The volume of patients that you have at different times of the day
   C. The timing and volume of nurse-intensive activities such as administration of chemotherapy and blood
   D. The skill mix of your staff and the patient care requirements throughout a 24-hour period

REVIEW ACTIVITIES

1. How do you know whether the outcomes of your staffing plan are positive? What measures do you have available in your organization that indicate your staffing is adequate or inadequate?

2. You are a nurse on a new unit for psychiatric patients. What should be considered in planning for FTEs and staffing for this unit?

3. You are a new nurse and you have increasing concerns regarding the staffing levels on your unit. You are becoming increasingly anxious each time you go to work. What would you do?

EXPLORING THE WEB

- To get more information on mandated staffing levels, go to *http://www.ana.org*. Go to staffing issues on the menu and review the legislative agenda for the ANA regarding staffing. Also review data on the ANA's latest staff survey.

- To get more information on nursing quality measures, go to *http://www.mriresearch.org*. Review the quality measures.

REFERENCES

Baker, C. M., Lamm, G. M., Winter, A. R., Robbleloth, V. B., Ransom, C. A., Conly, F., et al. (1997). Differentiated nursing practice: Assessing the state-of-the-science. *Nursing Economic$, 15*(5), 253–261.

Buerhaus, P. I. (2000, May/June). Why are shortages of hospital RNs concentrated in specialty care units? *Nursing Economic$, 18*(3), 111–117.

Dearholt, S., & Feathers, C. A. (1997). Self-scheduling can work. *Nursing Management, 28*(8), 47–48.

Del Togno-Armanasco, V., Hopkin, L. A., & Harter, S. (1995). How case management really works. *American Journal of Nursing, 5*, 24i, 24j, 24l.

Diers, D., Bozzo, J., & RIMS/Nursing Acuity Project Group. (1997). Nursing Resource Definition in DRGs. *Nursing Economics, 15*(3), 124–130.

Differentiated nursing practice in all care settings. (1995). *Journal of Nursing Administration, 25*(7/8), 5, 6, 11.

Epstein, R. S., & Sherwood, L. M. (1996). From outcomes research to disease management. A guide for the perplexed, *Annals of Internal Medicine, 124*, 835–837.

Hill-Popper, M. (2000, January). *Reversing the flight of talent.* Symposium at the Nursing Executive Center annual meeting, The Advisory Board Company, Washington, DC.

Joint Commission on Accreditation of Healthcare Organizations. (2000). *2000 hospital accreditation standards.* Oakbrook Terrace, IL: Author.

Lagoe, R. J. (1998). Basic statistics for clinical pathway evaluation. *Nursing Economic$, 16*(3), 125–131.

Lichtig, L. K., Knaug, R. A., Rison-McCoy, R., & Wozniak, L. M. (2000). *Nurse staffing and patient outcomes in the inpatient hospital setting.* Washington, DC: American Nurses Association.

Malloch, K., & Conivaloff, A. (1999). Patient classification systems, part 1. *Journal of Nursing Administration, 29*(7/8), 49–56.

Manthey, M. (1980). *The practice of primary nursing.* Boston: Blackwell Scientific.

Needleman, J., Buerhaus, P., Mattke, S., Stewart, M. & Zelinski, (2002). Nurse-staffing levels and the quality of care in hospitals. *New England Journal of Medicine, 346*(22), 1715–1722.

Rich, M. W., Beckham, V., Wittenberg, C., Leven, C. L., Friedland, K., & Carney, R. M. (1995). A multidisciplinary intervention to prevent readmission of elderly patients with congestive heart failure. *New England Journal of Medicine, 333,* 1190–1195.

Shullanberger, G. (2000). Nurse staffing decisions: An integrative review of the literature. *Nursing Economic$, 18*(3), 124–126.

Steefel, L. (2003, March). Walk the ratio talk. *Nursing Spectrum Southern Edition.*

Swansburg, R. C. (1996). *Management and leadership for nurse managers* (2d ed.). Sudbury, MA: Jones & Bartlett.

Zimmermann, P. G., (2003). Cutting-Edge Discussions of management, policy, and program issues in Emergency Care. *Journal of Emergency Nursing, 28,* 453–462.

SUGGESTED READINGS

Abraham, A. (2003). Poor nursing systems and staffing problems led to poor patient outcomes. *Professional Nurse, 18*(10), 576–577.

Benko, L. B. (2003). Workforce report 2003. Ratio daze in California. *Modern Healthcare, 33*(24), 30–31.

Buckingham, M., & Coffman, C. (1999). *First break all the rules—what the world's greatest managers do differently.* New York: Simon & Schuster.

Falco, J., Wenzel, K., Quimby, D., & Penny, P. (2000). Moving differentiated practice from concept to reality. *Aspen Adviser for Nurse Executives, 15*(5), 6–9.

McCue, M., Mark, B. A., Harless, D. W. (2003). Nurse staffing, quality, and financial performance. *Journal of Health Care Finance, 29*(4), 54–76.

Nelson, J. W. (2000). Consider this . . . Models of nursing care: A century of vacillation. *Journal of Nursing Administration, 30*(4), 156, 184.

Seago, J. A. (1999). Evaluation of hospital work redesign: Patient focused care. *Journal of Nursing Administration, 29*(11), 31–38.

Tuttas, C. A. (2003). Decreasing nurse staffing cost in a hospital setting: Developing stability. *Journal of Nurse Care Quarterly, 18*(3), 226–240.

White, K. (2003). Effective staffing as a guardian of care. *Nurse Management, 34*(7), 20–24.

CHAPTER 7

Budgeting

OBJECTIVES

Upon completion of this chapter, the reader should be able to:

1. Discuss perspectives on the cost of health care.
2. Identify at least three reasons why cost is an important consideration in health care discussions.
3. Discuss budgets commonly used for planning and management.
4. Describe key elements that influence budget preparation.
5. Identify revenue and expenses associated with the delivery of service.
6. Discuss budget monitoring.

You are assigned to a patient care unit for your clinical experience. You are wondering what types of services are provided to patients on this unit. You talk with your instructor and the nursing manager of the unit. Together, you review the unit's scope of service and budget.

What kinds of services are provided to patients on this unit?

How does the unit's budget help ensure provision of care for patients on this unit?

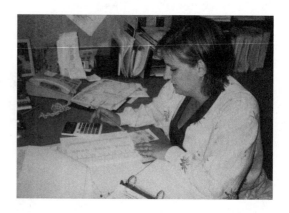

Regardless of how expert, creative, collaborative, and altruistic a health care system may be, it cannot function without money. Securing the bottom line is basic to achieving the mission of providing health care. Nurses need to understand concepts of budgeting and economics to help secure this bottom line. **Economics** is the study of how scarce resources are allocated among possible uses in order to make appropriate choices among the increasingly scarce resources.

The study of economics is based on three general premises: (1) scarcity—resources exist in finite quantities and consumption demand is typically greater than resource supply; (2) choice—decisions are made about which resources to produce and consume among many options; and (3) preference—individual and societal values and preferences influence the decisions that are made. In a traditional market economy, the sellers sell to the buyers who buy, with each trying to maximize their gains from the transactions. Health care does not fit well in this model. For example, consider the concept of price elasticity, which is related to the price that an individual is willing to pay for a given item. Normally, as the price goes up, the demand goes down. When the purchase is health care, however, the price may be viewed as irrelevant to the decision to purchase. Think of a wristwatch that you might always purchase for $5, would likely not buy at $50, and would never consider at $500. Now, imagine that instead of a wristwatch, the item in question is a medication or therapy needed to save your sick child. Now the consideration of price in the decision-making process is likely quite different. Thus, health care is much less "elastic" with reference to price than many other consumer goods.

Another aspect of health care's difference from the traditional economic model relates to the knowledge of options and payment mechanisms available to the consumer. In a typical market, the buyer is also the payer. In health care, the health care provider (buyer) ordering a hospitalization or treatment is a doctor or nurse. The provider is not the payer, nor is the patient (buyer) using the hospital or treatment the payer. The actual **payer** is the third-party reimburser (insurance company or government). Consequently, the financial impact of the decision on the provider (buyer) and the patient user (buyer) is skewed. Neither of these buyers is the payer.

This chapter presents basic health care budgeting and economics concepts that are important to the novice nurse entering clinical practice. Included are perspectives on the role cost has played and will play in directing health care delivery, the methods for determining the cost of delivering nursing care, and the effect of health care policy on the delivery of nursing care. Common financial language and tools are discussed so nurses can understand the elements of cost-effective care.

SOME PERSPECTIVES ON THE COST OF HEALTH CARE

It may come as a surprise to note in Figure 7-1 that 1999 statistics show that the federal government, through the Medicare and Medicaid programs, paid for 33.6%, and other public sources paid for 12.7%, of all health care costs in the United States that year. In addition to the Medicare and Medicaid programs, government tax funds pay for the health care of members of the military, eligible veterans, Native Americans, federal prisoners, selected vulnerable or at-risk populations, and developmentally disabled and mentally ill patients who are institutionalized (Finkler & Kovner, 2000). Such funding bears some resemblance to the socialized health care programs of other nations.

Socialized Health Care

Socialized systems of providing health care are in place around the world. Philosophically, under such systems, complete health care and hospital care are provided to all the citizens in a community, district, or nation (universal access). However, it is important to realize that the term socialized health care refers to a variety of health care programs, each specific about what coverage is provided and how it is funded. Savage, Hoelscher, and Walker (1999) studied seven industrialized European countries and Canada for commonalities in coverage and funding. Their work reveals both centralized and decentralized compulsory single-payer systems with fee-for-service components, as well as some private insurance components.

Funding for the programs under study also varied. In general, care is funded through public taxation of citizens, who are then eligible for care but who may or may not use it. Programs in Canada, Sweden, and the United Kingdom are funded from income taxes and selected other taxes. Germany and the Netherlands rely on payroll taxes for funding. The authors of the study pointed out that the countries studied face similar challenges of aging populations with chronic disease, the need to ration costly technology, severe budget shortages, managed competition, and decentralization. Compare the study findings to the 13.6% of gross national product spent the same year by the United States (more than any other country in the world and nearly twice that of many of the European countries studied) and to the $3,759 spent per capita in the United States, as shown in Table 7-1. Still, there are approximately 44 million people in the United States without health insurance, and the United States continues to experience a stubbornly high infant mortality rate.

With U.S. life expectancy for males at 72.5 years and for females at 79.2 years, the benefits reaped in the U.S. health care system seem to be those of enhanced quality of life rather than enhanced longevity. Quality of life must be defined within the specific cultures and value systems of each country. In the United States, qualities of life highly valued by Americans include prompt access to diagnostic and treatment services, even when health problems are not life threatening; ready availability of cutting-

Where It Came From

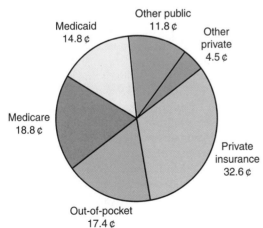

Figure 7-1 The Nation's Health Care Dollar: 1999 (From: "The Nation's Health Dollar: 1999," Health Care Financing Administration. Retrieved 12/17/01, from http://www.cms.hhs.gov.)

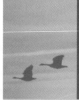

TABLE 7-1

COMPARISON OF HEALTH CARE SPENDING AND LIFE EXPECTANCY ACROSS FOUR INDUSTRIALIZED COUNTRIES

Country	% GNP	Per Capita Spending	Male Life Expectancy (years)	Female Life Expectancy (years)
United States	13.6	$3,759	72.5	79.2
Germany	10.5	$2,222	73.0	79.5
Canada	9.2	$2,002	75.3	81.3
United Kingdom	6.9	$1,304	74.3	79.7

edge technology and pharmaceuticals; the ability to choose among health care practitioners and sites for care; and participation in health care decisions. All these contribute to the cost of health care. Is that enough to justify spending more than any other country in the world (Pantel, 2001) and nearly twice as much as European countries with similar health and financial circumstances? Perhaps.

THE COST EQUATION: MONEY = MISSION = MONEY

The mission statement of any health care business or unit describes the purpose for existence of the business or unit and the rationale that justifies that existence (Finkler & Kovner, 2000). The mission directs decision making about what is or is not within the purview of the business or unit. The vision statement is a logical extension of the mission into the future and establishes long-range goals for the business or unit. Once the vision is established and the business can articulate where it wants to go, a strategic plan that identifies how to achieve the vision or how to get to the goals is developed.

There must be cohesion and consistency across the mission, vision, and strategic plan for the business or unit to successfully achieve its mission. There must also be money, for without it no mission can be accomplished.

Business Profit

Revenue (income) minus cost (expense) equals profit. Profit is not restricted to for-profit businesses. Profit is not a dirty word. All businesses must realize a profit to remain in business. In for-profit businesses, a portion of the profit is distributed to stockholders in appreciation for their investing in the business and the remainder is used to maintain and grow the organization. In nonprofit businesses, there are no stockholders to share the profit, so all of it is fed back into the business for maintenance and growth.

Not-for-profit organizations desiring a purer image than the term *profit* engenders refer to their profit as contribution to margin, with the rule of thumb being to secure 4% to 5% of the total budget as profit or margin. Mission and margin are strategically and operationally linked by the reality that resources are required to carry out the organization's strategic plan and achieve its mission. Without margin, or with limited margin, there would be a lack of money to replace

REAL WORLD INTERVIEW

The age of "volume" as a measure of anything is long past. In health care, for so many years, the notion of unparalleled growth and expansion and anything for anyone was common. Subsequent introduction of broader concepts reflecting an understanding of value and sustainability now drive rational thinking about availability and delivery of health services. The issue of "value" now drives all elements of health service from access to delivery and, ultimately, to making a difference. Now we can more clearly enumerate the relationship between inputs and outcomes, process and product. Health services now must be able to establish the connection between what is done and what is achieved. Professions' addictions to what they do now gives way to tightening the connection between what is done and what difference it makes. The noise for both nurses and physicians is a closer look by everyone at the "value" of action in the light of the promise it holds. The issue: either deliver, or rethink why you're doing what you're doing. This critical examination and expectation will radically alter the economics and values of health care for the next two decades.

Tim Porter-O'Grady, EdD, PhD, RN, FAAN
Prolific Nurse Author and Speaker on New-Edge Health Care

worn-out equipment, to establish new services or enlarge existing services in response to changing community needs for health care, to purchase state-of-the-art technology, to improve salaries, to maintain existing buildings or undertake new construction, to replace heating and lighting systems. Failure to maintain such infrastructure can impair the organization's ability to be competitive, resulting in failure to meet its mission and eventual organizational failure.

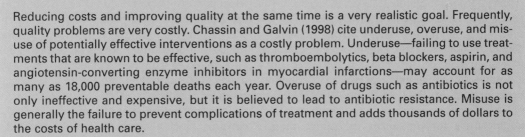

STOP AND THINK

Reducing costs and improving quality at the same time is a very realistic goal. Frequently, quality problems are very costly. Chassin and Galvin (1998) cite underuse, overuse, and misuse of potentially effective interventions as a costly problem. Underuse—failing to use treatments that are known to be effective, such as thromboembolytics, beta blockers, aspirin, and angiotensin-converting enzyme inhibitors in myocardial infarctions—may account for as many as 18,000 preventable deaths each year. Overuse of drugs such as antibiotics is not only ineffective and expensive, but it is believed to lead to antibiotic resistance. Misuse is generally the failure to prevent complications of treatment and adds thousands of dollars to the costs of health care.

Identify some ways in which nurses can participate in reducing underuse, overuse, and misuse to improve quality. Is keeping current with the literature in your specialty necessary to be effective in doing this? Do you underuse any health care promotion activities? What is the cost to your health of poor exercise habits? Do you overuse good nutrition?

REAL WORLD INTERVIEW

Nursing is a collaborative profession existing in a complex health care system. At one time it was influenced by three factors: cost, access, and quality. Today there are five influencing factors: cost, access, cost, quality, and cost.

John M. Lantz, RN, PhD, Dean and Professor, School of Nursing,
University of San Francisco

DIAGNOSTIC, THERAPEUTIC, AND INFORMATION TECHNOLOGY COST

Close examination of a health care budget often reveals that although the nursing payroll is the most expensive payroll item and the most expensive operating budget item, the most expensive item on the total budget is often diagnostic, therapeutic, and information technology.

The high cost of technology has been recognized by regulatory agencies for many years. In pursuit of cost control in hospitals, the states independently established laws more than 30 years ago creating Certificate of Need (CON) agencies to oversee, regulate, and approve major technology and construction expenditures (Chang, Price, & Pfoutz, 2001). A secondary goal was to ensure equitable distribution of and access to high-end technology across the state. The CON approach was not successful because it focused only on hospitals and provided no incentives to change either physician or patient behavior (Chang, Price, & Pfoutz, 2001). Hospitals were given spending limits, but there was no incentive for physicians to change their practice, so they didn't. Without incentives, patients' expectations and demands for care also remained unchanged.

Cost of Medications and Health Care Executive Salaries

Medications are a significant item in the overall budget. A recent visit to New York City in April 2003 identified these drug charges. See Table 7-2. Note that the high cost of medications in the United States is driving many Americans to go to Canada or Mexico for less expensive medications. Also note the health care executive compensation shown in Table 7-3.

NURSING COST

Fiscally, most organizations view nursing as a cost center that does not independently generate revenue. Although some deviation from that fiscal philosophy may occur when selected nursing practitioners are permitted by law to bill directly for their unique professional services, the cost of providing nursing care (wages, benefits, selected supplies and equipment, overhead) is commonly bundled into a catchall, room, or per diem, cost that assumes that every patient consumes identical nursing resources each day. Such a view is not only antiquated, it is incorrect. Nursing care is not an identical product delivered in assembly-line fashion. It varies remarkably in intensity, in depth, and in

TABLE 7-2
COST OF SELECTED MEDICATIONS

Medication	Number of Doses	Cost
Cipro 250 mg	30	$135.59
Coumadin 5 mg	30	33.59
Diabeta 5 mg	90	79.89
Lanoxin 0.25 mg	100	23.69
Paxil 20 mg	30	101.89
Pepcid 40 mg	60	245.49
Prilosec 20 mg	30	157.99

breadth across patients, consistent with their unique, individual dependency needs.

Access to a high degree of nursing care is accepted as second only in importance to access to medical technology as a reason for hospitalization. When access to both nursing care and medical technology is needed, hospitalization is unquestionably appropriate. Consequently, the revenue generated from hospitalization is, in fact, payment, primarily, for consumption of medical technology and nursing services and should be recognized as such.

TYPES OF BUDGETS

Health care organizations use several types of budgets to help with future planning and management. A **budget** is a plan that provides formal quantitative expression for acquiring and distributing funds over the ensuing time period (generally 1 year). A budget is based on what is known about how much was spent in the past and how that will inevitably change in the coming year. The types of budgets are operational, capital, and construction.

TABLE 7-3
HEALTH CARE EXECUTIVE COMPENSATION

Executive	Annual Salary
Jeff Barbakow, Tenet Healthcare	$35 million
Miles White, Abbott Laboratories	$30.4 million
Richard Jay Kagan, Schering-Plough	$24.4 million

Useem, J. Have they no shame. *Fortune,* April 28, 2003, 56–64.

Operational Budget

An **operational budget** accounts for the income and expenses associated with day-to-day activity within a department or organization. Revenue generation is based on billable services and expenses associated with equipment, supplies, staffing, and other indirect costs. Revenue may be based on the number of days that a patient stays on an inpatient unit or the number of hours spent in a procedure room. Revenue may be also based on the types of procedures delivered to a patient. Depending on reimbursement rates and requirements, expenses are sometimes bundled or included into a procedure or room charge, for example, an admission packet that includes a washbasin, cup, soap holder, and so on. In other situations, supply items may be billed separately, such as IV start kits, leukocyte removal filters, and so on.

Capital Budget

A **capital budget** accounts for the purchase of major new or replacement equipment. Equipment is purchased when new technology becomes available or when older equipment becomes too expensive to maintain because of age-related problems such as inefficiencies resulting from the decreased speed of equipment or downtime (amount of time it is out of service for repairs). Sometimes the expense and availability of replacement parts make it prohibitive to maintain equipment. Other times equipment may become antiquated because of its inability to deliver service consistently, meet industry or regulatory standards, or provide high-quality outcomes.

Construction Budget

A **construction budget** is developed when renovation or new structures are planned. The construction budget generally includes labor, materials, building permits, inspections, equipment, and so on. If it is anticipated that a department will need to close during construction, then projected lost revenue is accounted

for in the budget. Revenue and expenses may also be shifted to another department that absorbs the services on a temporary basis.

BUDGET OVERVIEW

A budget is a financial tool that outlines anticipated revenue and expenses over a specified period. A process called **accounting**, which is an activity that managers engage in to record and report financial transactions and data, assists with budget documentation. Budgets serve as standards to plan, monitor, and evaluate the performance of a health care system. Budgets account for the income generated as compared to the expenses needed to deliver the service. **Profit** is determined by the relationship of income to expenses. Profitability results when the income is higher than the expenses.

Budgets make the connection between operational planning and allocation of resources. This is especially important because health care organizations measure multiple key indicators of overall performance. These key indicators can be illustrated in a dashboard. A **dashboard** is a documentation tool providing a snapshot image of pertinent information and activity at a particular point in time. A dashboard or balanced scorecard identifies any of four perspectives about an organization: finances, customer satisfaction and services, internal operating efficiency, and learning and growth (Norton & Kaplan, 2001). Figure 7-2 shows the dashboard of two separate units: gastrointestinal laboratory (GI lab) and a medical nursing unit. **Variance**, or the difference between what was budgeted and the actual result, can be tracked (Grohar-Murray & DiCroce, 1997).

Budget Preparation and Scope of Service

Formulating a budget involves a systematic approach that begins with preparation (Grohar-Murray & DiCroce, 1997). Budgets are generally developed for a 12-month period and are

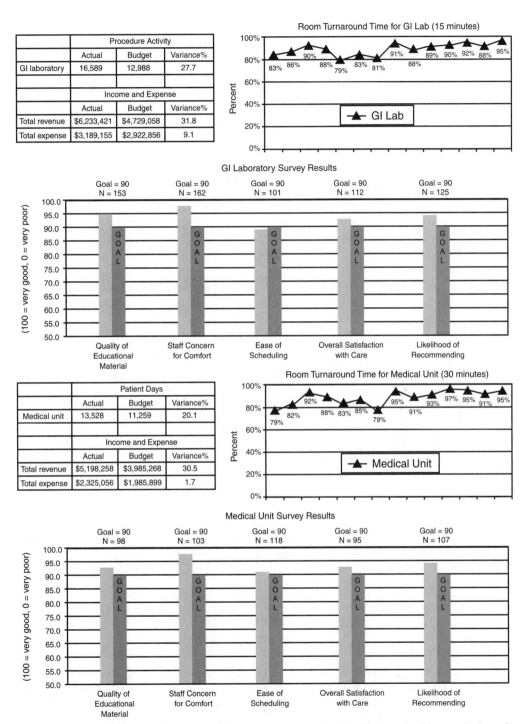

Figure 7-2 Patient Satisfaction, Turnaround Time, and Budget Activity (Adapted with permission of Northwestern Memorial Hospital, Chicago, IL)

monitored monthly. The yearly cycle can be based on a fiscal year as determined by the organization (e.g., September 1 through August 31) or a calendar year (e.g., January 1 through December 31). Shorter- or longer-term budgets may also be developed depending on the organizational planning process.

Prior to the beginning of the budget year, most organizations devote approximately 6 months to preparing and developing the operational budget. To prepare a budget, organizations gather fundamental information about a variety of elements that influence the organization, including patient demographic information such as age, race, sex, income, and so on; competitive analysis; regulatory influences; strategic plans; goals; and history. Additionally, it is helpful to review the department's scope of service. See Figure 7-3.

A medical nursing unit provides primarily inpatient care to patients with acute or chronic medical problems, such as congestive heart failure, diabetes, pulmonary disease, cancer, and so on. The unit, equipped with 30 private beds, a full kitchen, a lounge, and conference/consultation rooms, is operational 24 hours per day, 7 days per week. Patient education and support groups are held routinely in the library located directly on the unit. Team nursing is employed as the model of care. Nurses, patient care technicians, and unit secretaries are employed, with a social worker and diabetes educator providing additional patient support. Patients admitted to the unit for longer than 48 hours are discussed during daily multidisciplinary rounds. The rounds include case management personnel; psychosocial counselors; and nutrition, nursing, and medical staff. Staff discuss patient problems to facilitate future care, including discharge planning.

Figure 7-3 Medical Nursing Unit, Scope of Service

Competitive Analysis

A competitive analysis is important because it probes how the competition is performing as compared to other health care organizations. A competitive analysis examines other hospitals or practices' strengths and weaknesses, in addition to other details such as location and new or existing services and technology. Figure 7-4 presents a competitive analysis of three different hospitals.

Regulatory Influences

Regulatory requirements and reimbursement rates have an effect on financial performance. Regulatory changes are influenced by several governing bodies. A government agency that has high visibility in the area of reimbursement is the Centers for Medicare and Medicaid Services (CMS), whose mission is to

CASE STUDY 7-1

The manager from an inpatient units asks for staff input into identifying ways to decrease use of health care supply and paper items. These items have been identified as in excess of the budget by 10% to 20% during the past 3 months. This is the first time that the staff have been involved in helping with cost containment. Clinical nurses and assistants have been invited to participate.

When approaching an analysis of health care supply use, what might be the first step in the process? If you were to break the staff into work groups, which members should be chosen to analyze the use of clerical supplies? How would you proceed if you were trying to determine the supply costs associated with starting an IV with continuous intravenous infusions and medications. Would the pharmacist be helpful in this process?

Competitive Analysis: Hospital A

Location: Rural—100 miles from metropolitan area
Affiliation: Currently negotiating with three academic hospitals
General clinical description:
- Scattered bed approach to inpatient oncology
- Ambulatory chemotherapy clinic
- Many of the same physicians on staff at Hospital J
Radiation capability: None—refers to Hospital J
Support services: Cancer screenings offered sporadically
Miscellaneous:
- Tumor board
- Cancer committee

Competitive Analysis: Hospital C

Location: Urban city with a population of 150,000
Affiliation: For-profit corporation
- Medical oncology affiliation with University K
- Radiation Therapy Department affiliation with University K Radiation Therapy Department
General clinical description:
- Dedicated inpatient medical oncology unit
- Dedicated inpatient surgical oncology unit
- Four-bed autologous and stem cell bone marrow transplant unit (Eastern Cooperative Oncology Group Referral Center for autologous bone marrow transplants)
- Coagulation laboratory
- Therapeutic pheresis
- Pain clinic
- Oncology clinic
- Oncology rehabilitation
- Breast cancer rehabilitation program
- Ambulatory care chemotherapy unit
- Medical oncologist on staff at two hospitals
Radiation therapy:
- Linear accelerator
- Stereotactic radiosurgery
- Hyperthermia
- Brachytherapy
Support services:
- Home health and hospice program
- Cancer registry
- Cancer committee
- Physician update—quarterly cancer newsletter
- Cancer information line
- Cancer advisory council
- Cancer Survivor's Day offered annually
- Cancer screenings offered routinely
- Cancer support group—general cancer patients

Competitive Analysis: Hospital B

Location: Suburb of large metropolitan city
Affiliation: University hospital
General clinical description:
- Dedicated oncology inpatient unit
- Ambulatory chemotherapy department
- Comprehensive breast center
- Head and neck oncology team
Radiation therapy:
- Linear accelerator—two units
- High dose rate
- Intraoperative radiation therapy
- Stereotactic radiosurgery
Support services:
- Home infusion and home care program
- Hospice care program
- Annual cancer awareness fair
- Support group—general cancer patients
Miscellaneous:
- Tumor registry
- Tumor board
- Committee on cancer
- Head and neck patient conferences
- Stereotactic radiosurgery conferences

Figure 7-4 Competitive Analysis of Three Hospitals

ensure health care security for beneficiaries. CMS (www.cms.hhs.gov) administers federal control, quality assurance, and fraud and abuse prevention for Medicare, Medicaid, and the State Children's Health Insurance Program (SCHIP). Under the aegis of the Department of Health and Human Services, it is also responsible for coordinating health care policy, planning, and legislation.

Other regulatory bodies play a role in reimbursement by ensuring that federal and state laws are adhered to through approval and accreditation. For example, the Food and Drug Administration (www.fda.gov) regulates the use of drugs, food products, and medical devices in the United States. If equipment or drugs under its jurisdiction are not approved, then organizations cannot bill for their use, by law. The JCAHO (www.jcaho.org) accredits hospitals and health care agencies to ensure that they meet specific standards. Medicare and Medicaid will not reimburse for services unless a hospital is accredited by JCAHO.

Cost Centers

During the budget preparation phase, it is important to examine the individual nursing or hospital department or section thoroughly. Hospital systems are frequently divided into sections, departments, or units to compartmentalize

them for organizational purposes. These subsections or units, commonly called cost centers, are used to track financial data. Each department or cost center defines its own scope of service and goals.

Revenue Projections

Revenue is income generated through a variety of means, including billable patient services, investments, and donations to the organization. Specific unit-based revenue is generated through billing for services such as x-rays, invasive diagnostic or therapeutic procedures, drug therapy, surgical procedures, physical therapy, and so on. Revenue can also be generated through the delivery of multiple services over time, such as hourly rates for chemotherapy administration or blood transfusions. The specific number and

REAL WORLD INTERVIEW

The Joint Commission on Accreditation of Healthcare Organizations is a nonprofit organization that is committed to continuously improve the safety and quality of care provided to the public through the provision of health care accreditation and related services that support performance improvement in health care organizations. JCAHO currently evaluates and accredits nearly 19,000 health care organizations in the United States, including burn hospitals and home care organizations, more than 8,000 organizations that provide long term care, behavioral health care, laboratory and ambulatory services, as well as health plans and integrated delivery networks.

The JCAHO is a voluntary accreditation service with organizations surveyed on site every 3 years. The status of accreditation is reported to the public and to the payers who require a JCAHO quality evaluation or a federal inspection prior to paying for services provided under Medicare. The cost of this accreditation is borne by the organization on a sliding scale, dependent on its size and the extent of its services.

Health care organizations commit a great deal of time and energy to preparing for the on-site survey to successfully comply with the standards and receive a favorable accreditation status. The JCAHO standards are developed through a definitive process of input from the field, expert consultation, and research to validate the standard as a measure of quality.

Sally A. Sample, RN, MN, ND, DSc, FAAN

Nurse at Large, Board of Governors,
Joint Commission on Accreditation of Healthcare Organizations

types of services and procedures have to be projected for the budget. The reimbursement rates or payments received by hospitals often do not equal the actual hospital or unit charges for the services rendered. For example, there may be a fixed or flat reimbursement rate per case regardless of how long the patient stays in the hospital or how much the hospital pays for the service. If the costs exceed the reimbursement rate, then the provider absorbs the remaining costs. See Figure 7-5.

Expense Projections

Expenses are determined by identifying the costs associated with the delivery of service. Expenditures are resources used by an organization to deliver services and may include supplies, labor,

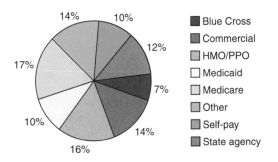

The reimbursement rates vary depending upon the payor. For example, Medicare may reimburse 40% of charges, Medicaid's rate may be 30%, and managed care may be at 60%. Factoring in reimbursement rates leads to profit and loss calculations for an organization.

Figure 7-5 Inpatient Payer Mix

LITERATURE APPLICATION

Citation: Elser, R., & Nipp, D. (2001). Worker designed culture change. *Nursing Economic$*, *19*(4), 161-163, 175.

Discussion: To effect operational efficiency and to improve employee performance, these authors proposed specific actions to change nursing culture. Work groups called resource utilization teams were organized to evaluate the unit values and the emotional components that affect relationships. Staff received educational support regarding communication and relationships so that differences and conflicts could be resolved. The staff was surveyed to determine their perceptions of their work environment based upon the cumulative responses. The team formulated a plan to staff the unit using the knowledge that they had gained and budgetary dollars that had been allocated. The team further identified role responsibilities and tasks that should be assigned to change the unit operations.

The strength of this article was in the creative proposal to capitalize on the knowledge and insight of staff to influence unit productivity. Every department or unit has its own unique characteristics and culture that influence the ability to produce and deliver quality care. Engaging staff in problem solving and role development is key to successful financial and operational management.

Implications for Practice: There are many creative ways to analyze expenses and productivity by using the workforce to improve operations and care. Imagine the potential if a work group were continually analyzing quality data points over time. The power of these work groups lies in their diverse members, who can see the department from different perspectives. When the work group is empowered, constructive measures can be identified to address problems that challenge departmental productivity, patient flow, and expenses.

STOP AND THINK

You work in an ED that sees 2,000 patients a month. Patients are charged $200 per visit plus charges for test and medications. Thus, these 2,000 patients can generate $400,000 per month in gross revenue for the hospital. Consider that there are five registered nurses (RNs) making $20 per hour and 2 medical doctors (MDs) making $100 per hour working each shift. Salaries for the RNs total $2,400 per day. Salaries for the MDs total $4,800 per day. The total salary for these two groups is $7,200 per day or $216,000 per month ($7,200 x 30 days).

Fifty percent of these patients have Medicare/Medicaid, and 45% of the patients are covered by managed care or insurance. Five percent of these patients have no insurance. Thus, 95% of patients can pay their bills. The other 5% of patients' bills are written off by the hospital as bad debt. Medicare/Medicaid/managed care/insurance companies often pay only 55% of the bills for these patients. They often deny payment for 45% of the bills. Thus, for the $380,000 (95% of $400,000) billed, the hospital will receive approximately $209,000 (55% of the $380,000 billed). Approximately $171,000 of the bill will not be paid by Medicare/Medicaid/managed care/insurance. Consider the following:

What other expenses besides salary must the hospital pay out of the $209,000 that it receives? Consider hospital space, liability insurance, technology costs, and so on.

Notice the effect that increasing the volume of patients has on budget figures. What happens to the budget if the patient volume goes to 2,500 patient ED visits per month and staffing stays the same? What happens if the fee rises to $300 per visit?

Are patients receiving useful information about future illness prevention and healthy living practices in the ED?

Is this a cost-effective way to deliver health care? How could we better serve the health care needs of 44 million Americans?

---

equipment, utilities, and miscellaneous items. See Figure 7-6.

Staffing. The amount and types of staff are often accounted for in a staffing model. The model outlines the number of staff required based upon the primary statistic such as procedures or patients. Figure 7-7 illustrates a sample staffing model.

Staffing ratios and salary data are particularly important because of the cost factor. Specialty salaries fluctuate, depending upon supply and demand. When there are shortages of certain staff, the salary tends to increase. Additionally, a health care organization may change its benefits, offering a more attractive package that includes

continuing education; paid time off for education, vacation, sick time, or personal needs; or professional membership expenses. Institutions may also look for alternative ways to supplement or deliver services during staff shortages. This means that supplemental staff—professional agency nurses, nurses from in-house registries, or patient care technicians—may be hired at a different salary rate. It is important to note whether a unit has had historical difficulty retaining or recruiting staff. Recruitment and retention, especially attracting, interviewing, hiring, and orienting staff, require dollars. For example, it has been estimated that the turnover cost per nurse, including advertising, recruitment, orientation, and time to fill the vacancy,

NET EXPENSE WORKSHEET
2004 BUDGET

DESCRIPTION	GI Lab	Medical Unit
Out Patient	8,290,564	33,450
In Patient	3,400,678	10,162,875
CORPORATE BILLING REVENUE	17,806	10,419
TOTAL OPERATING REVENUE	**11,709,048**	**10,206,744**
EXPENSES		
Salary Expense		
BUDGET REDUCTION SALARY	0	24,932
SALARIES	1,398,630	2,098,150
SALARIES OVERTIME	219,878	142,359
PROFESSIONAL AGENCY FEE	106,608	166,456
TOTAL SALARY	**1,725,116**	**2,431,879**
TRANSPORTATION EXPENSE	4,190	3,870
TOTAL	**4,190**	**3,870**
NON-SALARY EXPENSE		
NONMEDICAL SUPPLIES		
SUPPLIES CLERICAL	12,924	8,524
PRINTED FORMS	31,486	28,854
SOAP AND CLEANING	6,092	8,950
PAPER GOOD SUPPLIES	1,192	930
FILM SUPPLY PHOTO	3,836	
PACKAGING SUPPLIES	94	
TOTAL	**55,624**	**47,258**
FOODS		
MEETING AND LUNCHEONS BANQUETS	0	495
SUNDRY FOOD ISSUES	5,872	8,990
TOTAL	**5,872**	**9,485**

MEDICAL SUPPLIES

MEDICAL SUPPLIES	1,480,840	865,872
DIAG TEST CTR/IONIC CONTRST	2,798	
SUTURES	4,064	
DRUG SUPPLIES	120,120	569,088
IV & IRRIGATION SOLUTIONS	13,994	11,431
IV & IRRIGATION SETS	56,280	30,649
MEDIA	48	
PHLEBOTOMY SUPPLIES	680	
LAB GLASSWARE & INSTRUM	3,948	
LABORATORY SUPPLIES	156	
CHEMICALS	158	
TOTAL	**1,683,086**	**1,477,040**
TOTAL SUPPLIES	**1,744,582**	**1,533,783**
PURCHASE SERVICES		
PURCHASED SERVICES	41,436	15,678
TOTAL	**41,436**	**15,678**
UTILITIES		
TELEPHONE CHARGES-Long Distance	1,480	1,500
TELEPHONE CHARGES	13,608	15,238
TOTAL	**15,088**	**16,736**
OTHER EXPENSES		
CONTINUING ED	6,715	4,127
AUDIO VISUAL	500	0
TRAVEL EXPENSE	6,120	5,100
DISCOUNTED PARKING	190	150
MISCELLANEOUS	730	500
SM FIXTURES & EQUIPMENT	728	410
EQUIP RENTAL GENERAL	1,342	1,071
COPY MACHINE EXPENSES	13,440	6,424
BOOK LIBRARY	250	320
SUBSCRIPTION MAGAZINE	200	150
REPAIR REPL PARTS EQUIP	1,070	125
REPAIRS & REPL PARTS MED EQUIP	146,498	
FILM PROCESSING EXPENSE	220	
TOTAL	**178,003**	**18,377**
TOTAL NON-SALARY EXPENSE	**1,983,299**	**1,588,446**
TOTAL EXPENSE	**3,708,415**	**4,020,343**
TOTAL NET EXPENSES	**1,983,299**	**1,588,446**

Figure 7-6 Net Expense Worksheet (Adapted with permission of Northwestern Memorial Hospital, Chicago, IL)

STOP AND THINK

Talk with a nurse manager of the unit where you have your clinical experience. Ask to look at the budget for the nursing unit. How are salary supplies, utilities, and so forth monitored? How can nurses work to decrease expenses and increase quality of this unit? What kind of effect might that have on patient care?

can equate to $65,000 (The Advisory Board Company, 1998). The average cost to educate a nurse during a 6-week orientation period is more than $5,000. Not only the salary but also benefits are frequently factored into a salary package, and they need to be included in the budget.

Direct and Indirect Expenses. Expenses can be further broken down into direct and indirect. Direct expenses are those expenses directly associated with the patient, such as medical and surgical supplies, wages, and drugs. Indirect expenses are expenses for items such as utilities—gas, electric, and phones—that are not directly related to patient care but are necessary to support care. Other support functions frequently charged to a department that are not specifically related to patient care delivery are housekeeping, maintenance, materials management, and finance.

Fixed and Variable Costs. Fixed costs are those expenses that are constant and are not related to productivity or volume. Examples of these costs are building and equipment depreciation, utilities, fringe benefits, and administrative salaries. Variable costs fluctuate depending upon the volume or census and types of care required. Medical and surgical supplies, drugs, laundry, and food costs often increase the volume.

BUDGET APPROVAL AND MONITORING

Once developed, budgets are submitted to administration for review and approval, and the entire health care team is then responsible for ensuring that expenses are kept within the budgeted amount. The manner in which this is accomplished depends on the organization. Some institutions request that budget dashboards (see Figure 7-8) be developed reflecting departmental activity at a glance monthly. Variance reports or dashboards may be posted so that all staff members have an opportunity to review the budget and participate in any improvement needed.

THE FUTURE

Authors of the two seminal magnet hospital studies (McClure, Poulin, Sovie, & Wandelt, 1983; Kramer, 1990) and the authors of the study on nurse sensitive outcomes (Needleman, Buerhaus, Mattke, Stewart, & Zelevinsky, 2001) eloquently concluded that care by registered nurses is inseparable from high-quality patient care. Christensen, Bohmer, and Kenagy (2000), protagonists of disruptive innovation as the answer to the health care crisis, believe that most

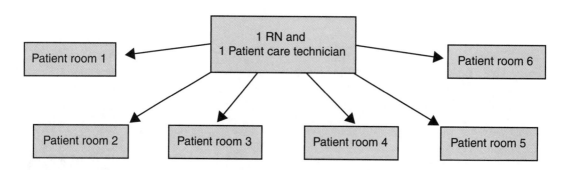

Figure 7-7 Inpatient Staffing Model

Year to Date					
		Volume/Access			
Department	**Cost Center**	**Volume Year to Date**	**Percentage Budget Variance**	**Percentage Variance from Last year**	**Days to Next Appointment/ Available Bed**
GI Laboratory	1265	6,706	16	23	3
Medical Unit	7095	9,705	18	28	1
Patient Satisfaction					
	Overall Score		**Percentile**	**Percentile**	**Results Reporting**
Department	**Actual**	**Target**	**Actual**	**Target**	**Average Report Turnaround Time** / **Reports > 24**
GI laboratory	90.5	91.70	90	95	28 / 20%
Medical unit	89	90.00	88	92	NA / NA
Human Resources					
					Employee Performance
		Actual	**Vacancies**	**Turnover**	**Staff Performance Reviews on Time**
Department	**Manager**	**FTEs Year to Date**	**Year to Date**	**Rate**	**> 30 Days**
GI laboratory	1	33.00	0.4	8%	0
Medical unit	1	45.00	6	12%	1
Expenses					
				Supply	**Productivity**
		Percentage of Budget Compared to Actual	**Percentage Variance from Budget Year to Date**	**Variance from Budget Year to Date**	**Variance from Last Year**
Department					
GI laboratory	250	(5.00)	11.00	unfavorable	unfavorable
Medical unit	118	8.00	12.00	favorable	unfavorable
Capital Budget					
Line Items	**Number**	**Year**	**Budgeted**	**Expensed**	**Balance**
GI lab					
7 Video endoscopes	10002895	2001	112,550.00	109,389.19	14,226.00
Endoscopy travel cart	30256409	2001	2,750.00	0.00	32,750.00
Scopes	89756452	2001	38,255.00	35,225.00	1,199.00
Comments					
Financial improvement plan ongoing in GI lab: Interventional charges have been adjusted and cost reduction/inventory control is being explored with materials management.					
Medical nursing unit has achieved highest overall patient satisfaction goal. Multidisciplinary conferences are being held every other day to focus on patient care issues.					

Figure 7-8 G1 Laboratory and Medical Unit Dashboard (Adapted with permission of Northwestern Memorial Hospital, Chicago, IL)

ailments are relatively straightforward disorders whose diagnosis and treatment tap but a small fraction of what physicians are educated to do and what nurse practitioners do so capably. They point out that most of the powerful innovations that disrupted other industries did so by enabling a larger population of less-skilled people to do, in a more convenient and less expensive way, things that historically were carried out only by a defined group of "experts." Nurses are poised to step into this role.

KEY CONCEPTS

- Nurses play an integral role in the development, implementation, and evaluation of a unit or department budget.
- If nurses are not conscious of revenue and expenses, then deviation from financial performance will occur.
- Overall, organizational performance is dependent upon the insight and skills of

staff members regarding patient care quality and financial outcomes.

- There are several types of budgets that hospitals use to help with future planning and management. These include operational, capital, and construction budgets.
- The budget preparation phase is one of data gathering related to a variety of elements that influence an organization, including demographic information, competitive analysis, regulatory influences, and strategic plans. Additionally, it is helpful to understand the department's scope of service, goals, and history.
- During the budget preparation phase, it is important to examine the individual nursing or hospital department or section thoroughly. Hospital systems are frequently divided into sections, departments, or units to compartmentalize them for organizational purposes. These subsections or units, commonly called cost centers, are used to track financial data.
- Organizations typically use history or past performance as a baseline of experience and data to better understand activity in a department or unit.
- Once background data have been gathered, the development of the budget can follow. This includes projecting revenue and expenses.
- Expenses are determined by identifying the cost associated with the delivery of service. Expenditures are resources used by an organization to deliver services and may include labor, supplies, equipment, utilities, and miscellaneous items.
- Once developed, budgets are submitted to administration for review and final approval. The approval process may take several months as the unit budgets are combined to determine the overall budget for the health care organization.
- Health care economics is grounded in past values and culture. Nearly 150 years ago, Florence Nightingale recognized that the

resources being used to care for sick people ought to be tracked and analyzed to improve clinical and business outcomes.

- Contemporary health care is characterized as a business struggling to balance cost and quality.
- In the United States, multiple programs exist to pay for health care.
- Industrialized countries around the world offer tax-supported socialized health care to every citizen through centralized or decentralized programs at about half of the U.S. per capita cost.
- The ability to track and manage both cost and quality is critical to achieve the organization's economic and quality goals.

 KEY TERMS

accounting	mission
budget	operational budget
capital budget	payer
construction budget	profit
cost centers	revenue
dashboard	socialized health care
direct expenses	strategic plan
economics	variable costs
fixed costs	variance
indirect expenses	vision
margin	

 REVIEW QUESTIONS

1. An operational budget accounts for
   A. the purchase of minor and major equipment.
   B. construction and renovation.
   C. income and expenses associated with daily activity within an organization.
   D. applications for new technology.

2. Cost centers are used to
   A. develop historical and demographic information.

B. track expense line items.
C. plan for strategic growth and movement.
D. track financial data within a department or unit.

3. Economics is the study of
   A. the cost:quality interface.
   B. cost accounting.
   C. the cost of doing business.
   D. how to manage scarcity of resources.

4. Profit is synonymous with
   A. dividends.
   B. billing privileges.
   C. margin.
   D. certificate of need.

REVIEW ACTIVITIES

1. Look around your clinical agency. Do you see any dashboards? What do they reveal about your agency?

2. Using the tables in this chapter as a guideline, construct a competitive analysis of one or more of the agencies in your community.

3. Interview the nurse manager of a health care organization to gain an understanding of how various costs are managed. Use the following questions to guide the interview:

   What method is used to measure nursing cost?

   What level of confidence does Fiscal Services have in its accuracy and why?

   How are contracts with various insurers such as Medicare, Medicaid, Blue Cross and managed care discounted?

   What percentage of profit did the organization make last year and how was it allocated? How typical was this?

   Which therapists' services are billed directly?

EXPLORING THE WEB

- Go to the site for the Joint Commission on Accreditation of Healthcare Organizations at *http://www.jcaho.org*. What information did you find there?

- Review the site for the American Organization of Nurse Executives, *http://www. aone.org.* Was the information helpful?

- Review the site for nurse sensitive outcomes at *http://www.nursingworld.org.* Search for nurse sensitive outcomes at this site.

- Review these sites for helpful information. What did you find there?

   Healthcare Financial Management Association: *http://www.hfma.org*

   American College of Healthcare Executives: *http://www.ache.org.*

   The Advisory Board Company: *http://www.advisoryboardcompany.com*

   Centers for Medicare and Medicaid Services: *http://www.cms.hhs.gov*

   Agency for Healthcare Research and Quality: *http://www.ahcpr.gov*

   Food and Drug Administration: *http://www.fda.gov*

- Go to the site for the Centers for Medicare & Medicaid Services: *cms.hhs.gov*

- Search an alternate government bureau site. What does the Bureau of Labor Statistics offer at *http://www.bls.gov*

- Search the following Web sites for information of interest to nurses:
   http://www.florence-nightingale.co.uk
   http://www.aahn.org
   http://www.my.webmd.com
   http://www.medexplorer.com
   http://www.healthology.com
   http://www.medicarerights.org

REFERENCES

The Advisory Board Company (1998). *Reversing the flight of talent: Executive briefing.* Washington, DC: Nursing Executive Center.

Chang, C., Price, S., & Pfoutz, S. (2001). *Economics and nursing: Critical professional issues.* Philadelphia: F. A. Davis.

Chassin, M. R., & Galvin, R. W. (1998). The urgent need to improve health care quality. Institute of Medicine National Roundtable on Health Care Quality. *Journal of the American Medical Association, 280*(11), 1000–1005.

Christensen, C., Bohmer, R., & Kenagy, J. (2000, September/October). Will disruptive innovations cure health care? *Harvard Business Review,* 102–112, 199.

Elser, R., & Nipp, D. (2001). Worker designed culture change. *Nursing Economic$, 19*(4) 161–163, 175.

Finkler, S., & Kovner, C. (2000). *Financial management for nurse managers and executives* (2nd ed.). Philadelphia: Saunders.

Grohar-Murray, M. E., & DiCroce, H. R. (1997). *Leadership and management in nursing.* Stamford, CT: Appleton & Lange.

Kramer, M. (1990, June). Trends to watch at the magnet hospitals. *Nursing90,* 67–74.

McClure, M., Poulin, M., Sovie, M., & Wandelt, M. (1983). *Magnet hospitals. Attraction and retention of professional nurses.* Kansas City, MO: American Academy of Nursing.

Needleman, J., Buerhaus, P., Mattke, S., Stewart, M., Zelvinsky, K. (2001, February 28). *Nurse staffing and patient outcomes in hospitals* (Final Report). U.S. Dept. of Health & Human Services, Health Resources & Services Administration.

Nightingale, F. (1859). *Notes on hospitals; being two papers read before the National Association for the Promotion of Social Science, at Liverpool in October, 1858. With evidence given to the Royal Commissioners on the State of the Army in 1857* (2nd ed.). London: Parker.

Norton, D., & Kaplan, R. (2001). *The strategy-focused organization: How balanced scorecard companies thrive in the new business environment.* Boston: Harvard Business School Press.

Pantel, E. (2001). Why does healthcare cost so much? Retrieved April 2, 2002, from the Healthology Web site: http://www.healthology.com.

Savage, G., Hoelscher, M., & Walker, E. (1999). International health care: A comparison of the United States, Canada, and Western Europe. In L. Wolper (Ed.), *Health care administration: Planning, implementing, and managing organized delivery systems* (3rd ed). Gaithersburg, MD: Aspen.

SUGGESTED READINGS

Camp, R. C. (1989). *Benchmarking: The search for industry best practices that lead to superior performance.* Milwaukee, WI: ASQC Quality Press.

Carruth, A., Carruth, P., & Noto, E. (2000). Nurse managers flex their budgetary might. *Nursing Management, 31*(2), 16–17.

Christman, L. (2001). The future of the nursing profession. In E. Hein (Ed.), *Nursing issues in the 21st century: Perspectives from the literature.* Philadelphia: Lippincott.

Copeland, T. (2001, September/October). Cutting costs without drawing blood. *Harvard Business Review,* 155–156, 159–160, 162, 164.

DiJerome, L., Dunham-Taylor, J., Ash, K., & Brown, R. (1999). Evaluating cost center productivity. *Nursing Economic$, 117*(6), 334–340.

Finkler, S. (2001). *Budgeting concepts for nurse managers* (3rd ed.). Philadelphia: Saunders.

Hoppszallern, S. (2001, January). 2001 benchmarking guide. *Hospitals and Health Networks,* 43–50.

Iowa Intervention Project. (2001). Determining cost of nursing instrumentations: A beginning. *Nursing Economic$, 19*(4), 146–160.

Joint Commission on Accreditation of Healthcare Organizations. (2001). *Comprehensive accredi-*

tation manual for hospitals (CAMH): The official handbook. Oakbrook Terrace, IL: Author.

Jones, K. R. (1999). The capital budgeting process. *Seminars for Nurse Managers, 7*(2), 55–56.

Keeling, B. (2000). How to establish a position and hours budget. *Nursing Management, 31*(3), 26–27

McCullough, C. (2001). *Creating responsive solutions to healthcare change*. Indianapolis, IN: Sigma Theta Tau International.

Nosek, L. (1986). Explanation of hospital stay by nursing diagnoses, medical diagnoses, and social position. (Doctoral dissertation, Case Western Reserve University, 1986). *Dissertation Abstracts International, 47*(07B), 00215. (University Microfilms No. AAG8622844).

Robnett, M., & Schaub-Rimet, A. (1999). *Nursing administration; Managing patient care financial skills for department managers* (pp. 293–312). Stamford, CT: Appleton & Lange.

Sullivan, E. J., & Decker, P. (Eds.) (2000). *Effective leadership and management in nursing: Key skills in nursing management* (pp. 90–104). Menlo Park, CA: Addison Wesley.

Wolper, L. (1999). *Health care administration planning, implementing, and managing organized delivery systems* (3rd ed.). Gaithersburg, MD: Aspen.

CHAPTER 8

Performance and Quality Improvement

The best outcomes evaluation is likely to come from partnerships of technically proficient analysts and clinicians, each of whom is sensitive to and respectful of the contributions the other can bring. (Robert L. Kane, Professor of Public Health, University of Minnesota)

OBJECTIVES

Upon completion of this chapter, the reader should be able to:

1. Articulate major principles of performance and quality improvement, including customer identification; the need for participation at all levels; and a focus on improving the process, not criticizing individual performance.

2. Discuss the University of Colorado Model for Evidence-Based Practice.

3. Discuss the Model for Improvement and the FOCUS-PDCA Method.

4. Identify how data are utilized for performance and quality improvement (time series data, Pareto charts).

During report, the staff nurse tells you about a 60-year-old woman, Miss Kelly, who was admitted to the unit today with left hip and sciatic pain after a recent fall at home. You immediately begin to think she has a hip fracture. The staff nurse interrupts your thoughts and says, "Wait, there is more. This woman has a new diagnosis of breast cancer and has also developed a pleural effusion, which necessitated the insertion of a chest tube this morning. Her dyspnea has improved since this morning, and her pulse oximetry on 2 liters of oxygen via nasal cannula is 99%."

Miss Kelly has lymphedema of her right hand and arm, and the right breast mass is a very large, open, foul-smelling lesion that bleeds intermittently. She appears anxious and has indicated that she is uncomfortable and afraid to move. She has Tylenol with codeine ordered orally every 4 hours as needed for pain but has been very reluctant to use the medication because she thought it would alter her ability to think and make decisions regarding her care. Results of a bone scan and CT scan of the abdomen and pelvis indicate that she has further metastatic involvement of the left acetabulum. This could be the cause of her left hip pain—tumor replacing the bone. Although the CT scan does not reveal a fracture, Miss Kelly is at high risk for developing a pathological fracture.

Miss Kelly is single, has no children, and lives with her brother and five cats. She does not smoke or drink. She is a retired clerk for the state Department of Labor. She has been followed by a cardiologist for hypertension for several years. She would call for

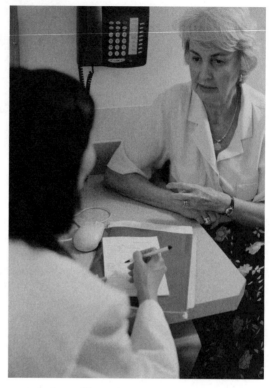

prescription refills and then cancel her appointments because she feared what the doctor would find or say.

What are your thoughts about how you will approach this patient?

What additional data do you need to develop a protocol of care to improve Miss Kelly's outcomes?

What priorities should be addressed to manage Miss Kelly's care?

Performance and quality improvement have been shown to be powerful tools to help make health care organizations more effective. Plsek (1993) notes that without strong, effective leadership and an infrastructure to support quality management, improvements may or may not happen, and they may quickly dissipate because of neglect and lack of integration with other activities within the organization. The improvement philosophies of quality experts such as Deming (1986) and Crosby (1989) also emphasize the importance of the commitment of management.

Deming's concepts of appreciating a system, understanding variation, and applying knowledge and psychology are fundamental improvement principles. Performance improvement is also described as an art that taps into creative, "out of the box" ideas. It is about systematically testing new ideas to improve customer care and outcomes. Health care customers are patients, families, staff, and so forth. This chapter discusses and provides examples of the application and implementation of performance and quality improvement principles in a health care setting. The use of evidence-based practice (EBP) is also illustrated.

SELECTED HISTORY OF QUALITY

Quality assurance (QA) emerged in health care in the 1950s, about the same time as hospital-accrediting organizations were founded (AMC Q Series, 1998). QA began as an inspection approach to ensure that health care institutions—mainly hospitals—maintained minimum standards of care. QA's methods consisted primarily of chart audits of various patient diagnoses and procedures. The method emphasized "doing it right," and did little to sustain change or proactively identify problems before they occurred. It did, however, encourage monitoring minimum standards of performance and improving performance when standards were not met.

Quality Health Care

Donabedian (1966) conceptualized a framework for quality (Bull, 1997). This framework is composed of the elements of structure, process, and outcome.

Structure, Process, Outcome

Using Donabedian's framework, a health care organization that wishes to develop quality will organize or structure itself for quality. Donabedian's framework has three elements: structure, process, and outcome.

Structure elements of quality lay a foundation for quality health care by identifying what structures must be in place in a health care system to deliver quality. Structure elements consist of such things as a well-constructed hos-

pital, quality patient care standards, quality staffing policies, environmental standards, and the like.

Process is the next element of the quality framework. Process elements of quality build on the structure elements and take quality a step further. Process elements identify what nursing and health care interventions must be in place to deliver quality. Process elements are such things as managing the health care process and utilizing clinical practice guidelines and standards for nursing and medical interventions—passing medications and the like.

Finally, an outcome element completes the quality framework. Outcome elements of quality are the end results of quality care. Outcome elements review the status of patients after health care has been delivered. Outcomes reflect the presence of structure and process elements of quality. Outcomes ask whether the patient is better as a result of health care. If a quality hospital (structure) and quality standards (process) are in place, patients should experience good quality health (outcome). See Table 8-1 for examples of structure, process, and outcome quality performance measures in three domains of activity: clinical care, financial management, and human resources management.

TOTAL QUALITY MANAGEMENT AND QUALITY AND PERFORMANCE IMPROVEMENT

Total quality management (TQM), also referred to as quality improvement (QI) and performance improvement (PI), began in the manufacturing industry with W. Edwards Deming and Joseph Juran in the 1950s. TQM, QI, and PI are terms that are frequently interchanged. For the purposes of this chapter, performance improvement (PI) will be referred to as a systematic process to improve outcomes based on customers' needs. This proactive approach emphasizes "doing the right thing" for customers, and

TABLE 8-1
EXAMPLES OF PERFORMANCE MEASURES BY CATEGORY

Domain of Activity

	Clinical Care	Financial Management	Human Resources Management
Structure	*Effectiveness* • Percent of active nurses and other practitioners who are certified • JCAHO accreditation • Number of filled positions • Presence of council for quality improvement planning • Magnet status of hospital	*Effectiveness* • Qualifications of administrators in finance and all hospital departments • Use of preadmission criteria • Presence of an integrated financial and clinical information system	*Effectiveness* • Ability to attract desired registered nurses and other health professionals • Size (or growth) of active physician staff • Salary and benefits compared to competitors • Quality of inhouse staff education • Clear policy on no staff or patient abuse, chain of command, reporting, and ethical issues
Process	*Effectiveness* • Rate of medication error • Rate of nosocomial infection • Rate of postsurgical wound infection • Rate of normal tissue removed *Productivity* • Ratio of total patient days to total full-time equivalent (FTE) nurses • Ratio of total admissions to total FTE staff	*Effectiveness* • Days in accounts receivable • Use of generic drugs and drug formulary • Market share *Productivity* • Ratio of collection to FTE financial staff • Ratio of total admissions to FTE in finance department • Ratio of new capital to fund-raising staff	*Effectiveness* • Grievances • Promotions • Organizational climate *Productivity* • Ratio of line staff to managers

(continues)

Table 8-1 *(continued)*

	Clinical Care	Financial Management	Human Resources Management
		Domain of Activity	
	Efficiency	*Efficiency*	*Efficiency*
	• Average cost per patient • Average cost per admission	• Cost per collection • Debt/equity ratio	• Cost of recruiting
Outcome	*Effectiveness*	*Effectiveness*	*Effectiveness*
	• Case-severity-adjusted mortality • Patient satisfaction • Patient functional health status • Incidence of nurse sensitive outcomes	• Return on assets • Operating margins • Size (or growth) of federal, state, or local grants for teaching and research • Bond rating	• Turnover rate • Absenteeism • Staff satisfaction

Adapted from Shortell, S. M., & Kaluzny A. D. (1997) *Essentials of health care management,* Clifton Park, NY: Delmar Learning.

the end result of this method is to satisfy customer needs. This approach was integrated into the health care industry in the 1980s (AMC Q Series, 1998). Movement into PI is an overall management approach. PI logic suggests that high quality could lead to a higher volume of use of the organization by patients and providers who have the flexibility to make choices about where they seek health care. Higher volume generally leads to higher profits which, in turn, may be directed toward improving programs and services, thus achieving higher quality, a very positive spiral that can result in the organization's thriving.

Increased quality > Increased volume > Increased profit > Enhanced programs/services > Increased quality

The obverse spiral is more likely when quality is shoddy, a very negative and potentially fatal spiral.

Decreased quality > Decreased volume > Decreased profit > Cutting corners > Decreased quality

General Principles of Performance Improvement

Performance improvement (PI) is a structured system for creating organization-wide participation and partnership in planning and implementing continuous improvement methods to understand and meet or exceed customer needs and expectations. PI principles include the following:

1. The priority is to benefit patients and all other internal and external customers.
2. Quality is achieved through the participation of everyone in the organization.
3. Improvement opportunities are developed by focusing on the work process used to achieve outcomes.
4. Decisions to change or improve a system or process are made based on data. Data are used for learning, not judgment.
5. Improvement of the quality of service is a continuous process.

Elements of Performance Improvement

Performance improvement is not about being perfect. First, it is about being better, doing things right the first time, and being better than the competition. This increases an organization's chances of survival during highly turbulent and competitive times.

Second, PI is about health care professionals seeing themselves as having customers. A customer is anyone who receives the output of a nurse's efforts. There are internal and external customers. An internal customer is anyone who

STOP AND THINK

Securing a profit might suggest that high quality is also secured because it facilitates purchase of state-of-the-art equipment and expert practitioners. Quality and profit do not necessarily go together. The Nosek-Androwich Profit:Quality (NAPQ) Matrix shown in Figure 8-1 models four possible relationships between profit and quality that may exist in a health care organization. Any organization can fit into any quadrant and a single organization may shift among quadrants from time to time in response to market forces. The challenge for the organization is to maintain existence in the high-profit, high-quality quadrant to be best positioned for clinical success and for business success, the mission of the organization. A common mission, consistent vision, collaboration, and constant vigilance to the elements of quality and profit by all employees and stakeholders together are keys to maintaining organizational positioning and achieving economic and quality success.

Into which quadrant of the NAPQ Matrix does a health care organization with which you are familiar fit? What kind of fiscal practices would you expect to find in each quadrant? What kind of clinical practices would you expect to find in each quadrant? How does patient choice influence the quadrant an organization occupies?

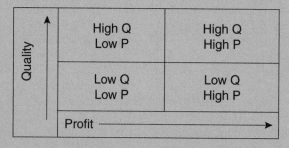

Figure 8-1 Nosek-Androwich Profit:Quality (NAPQ) Matrix from Nosek-Androwich, 2003, in Kelly-Heidenthal, Nursing Leadership and Management, Delmar.

works within the organization and receives the output of another employee. Internal customers include health care staff such as physicians, nurses, pharmacists, physical therapists, respiratory therapists, occupational therapists, pastoral caregivers, and so on. An external customer is anyone who is outside the organization and receives the output of the organization. The patients are external customers, but they are not the only external customers. Other external customers include private physicians, insurance payers, regulators such as the Department of Health, the Joint Commission on Accreditation of Healthcare Organizations (JCAHO), and the community you serve.

Third, PI directs health professionals to give their customers more than the basics so that customers will recommend and demand these services. This is achieved by proactively seizing opportunities to perform better, driving for quality consistently and continuously, and not waiting for a problem to be pointed out or for pressure from a competitor to improve. Improve-

ments are sustained over time when interdisciplinary teams collaborate and decisions about change are supported by data. A key in determining who participates in PI teams is including the point-of-service staff: the workers on the front line who do the direct care involved in the work process you are trying to change. They are the people who have the most knowledge of the work process so they can look for potential areas of improvement. There should be a clearly identified way for staff to suggest improvement opportunities that they see in their day-to-day work.

The primary benefits of adopting PI concepts and principles include discovering performance issues more quickly and efficiently by looking at every situation as an opportunity for improvement; involvement of staff in how the work is designed and carried out to improve staff satisfaction; and empowering staff to identify and implement change. Increasing the customer's perception that you care by designing health care work processes to meet the customer's needs, rather than the health care provider's, and

STOP AND THINK

On an orthopedic unit, when the original lengths of stay data by nursing unit were examined, one unit had a much shorter length of stay than the other. At first there was discussion about this variance and the idea emerged of just going to the floor with the longer length of stay and fixing things there. The group members decided that rather than approach the task from this limited perspective, they would study the care delivery process as a whole and determine whether there were steps they could take to improve the process before criticizing the staff on the floor with the longer length of stay. Several excellent opportunities for improvement were identified, for example, the need for preoperative home evaluation, increased physical therapy involvement, and shorter indwelling catheter use. All these areas contributed to the process improvement, and the outcome was that both units ended up reducing their lengths of stay. These opportunities would have been lost had the group members used the data only to say that one unit was doing a bad job. They needed to review the process as a whole to improve the length of stay on both units.

Describe a problem on a patient care unit with which you are familiar. What patient care process could be improved? Who would you ask to work on the improvements with you? How can you suggest ideas for PI to other staff without making them feel that the quality of their care is being criticized?

decreasing unnecessary costs from waste and rework, lost business, and not meeting regulations are also PI concepts. These PI concepts should be emphasized until they become work habits and part of an organization's daily operations.

USE OF AN EVIDENCE-BASED PRACTICE (EBP) MODEL IN PERFORMANCE IMPROVEMENT (PI)

Several EBP models are used in PI. The University of Colorado Hospital model is illustrated here. See full model in Chapter 2.

The University of Colorado Hospital Model

The University of Colorado Hospital model is an example of an evidence-based multidisciplinary practice model (Goode et al., 2000; Goode & Piedalue, 1999). This model presents a framework for thinking about how you use different sources of information to change or support your practice. The health care team or team member uses valid and current research from sources such as journals, conferences, and clinical experts as the basis for clinical decision making. The model depicts nine sources of evidence that are linked to the research core. This model provides a way for the nurse to organize information and data needed not only to care for a patient but also to evaluate the care provided. In other words, did this patient receive the best possible care not only that this institution can offer, but that is available in this world?

The elements of the University of Colorado's practice model can be applied to the case of Miss Kelly in the Opening Scenario of this chapter (Table 8-2). For example, to assess Miss Kelly's progress related to her diagnosis of breast cancer, it would be important to review evidence using institutional and national benchmarks comparing length of stay for Miss Kelly with that of other patients with breast cancer. **Benchmarking** is defined as the continuous process of measuring products, service, and practices against the toughest competitors or those customers recognized as industry leaders (Camp, 1994). The wound care regime related to nursing time and product use could be analyzed for quality and cost-effectiveness. How much time does it take for a nurse to complete a dressing? How much do the dressings, tape, and other supplies used for the dressing cost?

Pathophysiology would be analyzed by reviewing Miss Kelly's biopsy results, bone scan results, and CT scan results to rule out metastatic disease. These results could be discussed with a health care practitioner regarding implications related to the prognosis, treatment, and survival rates for breast cancer. A concurrent or ongoing review could be conducted using the Braden Scale for Predicting Pressure Sore Risk (Bergstrom, Braden, Laguzza, & Holman, 1987) and documenting the assessment score daily.

Data collected for quality improvement purposes could include information on the incidence and management of infection, bleeding, pressure ulcers, and pain. The pain and pressure ulcer guidelines from the Agency for Healthcare Research and Quality (AHRQ; formerly the Agency for Health Care Policy and Research) are examples of national standards that could be used to benchmark and manage cancer pain (AHCPR, 1994a), prevention of pressure ulcers (1992b), and treatment of pressure ulcers (1994b) for Miss Kelly. Research, literature, and the internet are reviewed for other sources of best practice. Infection control data could include a review of wound culture results and the use of appropriate institutional wound precautions. The nurse could discuss with Miss Kelly, document, and then implement Miss Kelly's wishes regarding advance directives. Utilization of clinical expertise could include consulting the acute care nurse practitioners (ACNPs) for input regarding wound, skin, and pain management initially and on an ongoing basis.

TABLE 8-2
PRACTICE APPLICATION TO ELEMENTS OF THE UNIVERSITY OF COLORADO HOSPITAL MODEL

Model Element	Application
Benchmarking data	Compare length of stay for Miss Kelly with that of other patients with breast cancer in this hospital and other hospitals nationally
Cost-effective analysis	Analyze cost-effectiveness of wound care regimens, including nursing time and use of actual products (e.g., hydrogel vs. normal saline dressings)
Pathophysiology	Review biopsy results/findings of testing for metastatic disease and implications
Retrospective/concurrent chart review	Assess changes in condition related to pressure ulcer development using the Braden Pressure Ulcer Risk Assessment Scale
Quality improvement and risk data	Review and analyze documentation regarding patient progress and risk assessment (e.g., infection, bleeding, pressure ulcer development); outcomes assessment (e.g., pain rating and dosage of narcotic administration)
International, national, and local standards	Assess effectiveness of care related to AHRQ guidelines for cancer pain and pressure ulcers
Infection control data	Review wound culture results and institute appropriate precautions and treatment
Patient preferences	Discuss, document, and implement patient's wishes regarding advance directives
Clinical expertise	Consult acute care nurse practitioner for wound, skin, and pain management

(By permission of University of Colorado Hospital Research Council, Denver, CO)

METHODOLOGIES FOR PERFORMANCE IMPROVEMENT

There are several models that outline methodologies for performance improvement. Two are reviewed here: the Model for Improvement and the FOCUS methodology. Improvement comes from the application of knowledge (Langley, Nolan, Nolan, Norman, & Provost, 1996). Thus, any approach to improvement must be based on building and applying knowledge.

The Model for Improvement

The Model for Improvement (Langley et al., 1966) (Figure 8-2) begins with these questions:

1. What are we trying to accomplish?

2. How will we know that a change is an improvement?

3. What changes can we make that will result in improvement?

These three questions provide the foundation for the Model for Improvement and will help focus the use of the Plan, Do, Study, Act (PDSA) Cycle (see Figure 8-3) to complete the Model for Improvement. We will apply the Model for Improvement to Miss Kelly, the patient in the Opening Scenario presented at the beginning of this chapter, in relation to pain. This process can also be applied to the patient's pressure ulcers and wound management.

Application of the Model for Improvement to Pain Management

Let's apply the Model for Improvement to Miss Kelly, the patient in the Opening Scenario.

1. *What are we trying to accomplish?* The overall objective is to reduce or alleviate Miss Kelly's pain, which may be related to a variety of physiological, psychosocial, and spiritual issues. Cancer pain may be related to the breast cancer compression of tissue and nerves, pressure from a pleural effusion, discomfort related to a chest tube, fear of diagnosis and prognosis, social isolation, and perceived lack of opportunity to participate in spiritual activities.

   The nurse can begin by asking Miss Kelly where her pain is and ask her to describe the quality and characteristics of

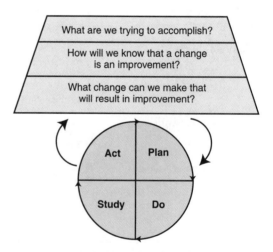

Figure 8-2 The Model for Improvement (From *A Practical Approach to Enhancing Organizational Performance* [p. 7], by G. J. Langley, K. M. Nolan, T. W. Nolan, C. L. Norman, and L. P. Provost, 1996, San Francisco: Jossey-Bass. Reprinted by permission of Jossey-Bass, Inc., a subsidiary of John Wiley & Sons, Inc.)

Figure 8-3 The PDSA Cycle (From *A Practical Approach to Enhancing Organizational Performance* [p. 3], by G. J. Langley, K. M. Nolan, T. W. Nolan, C. L. Norman, and L. P. Provost, 1996, San Francisco: Jossey-Bass. Reprinted by permission of Jossey-Bass, Inc., a subsidiary of John Wiley & Sons, Inc.)

her pain. Miss Kelly may express a range of sensations related to the different sources of her pain. The nurse will ask her to rate her pain on a scale from 0 to 10, with 0 meaning no pain and 10 meaning the highest pain possible. The nurse will then document the pain rating and the degree of relief that medications or other pain relief strategies provide and will also identify any alleviating or aggravating factors. The nurses in conjunction with the other members of the health care team will identify, implement, and document the best strategies that reduce, minimize, or alleviate her pain.

2. *How will we know that a change is an improvement?* Miss Kelly will state that her pain is decreased or relieved. Behaviors that may indicate decreased pain include her verbal or nonverbal expression of pain relief or improved comfort, her ability to reposition herself, and statements such as "I feel more rested," along with an improved mood.

3. *What change can we make that will result in improvement?* To standardize pain management for patients like Miss Kelly, the nursing staff created a protocol that includes a plan to use a trial pain management flow sheet to document the patient's reported pain status and pain interventions at various points in time.

Implementation of the PDSA Cycle

The PDSA Cycle can be individual or system focused. It can be used to solve a specific patient problem or to structure strategies to manage groups of patients with common problems. Based on our answers to the three questions, we will apply the PDSA Cycle as follows:

Planning Phase. Once the three Model for Improvement questions have helped staff identify what should be improved, the multidisciplinary staff (RN, MD, nurse practitioner, pharmacist, and so on) would develop a plan for improvement. The plan would include using the pain management flow sheet and implementing unit

standards for assessing, managing, evaluating, and documenting patient comfort.

Doing Phase. Nursing staff used the pain management flow sheet to collect data on Miss Kelly during her hospital stay. All nurses assigned to care for Miss Kelly were asked to complete the documentation tool. Data to be collected would include the patient's pain rating, her nonverbal behaviors, level of consciousness, respiratory rate, side effects, activity, nonpharmacological therapies, pharmacological interventions, and patient response to interventions and teaching.

Studying Phase. Data were collected for a period of 2 weeks. The nurses on the unit met and reviewed the documentation. Several improvements and issues were identified. Documentation of pain assessment and pain parameters had been completed 66% of the time during the 2-week period. Staff nurses reported that they referred to the pain management flow sheet when giving report to the doctor about Miss Kelly's pain status. Pain parameters commonly not documented included assessment and documentation of side effects, activity, and alternate therapy such as nonpharmacological interventions.

Acting Phase. After a meeting with the nurse manager, clinical nurse specialist, doctor, pharmacist, staff nurse, and other health care staff to discuss the findings, the staff agreed to continue to test the new pain management interventions and flow sheet for 4 months on all patients admitted to the oncology unit. This next step in the improvement process reflects the use of additional multiple PDSA cycles (Figure 8-4) to improve not only Miss Kelly's outcomes but also to improve the total care delivery system.

Multiple Uses of the PDSA Cycle

Multiple PDSA cycles were used to improve care, not just for Miss Kelly but for all patients.

Planning Phase. The inpatient oncology staff agreed to collect data for 4 months using the

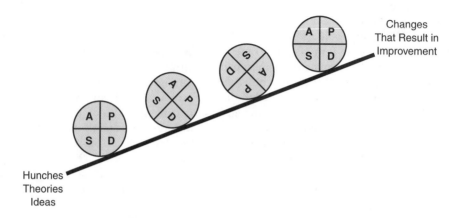

Figure 8-4 Use of Multiple PDSA Cycles (From *A Practical Approach to Enhancing Organizational Performance* [p. 5], by G. J. Langley, K. M. Nolan, T. W. Nolan, C. L. Norman, and L. P. Provost, 1996, San Francisco: Jossey-Bass. Reprinted by permission of Jossey-Bass, Inc., a subsidiary of John Wiley & Sons, Inc.)

pain management flow sheet on Miss Kelly and all new patients admitted to the oncology unit. A start date and stop date for the pilot study were identified. The pilot study also included a plan to orient the staff to the purpose, development, and procedures for using the tool and pain management standards. A plan was also developed to orient the pharmacist and all staff.

Doing Phase. All nursing staff working on the inpatient oncology unit attended an inservice reviewing the pain standards and the purpose, development, and procedures for using the pain management flow sheet. Once all the staff had completed the orientation, the data collection period was implemented. The pharmacist and practitioners were oriented individually by the clinical nurse specialists. Data were collected by the nurses for a period of 4 months on all patients admitted to the oncology unit.

Studying Phase. Pain management was reviewed on an ongoing basis and documentation practices were reviewed after 4 months. Documentation of pain assessment was completed on 78% of all patients' charts on admis-

sion to the inpatient unit, 67% were completed 24 hours after admission, and 50% were completed 48 hours after admission. The majority of the unit's nurses agreed that they were using the pain management flow sheet as a basis for their report to the practitioners regarding the patient's pain status. The pharmacist and the practitioners reported that they did review the pain management flow sheet approximately 50% of the time, but they most often relied on the staff to verbally share with them the information to improve the patient's pain status.

Acting Phase. A protocol for pain assessment, management, evaluation, and documentation was developed and integrated with the pain management flow sheet. Eventually, this process was published in the oncology literature (Jadlos, Kelman, Marra, & Lanoue, 1996).

This example using the Model for Improvement provides a framework to think about how to apply knowledge and increase the ability to make changes in individual patient care, ultimately resulting in improvement for many patients. This model for improvement can also be used to focus on other aspects of Miss Kelly's care.

The FOCUS Methodology

The FOCUS methodology describes in a step-wise process how to move through the improvement process (Figure 8-5).

F: Focus on an improvement idea. This step asks the question, "What is the problem?" During this phase, an improvement opportunity is articulated and data are obtained to support the hypothesis that an opportunity for improvement exists.

O: Organize a team that knows the process. This means identifying a group of staff members who are direct participants in the process to be examined—the point-of-service staff. A team leader is identified who will appoint team members.

C: Clarify what is happening in the current process. A flow diagram (see Figure 8-6) is very helpful for this.

U: Understand the degree of change needed. In this stage, the team reviews what it knows and enhances its knowledge by reviewing the literature, available data, and competitive benchmarks. How are other health care organizations doing the process?

S: Select a solution for improvement. The team can brainstorm and then choose the best solution. It can then use the PDSA Cycle to test

this solution. An implementation plan should be used to track progress and the steps required. This implementation plan can be in the form of a work plan or Gantt chart. This is a chart in the form of a table that identifies what activity is to be completed, who is responsible for it, and when is it going to be done. (See sample in Figure 8-7.) It outlines the steps needed to implement the change.

OTHER PERFORMANCE IMPROVEMENT STRATEGIES

Some other improvement strategies identified at the organizational level involve identifying opportunities for system changes following sentinel event review, using a balanced scorecard, and using a storyboard.

Sentinel Event Review

An adverse sentinel event is an unexpected occurrence involving death or serious physical or psychological injury to a patient (Joint Commission on Accreditation of Healthcare Organizations, 1998). Events are called sentinel because

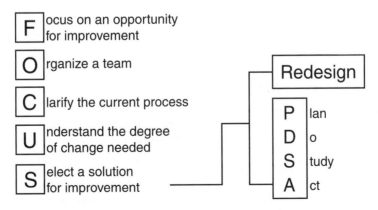

Figure 8-5 FOCUS Method (Adapted from Albany Medical Center, Albany, NY)

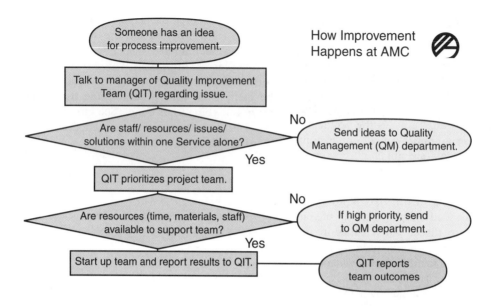

Figure 8-6 Flow Diagram—How Improvement Happens (Courtesy of Albany Medical Center, Albany, NY)

they require immediate investigation. During analysis of these sentinel events, opportunities for improving the system will arise and should be taken advantage of. Linkage of sentinel event review to the organization's performance improvement system will identify strategies for prevention of future sentinel events. An example of a sentinel event is surgery performed on the wrong extremity of a patient. Reviewing the surgical process and developing a system to mark the appropriate site is an example of a performance improvement to prevent future harmful occurrences.

Balanced Scorecard

To ensure value in care, measurement of progress has to be balanced. Generally, four cardinal domains of outcomes are measured (Caldwell, 1998).

Such an approach allows those reviewing data to examine a balanced approach to care (see Figure 8-8). For example, patient outcomes and access are reflected in a patient's functional status and clinical status. Patient satisfaction and

cost balance this to illustrate value. Data can be arranged to create a balanced scorecard, in an approach that uses the organization's priorities as categories for indicators. For example, three priorities might be customer service, cost-effectiveness, and positive clinical outcomes. These priorities help sort out what should be measured to give a balanced view of whether a strategy is working. Indicators are selected based on what they have in common, so that if a change occurs in the cost-effectiveness category, it will affect the data in another category. For example, if we decrease cost for orthopedic surgery, does that affect the customer's satisfaction positively or negatively? If we decrease the length of stay for these patients, does it increase or decrease complication rates? Once indicators are selected, data are tracked over time at regular intervals (every month or every quarter, for example). From the control charts on this orthopedic unit, you can see that the total hip pathway length of stay increased and then decreased. The satisfaction scores remained at around 90%, so even though the length of stay decreased, the satisfaction did not deteriorate. The ratio of complica-

Bed Access Improvement Team
Phase 2 Work Plan: Transition to Daily Management and Evaluation

Activity	Responsible Party	8/03	9/03	10/03	11/03	12/03
1.0 Modify the Team						
1.1 Identify Phase 2 tasks to be completed	Team	■				
1.2 Review & Modify Team Composition/membership	Team	■				
1.3 Develop Work Plan	Planning Team	■				
1.4 Review Work Plan with Team	Myers/Nolan		■			
2.0 Review/Modify Ideal Design						
2.1 Identify Modifications/Opportunities for Additional Change	Team			■		
2.2 Revise Ideal Flow Chart	Team					
3.0 Modify Structure & Supports: People/Forms Needed						
3.1 Revise Process Management Structure	Triage Management Subgroup				■	
• Modify job descriptions—triage Manager and Admitting Coordinator						
3.2 Assess Communication Needed with Nursing Units	Team				■	
4.0 Draft/Standardize Tasks						
4.1 Draft/Standardize Tasks					■	
5.0 Transition to Daily Operations, Develop Data Collection Process, Evaluate, Monitor						
5.1 Evaluate Bed Access Simulation	Team					■
• Review ED & PACU data						
• Identify accomplishments and opportunities of structure and ideal process						
5.2 Develop Plan to Transition Process and Structure to Daily Operations	Planning Team					■
5.3 Develop Data Collection Process	Planning Team					■
5.4 Evaluate Process & Structure (milestone meeting)	Team					■
5.5 Identify Subgroup of Pt Care Delivery System QIT to Monitor Progress	Team					■

Figure 8-7 Gantt Chart/Work Plan (Courtesy of Albany Medical Center, Albany, NY)

tions went down; the average number of physical therapy visits varied and then went up. This reporting mechanism offers a balanced view.

The balanced scorecard guides the development of a unit-based performance improvement plan (see Figure 8-9), and provides a tool with which to present the outcomes of performance improvement in the succinct visual format of an executive summary.

Storyboard: How to Share Your Story

Performance improvement teams share their work with others using a storyboard. The storyboard usually takes the major steps in the improvement methodology and visually outlines the progress in each step. The storyboard can be displayed in a high-traffic area of the organization to inform other staff of the QI efforts under way. Storyboarding can be done when an improvement process is complete, or used during the process to communicate information.

USING DATA

Several different types of charts are used to examine data in QI efforts. These include time series charts, Pareto charts, histograms, flowcharts, Ishikawa fishbone (root cause) diagrams, pie charts, and check sheets See Figure 8-10 and Figure 8-11. A full discussion of these tools is outside the scope of this chapter.

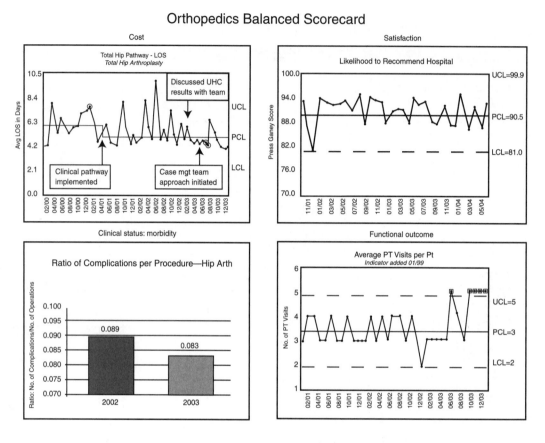

Figure 8-8 Orthopedic Balanced Scorecard (Courtesy of Albany Medical Center, Albany, NY)

ORGANIZATIONAL STRUCTURE FOR PI

Figure 8-12 is an organizational chart that shows a structure for quality improvement. Note that it includes staff from the board level to staff on individual quality improvement teams (QITs). Communicating priorities at all levels in the organization is key. Staff members must realize how their day-to-day work influences the accomplishment of strategic goals. Mission, vision, and value statements help accomplish this clarity of focus. This is discussed more in another chapter.

2000 PERFORMANCE IMPROVEMENT PLAN

As part of Bassett's commitment to quality, the Surgical Unit will strive to improve performance through a cycle of planning, process design, performance measurement, assessment and improvement. There will be ongoing assessment of important aspects of care and service and correction of identified problems. Problem identification and solution will be carried out using a systematic intra- and interdepartmental approach organized around patient flow or other key functions, and in concert with the approved visions and strategies of the organization. Priorities for improvement will include high risk, high volume and problem-prone procedures.

The Surgical Unit will:

- promote the Plan-Do-Check-Act methodology for all performance improvement activities
- provide staff education and training on integrated quality and cost improvement
- collect data to support objective assessment of processes and contribute to problem resolution

In identifying important aspects of care and service, the Surgical Unit will select performance measures in the following operational categories:

A. Clinical Quality
1. Patient safety

- Patient falls
- Indicator: # of patient falls per month/# of patient days with upper control limits set by the research department based on statistical deviation

- Medication and IV errors
- Indicator: # of patient IV/medication errors per month/# of patient days with upper control limits set by the research department based on statistical deviation

- Restraint use
- Indicator: % of compliance with policy for use of restraints and overall rate of restraint use

2. Pressure ulcer prevention
- Indicator: Rates of occurrence-quarterly tracking report

3. Surveillance, prevention and control of infection
- Indicator: Infection control statistical report of wound and catheter associated infections
- Indicator: Quarterly monitoring of compliance with standards for Acid Fast Bacilli (AFB) room use; evidence of staff validation in AFB practice

4. Employee safety
- Injuries resulting from
- Back and lifting-related injuries
- Morbidly obese patients
- Orthopedic patients
- Indicators: # of injuries sustained by employees and any resultant workmen's compensation (Human Resources quarterly report)
- 100% competency validation in lifting techniques and back injury prevention
- Respiratory fit testing
- Indicator: competency record of each employee

5. Documentation by exception
Indicators:
- 100% validation of RN/LPN staff
- Monthly chart audit (10% average daily census or 20 charts) meeting compliance with established standards

B. Access:
- Maintenance of the 30 minute standard for bed assignment of ED admissions
- Indicator: Quarterly review of ED tracking record

C. Service:
Patient Satisfaction
Indicator: Patient Satisfaction Survey: 90% or above response to, "Would return", and "Would recommend"

D. Cost:
- Nursing staff productivity will remain at 110% of target of 8.5 worked hours per adjusted patient day within a maximum variance range of 10%

For each of the above performance measures, this performance improvement plan will:

- address the highest priority improvement issues
- require data collection according to the structure, procedure and frequency defined
- document a baseline for performance
- demonstrate internal comparisons trended over time
- demonstrate external benchmark comparisons trended over time
- document areas identified for improvement
- demonstrate that changes have been made to address improvement
- demonstrate evaluation of these changes; document that improvement has occurred or, if not, that a different approach has been taken to address the issue

The Inpatient Surgical Unit will submit biannual status reports to the Bassett Improvement Council (BIC) through the Medical Surgical Quality Improvement Council (MSQIC).

I

Approved by:_____**Date:**_____

(Chief or Vice President)

Figure 8-9 Inpatient Surgical Unit, 2000 Performance Improvement Plan (Courtesy Patricia Roesch, BS, RN, Bassett Healthcare)

REAL WORLD INTERVIEW

We have developed a nursing practice quality scorecard. The scorecard is a tool to display data on our three organizational priorities: mission, customer orientation, and cost-effectiveness. By looking at measures in all three arenas, we can see how we are doing in these areas. We also can see if changes made in one arena positively or negatively affect the other measures. To look at nursing's mission for nursing practice, we track and trend several of the American Nurses Association national indicators. We track medication errors, patient falls, restraints, nosocomial pressure ulcers, and urinary tract infections. For customer satisfaction, we measure overall satisfaction with nursing care provided and how well patients' pain was controlled. For cost-effectiveness, we track nursing hours per patient day. All of these measures are tracked and trended on control charts every 3 months. The specific data is trended, and measures that are greater than 2 standard deviations of the target are identified as potential points to be reviewed for identification of opportunities for improvement.

One of the areas we chose to target for improvement was medication errors. It became evident that the most prominent reason for medication errors was delayed and omitted medications. Further investigation proved that the procedures for obtaining medications were unclear and outdated. We have written new procedures to specify responsibilities of the nursing staff and the pharmacy staff. We are now monitoring our rate of medication errors to see if our changes have made any improvement in the error rate.

Another example of use of the scorecard was in review of our pressure ulcer rate. We found there was an increase in the incidence of pressure ulcers in October 2000.

In review of causes, we found that the reporting system had been revised to include all stages of skin breakdown. Since the reporting change, we have seen an increase in the number of pressure ulcers reported. This is a positive change as we now have accurate data on which to target our improvement efforts.

Lessons that we have learned in the development of the scorecard is that we needed to set improvement targets earlier in the process to push the search for opportunities for improvement. We also learned that many of these measures are not well defined and therefore benchmarking to other organizations is difficult. We continue to strive for further improvement and utilize the scorecard to measure our success and look for opportunities for improvement. Reviewing nursing outcome data for the entire nursing division has been a powerful tool to ensure that care provided is meeting expected outcomes, and it allows us to benchmark our outcomes to other organizations.

Louann Villani, RN, BSN
Nursing Quality Specialist

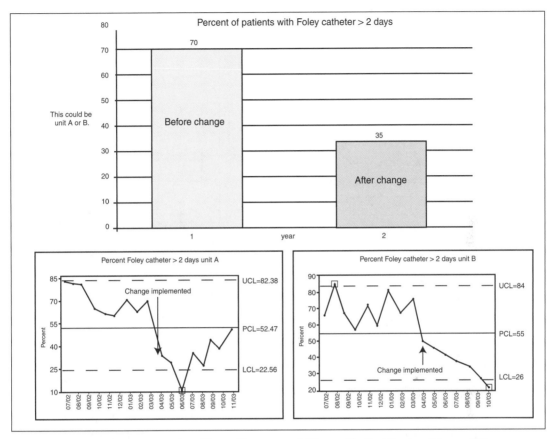

Figure 8-10 Time Series versus Bar Charts (Courtesy of Albany Medical Center, Albany, NY)

CASE STUDY 8-1

A group that was developing a clinical pathway for the care of patients with acute myocardial infarction noted evidence showing that these patients should receive acetylsalicylic acid (ASA) on admission. The research in this area was very clear, and most practitioners believed this was being done. When a chart audit was performed to determine whether this was, in fact, the practice on the unit, it was discovered that only 48% of the patients were receiving ASA within 8 hours of admission. The team added this to the clinical pathway. After this was implemented, 85% of the patients received ASA within the first 8 hours of admission.

What clinical practices do you see on your clinical unit that are based on an evidence-based clinical pathway? How can you participate in improving the care of more patients using evidence-based clinical pathways? Who should be involved in these efforts?

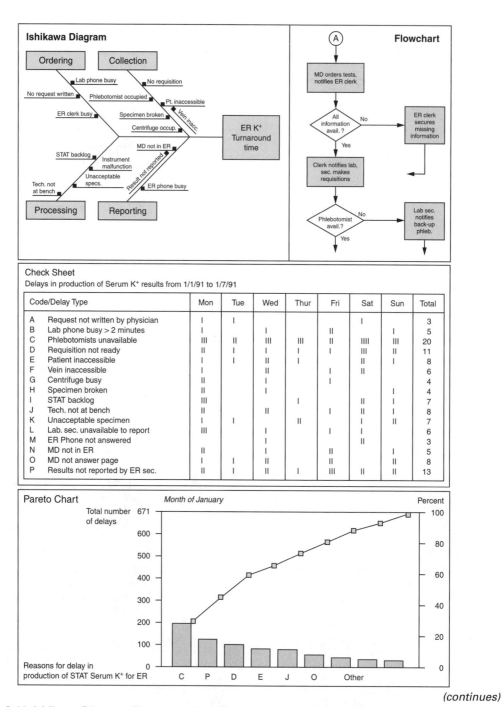

Ishikawa Diagram

Ordering · Collection
- Lab phone busy
- No request written
- No requisition
- ER clerk busy
- Phlebotomist occupied
- Pt. inaccessible
- Specimen broken
- Vein inacc.
- Centrifuge occup.

ER K⁺ Turnaround time

- MD not in ER
- STAT backlog
- Instrument malfunction
- Result not reported
- Tech. not at bench
- Unacceptable specs.
- ER phone busy

Processing · Reporting

Flowchart

A → MD orders tests, notifies ER clerk → All information avail.? — No → ER clerk secures missing information

Yes → Clerk notifies lab, sec. makes requisitions → Phlebotomist avail.? — No → Lab sec. notifies back-up phleb.

Yes ↓

Check Sheet

Delays in production of Serum K⁺ results from 1/1/91 to 1/7/91

Code/Delay Type	Mon	Tue	Wed	Thur	Fri	Sat	Sun	Total
A Request not written by physician	I	I				I		3
B Lab phone busy > 2 minutes	I		I		II		I	5
C Phlebotomists unavailable	III	II	III	III	II	IIII	III	20
D Requisition not ready	II	I	I	I	I	III	II	11
E Patient inaccessible	I	I	II	I		II	I	8
F Vein inaccessible	I		II		I	II		6
G Centrifuge busy	II		I		I			4
H Specimen broken	II		I				I	4
I STAT backlog	III			I		II	I	7
J Tech. not at bench	II		II		I	II	I	8
K Unacceptable specimen	I	I		II		I	II	7
L Lab. sec. unavailable to report	III		I		I		I	6
M ER Phone not answered			I			II		3
N MD not in ER	II		I		II		I	5
O MD not answer page	I	I	II		II		II	8
P Results not reported by ER sec.	II	I	II	I	III	II	II	13

Pareto Chart

Month of January

Total number of delays — 671

Reasons for delay in production of STAT Serum K⁺ for ER: C, P, D, E, J, O, Other

Percent scale: 0–100

(continues)

Figure 8-11 Ishikawa Diagram, Flowchart, Check Sheet, Pareto Chart, and Control Chart (Reprinted with permission from *Clinical Laboratory Management Review*, November/December 1991, 5[6]:448–462. ©Clinical Laboratory Management Association, Inc. All rights reserved)

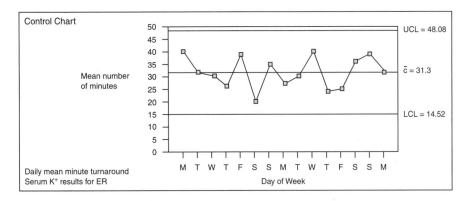

Figure 8-11 *(continued)*

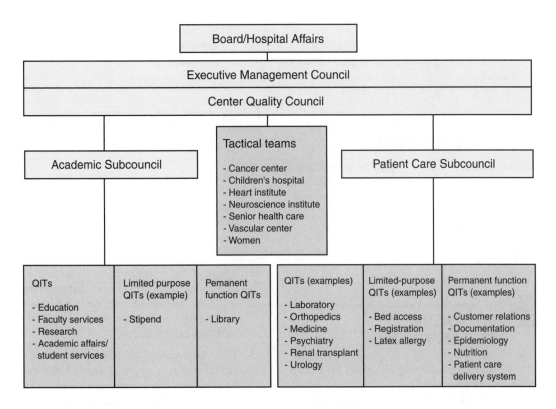

Figure 8-12 Structure for Quality Improvement (Courtesy of Albany Medical Center, Albany, NY)

KEY CONCEPTS

- Patient care needs should drive improvement opportunities.
- Decisions should be driven by data.
- Improvement initiatives should be linked to the organization's mission, vision, and values.
- Organizational goals and objectives should be communicated up and down the organization.
- There should be a balance in improvement goals focused on patient clinical and functional status, access, cost, and patient satisfaction outcomes.
- The University of Colorado Hospital model is an example of a multidisciplinary evidence-based practice model for using different sources of information to change or support your practice.
- The Model for Improvement and FOCUS-PDSA can be applied to a system or an individual.

KEY TERMS

benchmarking
outcome elements
  of quality
performance
  improvement
process elements
  of quality

quality assurance
sentinel event
structure elements
  of quality

REVIEW QUESTIONS

1. Which of the following describes the benchmarking process?
   A. Reviewing your own unit's data for opportunities
   B. Collecting data on an individual patient
   C. Reviewing data in the literature
   D. Comparing your data to that of other organizations to identify opportunities

2. Identifying opportunities in the health care arena is the responsibility of which group?
   A. Administration
   B. Practitioners
   C. Patients
   D. Everyone

3. Following a sentinel event, which step would be initiated first?
   A. No action
   B. Corrective action of personnel
   C. Reporting to health department/root cause analysis
   D. Immediate investigation

4. What tool could be used to track a change in a process over time?
   A. Flowchart
   B. Histogram
   C. Time series chart
   D. Pie chart

REVIEW ACTIVITIES

1. Risk management, infection control practitioners, and a benchmark study have revealed that your unit's utilization of indwelling catheters is above average. Brainstorm reasons why this may be occurring. Creating a fishbone (root cause) diagram may help.

2. Think about your last clinical rotation experience. Identify one process that you believe could be improved and describe how you would begin improving the process. Use the FOCUS methodology.

3. The University of Colorado Hospital model is one example of an evidence-based multidisciplinary practice model. This model presents a framework for thinking about how you use different sources of information to change or support your practice. Select a situation from your clini-

cal practice and apply the model. For example, if you were caring for an elderly patient, admitted with a hip fracture sustained during a fall at home, what benchmarking data would you review to compare the patient's length of stay with that of other patient with fractured hips? What standards of care would be used? Are these institutional specific or do they also incorporate any specific outside organizations' guidelines?

EXPLORING THE WEB

- Use these sites for potential benchmark data:
University HealthSystem Consortium (UHC): http://www.uhc.org
Institute for Healthcare Improvement (IHI): http://www.ihi.org
- These sites are recommended for a team that is looking for evidence-based guidelines or research studies for a particular diagnosis:
National Guideline Clearinghouse: http://www.guideline.gov
Cochrane Library: http://www.cochrane.org
PubMed's Clinical Queries: http://www.ncbi.nlm.nih.gov
Evidence-Based Practice Internet Resources: http://www-hsl.mcmaster.ca
- The Web site for the Agency for Healthcare Research and Quality (AHRQ), formerly the Agency for Health Care Policy and Research (AHCPR), has a clinical information index page that lists evidence reports for topics such as swallowing disorders in stroke patients, evaluation of therapies for stable angina, and access to agency-supported guidelines (e.g., cancer pain, cardiac rehabilitation, pressure ulcers, and so on).
http://www.ahrq.gov
- Go to http://www.nursingworld.org and find the information about the Nursing

Information and Data Set Evaluation Center. Note the ANA Recognized Classification Systems listed.
- Check this source of quality information: http://www.leapfroggroup.org

REFERENCES

Agency for Health Care Policy and Research. (1992b). *Pressure ulcers in adults: Prediction and prevention* (Clinical Practice Guideline, Pub. No. 92-0047). Rockville, MD: Author.

Agency for Health Care Policy and Research. (1994a). *Management of cancer pain* (Clinical Practice Guideline Pub. No. 94-0592). Rockville, MD: Author.

Agency for Health Care Policy and Research. (1994b). *Treatment of pressure ulcers* (Clinical Practice Guideline, Pub. No. 95-0652). Rockville, MD: Author.

AMC Q series curriculum. (1998). Albany, NY: Albany Medical Center, Quality Management Department.

Bull, M. J. (1997). Lessons from the past: Visions for the future of quality care. In Meisenheimer, C. G., *Improving quality* (2nd ed.). Gaithersburg, MD: Aspen.

Bergstrom, N., Braden, B. J., Laguzza, A., & Holman, V. (1987). The Braden Scale for Predicting Pressure Sore Risk. *Nursing Research, 36*(4), 205–210.

Caldwell, C. (1998). *Handbook for managing change in health care.* Milwaukee, WI: ASQ Quality Press.

Camp, R. (1994). Benchmarking applied to healthcare. *The Joint Commission on Quality Improvement, 20,* 229–238.

Crosby, P. B. (1989). *Let's talk quality.* New York: McGraw-Hill.

Deming, W. E. (1986). *Out of the crisis.* Cambridge, MA: Center for Advanced Engineering Study.

Donabedian, A. (1966). Evaluating the quality of medical care. *Milbank Memorial Fund Quarterly, 44,* 194–196.

Goode, C. J., & Piedalue, F. (1999). Evidence-based clinical practice. *Journal of Nursing Administration, 29,* 15–21.

Goode, C. J., Tanaka, D. J., Krugman, M., O'Connor, P. A., Bailey, C., Deutchman, M., & Stolpman, N. M. (2000). Outcomes from use of an evidence-based practice guideline. *Nursing Economic$, 18,* 202–207.

Jadlos, M. A., Kelman, G. B., Marra, K., & Lanoue, A. (1996). A pain management documentation tool. *Oncology Nursing Forum, 23,* 1451–1454.

Joint Commission on Accreditation of Healthcare Organizations. (1998). *Comprehensive accreditation manual for hospitals* (p. AC-5). Oakbrook, IL: Joint Commission on Accreditation of Healthcare Organizations.

Kane, R. L. (1997). *Understanding health care outcomes research* (1st ed.). Gaithersburg, MD: Aspen.

Langley, G. J., Nolan, K. M., Nolan, T. W., Norman, C. L., & Provost, L. P. (1996) *The improvement guide: A practical approach to enhancing organizational performance.* San Francisco: Jossey-Bass.

Plsek, P. E. (1993). Tutorial: Quality improvement project models. *Quality Management in Health Care, 1*(2), 69–81.

SUGGESTED READINGS

Agency for Health Care Policy and Research. (1992a). *Acute pain management: Operative or medical procedures and trauma* (Clinical Practice Guideline, Pub. No. 92-0032). Rockville, MD: Author.

Agency for Health Care Policy and Research. (1999, July 13). *Clinical information: Clinical practice guidelines online.* Retrieved January 30, 2002, from http://www.ahcpr.gov.

American Nurses Association. (1995). *Nursing report card for acute care settings.* Washington, DC: American Nurses Publishing.

Benner, P. E., Hooper-Kyriakidis, P., Hooper, P. L., Stannard, D., & Eoyang, T., (1998). *Clinical wisdom and interventions in critical care: A thinking-in-action approach.* Philadelphia: Saunders.

Berwick, D., & Plsek, P. (1992). *Managing medical quality videotape series.* Woodbridge, NJ: Quality Visions.

Duffy, J. R. (2000, July–September). Cardiovascular outcomes initiative: Case studies in performance improvement. *Outcomes Management in Nursing Practice, 4*(3), 110–116.

Gift, R. G., & Mosel, D. (1994). *Benchmarking in health care: A collaborative approach.* Chicago: American Hospital Publishing.

Kelly-Heidenthal, P., & Heidenthal, P. R. (1995, March-April). Benchmarking. *Nursing Quality Connections, 4*(5), 4.

King, K. M., & Teo, K. K. (2000, August). Integrating clinical quality improvement strategies with nursing research. *Western Journal of Nursing Research, 22*(5), 596–608.

Kitson, A. (2000, December). Towards evidence-based quality improvement: Perspectives from nursing practice. *International Journal of Quality in Health Care, 12*(6), 459–464.

Maleyeff, J., Kaminsky, F. C., Jubinville, A., & Fenn, C. (2001, July-August). A guide to using performance measurement systems for continuous improvement. *Journal of Healthcare Quality, 23*(4), 33–37.

Meisenheimer, C. G. (1997). *Improving quality: A guide to effective programs* (2nd ed.). Gaithersburg, MD: Aspen.

Sackett, D. L., Rosenberg, W. M., Gray, J. A., Haynes, R. B., & Richardson, W. S. (1996). Evidence based medicine: What it is and what it isn't. *British Medical Journal, 312*(7023), 71–72.

Wheeler, D. J. (1993). *Understanding variation: The key to managing chaos.* Knoxville, TN: SPC Press.

CHAPTER 9

Power

Significant progress has occurred over the years toward advancing nursing's presence, role, and influence in the development of health care policy. However, more nurses need to learn how to identify issues strategically; work with decision makers; understand who holds the power in the workplace, communities, state and federal level organizations; and understand who controls the resources for health care services. (Stephanie L. Ferguson, 2001)

OBJECTIVES

Upon completion of this chapter, the reader should be able to:

1. Define the concept of power.
2. Identify various sources of power, i.e., reward and coercion, legitimacy, expertise, reference or charisma, connection, and information.
3. Identify nurse sensitive patient outcomes.
4. Discuss the role of the American Nurses Association.
5. Discuss workplace advocacy, including collective bargaining.
6. Discuss professionalism.
7. Review a plan for developing power.

189

Nurse Pat, who just finished orientation, is working with a patient for whom a surgical consult has been written. The unit clerk and a long-time nurse on the unit remark that Dr. Killian, the physician doing the surgical consultation, should be named Dr. Killjoy because she humiliates new nurses to try to put them in their place. Based on previous reports by other nurses on the unit, Pat knows Dr. Killian has the reputation of being demeaning and inappropriately demanding when interacting with new nurses. Two hours later, Dr. Killian appears on the unit and asks to see the nurse who did the surgical admission sheet.

What would you do if you were Pat?

How would you approach Dr. Killian?

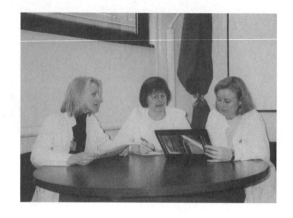

Effective nurses are powerful. They show objectivity, creativity, and knowledge throughout their practice and regardless of their work setting. They exert power by understanding the concept of power from multiple perspectives and using this understanding to change and improve care.

This chapter discusses power and how nursing power affects patient care.

DEFINITION OF POWER

Power has been defined in multiple ways, some not so positive. Commonly, **power** is described as the ability to create, get, and use resources to achieve one's goals. If the goals are self-determined, there is an implication of even greater power than if the goals are made by or with others. Power can be seen at various levels: personal, professional, and organizational. Power, regardless of level, comes from the ability to influence others or affect others' thinking or behavior.

SOURCES OF POWER

Most researchers agree that the sources of power are diverse and vary from one situation to another. They also agree that these **sources of power** are a combination of conscious and unconscious factors that allow an individual to influence others to do as the individual wants (Fisher & Koch, 1996). Articles and textbooks about nursing administration, educational leadership, and organizational management commonly include references to the work of Hersey, Blanchard, and Natemeyer (1979), an expansion of the power typology originally developed by French and Raven in 1959 (cited in Hersey, Blanchard, & Natemeyer, 1979). The typology helps nurses understand how different people perceive power and subsequently relate to others in the work setting and in attempts to achieve their goals. Power is described as having a basis in expertise, legitimacy, reference (charisma), reward and coercion, or connection. More recently, another power source—information—has been added to the typology (Wells, 1998). Generally speaking, nurses exert influence derived from one or a combination of these power sources. See Table 9-1.

Effective nurses use these sources of power and combine reference (charismatic) power and expert power from a legitimate power base, adding carefully measured portions of reward power and little or preferably no coercive power (Fisher & Koch, 1996). These leaders gather and use information in new and creative ways. They understand that power from all sources should

TABLE 9-1
PRINCIPLES FOR UNDERSTANDING AND USING DIFFERENT SOURCES OF POWER

Concept	How it works
Expertise (Fisher & Koch, 1996)	Power derived from the knowledge and skills nurses possess is referred to as expert power. The greater nurses' proficiency in performing their role, the greater their expert power. This power should be acknowledged by others to be most effective.
Legitimacy (Fisher & Koch, 1996)	Legitimate power is power derived from the position a nurse holds in a group, and it indicates the nurse's degree of authority. This legitimate power is based on such factors as licensure, academic degrees, certification, experience in the role, and title/position in the institution.
Reference (charisma) (Fisher & Koch, 1996)	Reference power is derived from the admiration, trust, and respect that people feel toward an individual, group, or organization. The referent person has the ability to inspire confidence. In any situation, strong referent leaders are considered charismatic and people of great vision, which may or may not be the reality.
Reward and coercion	The ability to reward or punish others as well as to create fear in others to influence them to change their behavior is commonly termed reward power and coercion power.
Connection	Both personal and professional relationships are part of a nurse's connections. People who are strongly connected to others, both personally and professionally, have enhanced resources, capacity for learning and information sharing, and increase their overall sphere of influence. Teamwork, collaboration, networking, and mentoring are some of the ways in which nurses can become more connected and, therefore, more powerful.
Information (Bower, 2000) (Wells, 1998)	Information power is power based on the information that any person can provide to the group. Authoritarian leaders attempt to control information. Charismatic leaders provide information that is seductive for many people. Information leaders provide a sense of stability with the use and synthesis of information. If one knows how to get it and what to do with it, the greatest power may be in information.

be a means to accomplish a goal instead of a goal in itself.

Use of Power

Many nursing authors support nurses' involvement in developing and using power in public policy and health care politics (Fagin, 1998; Williams, 1998; Mason & Leavitt, 1999; Milstead, 1999). Several other authors promote greater inclusion of the political process in nursing curricula (Brown, 1996; Gebbie, Wakefield, & Kerfoot, 2000; Jones, Jennings, Moritz, & Moss, 1997).

Nursing involvement in power and politics includes using power to improve the position of patients and nurses. Nurses use their power with colleagues, administrators, and subordinates. Nurses can also use power in the legal system, their professional nursing organizations, and the media to work to improve care. Nurses must grow in their ability to work with all of these groups. Many nurses believe that it is helpful to become active participants in some formal part of the nursing profession such as the American Nurses Association (ANA), the National League for Nursing (NLN), or one of the nursing specialty organizations.

Ultimately, health care will be defined and controlled by those wielding the most power. If nurses fail to exert political pressure on health policy makers, they will lose ground to others who are more politically active. It is unrealistic to believe that other stakeholders will take care of nursing while the competition for health care resources increases. It is not useful to complain about other nurses and members of the health care team in order to improve health care.

Nurses strengthen their power by taking ownership of their problems in serving patients. Leddy and Pepper (1998) stated, "When nurses blame others such as physicians, administrators, or politicians for the state of the health care delivery system, or constantly look to others for improvement of this system, they weaken their position and power base [p. 331]. . . . Historically, some stakeholders in health care have never supported nursing as a profession or acknowledged professional roles for nurses. Nurses, like other health care providers, must stand up and compete, negotiate, and collaborate with others who lobby for health care. See Table 9-2.

Nurse Sensitive Outcomes To be most politically effective, nurses must be able to clearly articulate at least four dimensions of nursing to any audience or stakeholder: what nursing is, what distinctive services nurses provide to consumers, how nursing benefits con-

STOP AND THINK

The Luck Factor, 2003, by R. Wiseman discusses research that illustrates luck as something that can be learned if one pays attention to four principles:

- Lucky people create, notice, and act on the chance opportunities in their life.
- Lucky people make successful decisions by using their intuition and gut feeling.
- Lucky people's expectations about the future help them fulfill their dreams and ambitions.
- Lucky people are able to transform their bad luck into good fortune.

Do you agree with Wiseman's findings? Can you use your "luck" to increase your power? Discuss.

TABLE 9-2
WASHINGTON'S MOST POWERFUL LOBBYING GROUPS

1. National Rifle Association
2. American Association of Retired Persons
3. National Federation of Independent Business
4. American Israel Public Affairs Committee
5. Association of Trial Lawyers
6. AFL-CIO
7. Chamber of Commerce
8. National Beer Wholesalers Association
9. National Association of Realtors
10. National Association of Manufacturers
11. National Association of Home Builders
12. American Medical Association
13. American Hospital Association
14. National Education Association
15. American Farm Bureau Federation

From "Fat & Happy in D.C.," *Fortune*, May 28, 2001, p. 95.

sumers, including improvement in nurse sensitive outcomes, and what nursing services cost in relation to other health care services. Although anecdotal stories and emotional appeals may be effective with certain audiences, it is far more powerful to present research-based evidence to support the political position of the nursing profession. Table 9-3 details responses to four essential dimensions of nursing.

American Nurses Association   The American Nurses Association (ANA) is a full-service professional organization representing the nation's entire registered nurse population. The ANA represents the 2.6 million registered nurses in the United States through its 54 constituent state and territorial associations. The ANA's mission is to work for the improvement of health standards and availability of health care services for all people, foster high standards for nursing, stimulate and promote the professional development of nurses, and advance their economic and general welfare (ANA, n.d.).

The ANA represents the interests of nurses in workplace advocacy and collective bargaining and in many other areas as well. The ANA advances the nursing profession by fostering high standards for nursing practice and lobbies Congress and regulatory agencies on health care issues affecting nurses and the general public. The ANA initiates many policies involving health care reform. It also publishes its position on issues ranging from whistle-blowing to patients' rights. See the ANA's Web site at http://www.nursingworld.org.

Workplace Advocacy.   In June 2000, the ANA created the Commission on Workplace Advocacy (WPA) to ensure that nurses who are not represented by collective bargaining have access to meaningful workplace advocacy strategies. The nine members of the commission are appointed by the ANA's board of directors. They represent constituent member associations that provide workplace advocacy programs or collective bargaining programs, or both, to their members.

TABLE 9-3
FOUR ESSENTIAL DIMENSIONS OF NURSING

1. *Nursing is* "attention to the full range of human experiences and responses to health and illness without restriction to a problem-focused orientation" (American Nurses Association, 1995, p. 6).

2. *Distinctive services nurses provide* include, but are not limited to, coordinating total patient care, completing ongoing health assessment, and advocating for quality care for patients. Nursing is perhaps the only profession whose focus is the patient's total health care.

3. *Benefits to consumers* include lower rates of nurse sensitive outcomes (defined in research study as death of a patient with one of the following life-threatening complications: pneumonia, shock, cardiac arrest, urinary tract infection, gastrointestinal bleeding, sepsis, or deep vein thrombosis, and "failure to rescue") (Needleman, Buerhaus, Mattke, Stewart, and Zelevinsky, 2002).

4. *Costs of nursing services* vary according to the care setting and role of the nurse. Primary care delivered by nurse practitioners and services provided by certified nurse midwives cost less than the same care delivered by physicians (Shi & Singh, 2001, pp. 138–139).

STOP AND THINK

As a beginning nurse, how does your nursing practice identify the four essential dimensions of nursing? How do you define nursing and how do you identify your distinctive services, benefits to consumers, and cost of your services? Have you ever witnessed a "failure to rescue" or witnessed a nurse "rescuing" a patient? Would the patient have lived if the nurse was not present?

Issues that are commonly the subject of workplace advocacy include poor wages, unsafe staffing, health and safety issues, mandatory overtime, poor quality of care, job security, and restructuring issues such as cross-training nurses for areas of specialty other than those in which they were hired to practice.

Collective Bargaining Agents. Different organizations act as **collective bargaining agents** for nurses. Some of these are the Teamsters Union, the General Service Employees Union, and the American Nurses Association. The largest collective bargaining agent for nurses is the United American Nurses AFL-CIO. The United Amer-

REAL WORLD INTERVIEW

I graduated from a diploma nursing program in 1962. I worked for 5 years and then was home for 15 years raising my children. I wanted to return to nursing and took a refresher course. It was very hard. So much had changed. I made it, though. I think that with the shortage of nurses now, hospitals would be smart to try to make it easier for nurses who have left nursing to return by offering reasonable, supportive refresher courses. I stayed at the hospital I went back to and later retired with just short of 19 years of service. When I retired, I was shocked to find out what my pension was going to be. It was $425 a month—this after almost 19 years of service. If it wasn't for my husband's pension, who, with a high school education, gets almost 10 times what I get, I would never be able to retire. My husband worked through a union. I understand that teachers who work through unions often get 75% of their salary when they retire. Some nurses who are single or divorced would like to retire but simply can't afford to do so. You keep hearing about the poor pay for teachers, and while I agree it should be better, at least they can afford to retire. Who thinks about nurses? It seems to me that more and more of the doctors' work is being given to the nurses and yet a survey I read said that the gap between the doctors' and nurses' pay is greater than what it was at the end of World War II. New nurses should start thinking about retirement benefits when they look for their first job. I know my 40 years as a nurse went fast.

Gerri Kane, RN

Retired Staff Nurse

ican Nurses (UAN) and its constituent member nurse associations, including state nurses associations, are a division of the American Nurses Association (ANA) that serves as a collective bargaining agent. The UAN represents approximately 400,000 nurses. The second largest collective bargaining agent for nurses is the National Union of Hospital and Health Care Employees. It represents 375,000 nurses and health care workers nationally. The third largest collective bargaining agent for nurses is the Service Employees International Union. It represents 110,000 nurses and health care workers nationally. Other nursing collective bargaining agents are part of the United Autoworkers of America and the United Steelworkers of America (Seltzer, 2001). See Table 9-4 for the pros and cons of collective bargaining.

PROFESSIONALISM

Experts in the social sciences are considered the authorities on what makes an occupation a profession. Although there is some variation in actual criteria, there is general agreement in several areas:

- Professional status is achieved when an occupation involves a unique practice that carries individual responsibility and is based on theoretical knowledge.
- The privilege to practice is granted only after the individual has completed a standardized program of highly specialized education and has demonstrated an ability to meet the standards for practice.
- The body of specialized knowledge is continually developed and evaluated through research.

TABLE 9-4
PROS AND CONS OF COLLECTIVE BARGAINING

Pros	Cons
The union contract guides standards.	There is reduced allowance for individuality.
Members are able to be a part of the decision-making process.	Other union members may outvote your decisions.
All union members and management must conform to the terms of the contract without exception.	All union members and management must conform to the terms of the contract without exception.
A process can be instituted to question a manager's authority if a member feels something was done unjustly. More people are involved in the process.	Disputes are not handled with an individual and management only; there is less room for personal judgment.
Union dues are required to make the union work for you.	Union dues must be paid even if individuals do not support unionization.
Unions give a collective voice for employees.	Employee may not agree with the collective voice.
Employees are able to voice concerns to management without fear of job security.	Unions may be perceived by some as not professional.

• The members are self-organizing and collectively assume the responsibility of establishing standards for education in practice. They continually evaluate the quality of service provided in order to protect the individual members and the public.

There has been a trend in recent years to call every occupation a profession. Have you heard of "professional baseball players" or "professional automobile mechanics"? There has been a tendency to confuse professionalism and profession. The term *professionalism* generally refers to an individual's commitment and dedication to the occupation. Professionalism often also refers to the attitude, appearance, and conduct of the individual. Whether an occupation is a profession requires more analysis. Figure 9-1 refers to some of the studies about the characteristics of a profession. Figure 9-2 lists some of the various values, behaviors, and attributes that may be exhibited by a "professional" (Mitchell and Grippando, 1993).

A Plan for Personal Power

There are three ways to imagine the future: (1) what is possible, (2) what is probable, and (3) what is preferred. A nurse who wants to experience a preferred future should think about what is happening to the nurse as a person and as a nurse, what possibilities the nurse faces as a person and as a nurse, and what the nurse is going to do about it. See Table 9-5.

Flexner, 1915	Bixler and Bixler, 1959
• Intellectual activities • Activities based on knowledge • Activities can be learned • Activities must be practical • Techniques are teachable • A strong organization exists • Altruism motivates the work	• Specialized body of knowledge • Growing body of knowledge • New knowledge used to improve education and practice • Education takes place in higher education institutions • Autonomous practice • Service above personal gain • Compensation through freedom of action, continuing professional growth, and economic security
Pavalko, 1971	**Public Law 93-360 on Collective Bargaining**
• Work based on systematic body of theory and abstract knowledge • Work has social value • Length of education required for specialization • Service to public • Autonomy • Commitment to profession • Group identity and subculture • Existence of a code of ethics	• Predominantly intellectual work • Varied work requirements • Requires discretion and judgment • Results cannot be standardized over time • Requires advanced instruction and study

Figure 9-1 Characteristics of a Profession

Professional Values:		
Caring	Freedom	Justice
Altruism	Esthetics	Truth
Equality	Human dignity	Ethical
Nonjudgmental		
Professional Behaviors and Attributes:		
Appearance Time-management skills Self-discipline Maintenance of licensure/certification Participation in institutional/community activities Participation in continuing education Political awareness Reading professional journals Participation in nursing research		Stress management Self-evaluation Initiative Motivation Creativity Effective communication

Figure 9-2 Possible Characteristics of a Professional

TABLE 9-5
A PLAN FOR DEVELOPING PERSONAL POWER

Background	A nurse can develop the power to discover what is important information and to use it to advantage, as well as to the advantage of patients.
Steps	Assess personal needs, patient and community needs, and professional needs. Get involved beyond direct patient care.
	Maintain and develop your expertise. Attend continuing education conferences, professional organizations, and community meetings.
	Read current journals and books in your clinical practice area. Consider returning to school for a higher degree. Review Internet sources of information. Participate in research.
	Network with others and ask questions. Listen to all sides of the story. Analyze the answers to your queries and set priorities for action. Get feedback from key people before taking action. Get their support.
	Make a plan with the information acquired. Know that there will always be more information to analyze.
	Take action and evaluate the outcomes. Recognize that choosing to make no decision is a decision and that information is never complete.
	Downplay rivalry and address conflict in a timely, constructive manner.
	Report, publicize, and lobby the group's political cause. Draw public attention to the needs of the patient. Work for health care regulations and guidelines that serve patient needs.
Information for providing care	Assess the patient's condition using relevant, objective measurements.
	Consult with other nurses, physicians, and other health care workers involved in the care of patients.
	Consult with significant others, friends, and members of the patient's family.
Information for becoming more effective in the work and community settings	Volunteer for committee assignments that will challenge you to learn and experience more than what is expected of you in a staff nurse role.
	Think about the following when involved with committees: • What is the committee trying to do? • Who are the leaders? • What specific information does the committee use to make decisions?

(continues)

Table 9-5 *(continued)*

	• How does the committee's work apply to my practice, my colleagues, my patients, my organizational unit, the organization, and the nursing profession as a whole? • How can you readily share information with others who will value it and use it to a good end?
Evaluation	Periodically reexamine your plans. Did you achieve your expected outcomes? If not, why? Were there staffing problems or patient crises? Were the activities that were necessary for outcome achievement carried out? What have you learned from this evaluation that you can apply to the future?

Adapted from Miller, T. (2003). In Kelly-Heidenthal, P. (2003) *Nursing Leadership & Management*

STOP AND THINK

You may use a Web site to contact your members of Congress. You may access these sites via

http://www.house.gov

or

http://www.senate.gov

or you may contact them through the U.S. Capitol at (202) 224-3121. How could you use these contact sites to improve care for your patients or advocate for an important health care issue?

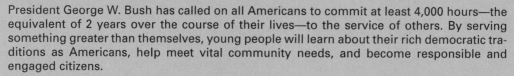

LITERATURE APPLICATION

Citation: Gebbie, K. M., Wakefield, M., & Kerfoot, K. (2000). Nursing and health policy. *Image: Journal of Nursing Scholarship, 32*(3), 307–314.

Discussion: The purpose of this qualitative study was to define ways nurses were or were not effectively involved in the development of health policy in the United States. The findings provide illustrations of world views that can be learned through nursing education and emphasize the importance of career decisions in moving nurses into policy roles. Participants in the study offered valuable suggestions about actions to strengthen the nurses' policy roles. Policy involvement is described as speaking for patients in arenas where patients' voices have been limited or absent. The authors discuss the need to change the way health care resources are allocated. They also discuss caring as a characteristic that distinguishes nurses in their policy roles from other stakeholders. The most important finding was that policy makers responded to nurses in the policy arenas when nurses presented their experiences regarding the determinants of health and illness.

Implications for Practice: "A nurse's knowledge of health issues and unmet needs, coupled with an understanding of what motivates people to get involved, is a potent combination in health policy. For example, a nurse can help policymakers understand the difference between regulations for physicians' decisions about home care and nurses' decisions in patients' homes" (p. 314). Nurses in practice and the patients they care for are directly affected by health care policy decisions. No one can represent nurses in practice to policy makers better than nurses themselves. Nurses in practice gain political power and help patients by offering experience-based perspectives of health and illness to policy makers. Neophyte nurses should not discount their need for understanding health care organizations, financing, and policy making.

CASE STUDY 9-1

President George W. Bush has called on all Americans to commit at least 4,000 hours—the equivalent of 2 years over the course of their lives—to the service of others. By serving something greater than themselves, young people will learn about their rich democratic traditions as Americans, help meet vital community needs, and become responsible and engaged citizens.

Sign up at *http://www.freedomcorps.gov*.

Are there any opportunities at this Web site in which you are interested? How can you exert your power as an individual and member of one of these organizations?

KEY CONCEPTS

- Effective nurses are powerful. They show objectivity, creativity, and knowledge throughout their practice and regardless of their work setting.
- Effective nurses have and exert power by understanding the concept of power from multiple perspectives, they then use this understanding to motivate others, accomplish organizational goals, and provide safe, competent care.
- Sources of power are reward and coercion, legitimacy, expertise, reference, information, and connection.
- Nurses who are unhappy in the workplace because of issues such as wages and unsafe staffing may want to consider workplace advocacy.
- The American Nurses Association is a full-service professional organization that represents the nation's entire registered nurse population. The ANA has a dual role of being a professional organization and a collective bargaining agent for nursing. The ANA is politically active and lobbies on issues affecting nursing and the general public.
- Nurse sensitive outcomes should be monitored in all health care settings.
- Nurses must articulate what nursing is, what distinctive services they provide, how these services benefit consumers, and how much these services cost in relation to other health care services.

 KEY TERMS

collective bargaining agent

power

sources of power

 REVIEW QUESTIONS

1. The most effective nurses use power
   A. in one primary way.
   B. to influence others or affect others' thinking or behavior.
   C. predominantly at an organizational level.
   D. only to gain the necessary resources to be a better nurse.

2. When a person fears another enough to act or behave differently than he would otherwise, the source of the other person's power is called
   A. coercive power.
   B. reward power.
   C. expert power.
   D. connection power.

3. What source of power has become increasingly important because of technological innovation in the past decade?
   A. Expert power
   B. Information power
   C. Connection power
   D. Legitimate power

4. A nurse's personal power can be enhanced by
   A. collaborating with colleagues on special projects outside the work setting.
   B. developing skills that do not apply directly to patient care.
   C. volunteering to serve on organizational committees with nonnurses.
   D. All of the above

 REVIEW ACTIVITIES

1. Identify a nursing leader. Observe them and note what type of power they use to meet their objectives.

2. Find out who your congresspeople are. Write or e-mail them and find out what health care legislation they are supporting.

EXPLORING THE WEB

- What site would you access to find out about the history of collective bargaining? *http://www.nlrb.gov*
- Which sites can you visit for information on nursing leaders, women, and nursing history? *http://members.tripod.com* and *http://www.members.aol.com*
- What site has a funny, not scholarly, synopsis of nursing power? *http://www.nursing-power.net*
- What site supports political power for patients? *http://www.healthcareform.net*
- Find two nurses identified on the following site: *http://dbois@distinguishedwomen. com*
- Identify some Web sites for consumer groups.
  http://www.aarp.org
  http://www.cchc-mn.org
  http://www.consumertips.com
  http://www.consumerwatchdog.org
  http://www.consumerunion.org
- Identify some sites for government bodies and health care agencies.
  U.S. Congress: *http://congress.org*
  U.S. Department of Health and Human Services: *http://hhs.gov*
- What sites would you recommend to someone inquiring about workplace advocacy, collective bargaining, and their state nurses association?
- Go to the site *http://www.nursingworld. org* and type in, workplace advocacy and collective bargaining and your state nursing association.

REFERENCES

American Nurses Association. (n.d.). Mission statement. Retrieved March 2, 2000, from http://www. nursingworld.org Charatan, F. (1999).

American Nurses Association. (1995). *Nursing's social policy statement.* Washington, DC: American Nurses Publishing.

Bower, F. L. (2000). *Nurses taking the lead:Personal qualities of effective leadership.* Philadelphia: Saunders.

Brown, L. D. (1996) *Health policy in the United States: Issues and options.* New York: the Ford Foundation.

DuBrin, A. J. (2000). *The active manager.* South Western College Publisher.

Fagin, C. (1998). Nursing research and the erosion of care. *Nursing Outlook, 46*(6), 259–261.

Fat & happy in D.C. (2001, May). *Fortune,* p. 95.

Ferguson, S. L. (2001). An activist looks at nursing's role in health policy development. *Journal of Obstetric, Gynoecologic, and Neonatal Nursing, 30*(5), 546–551.

Fisher, J. L., & Koch, J.V. (1996). *Presidential leadership: Making a difference.* Phoenix, AZ: American Council on Education and The Oryx Press.

Gebbie, K. M., Wakefield, M., & Kerfoot, K. (2000). Nursing and health policy. *Image: Journal of Nursing Scholarship, 32*(3), 307–314.

Hersey, P., Blanchard, K., & Natemeyer, W. (1979). Situational leadership, perception and impact of power. *Group and Organizational Studies, 4,* 418–428.

Jones, K., Jennings, B., Moritz, P., & Moss, M. (1997). Policy issues associated with analyzing outcomes of care. *Image: Journal of Nursing Scholarship, 29,* 261–268.

Leddy, S., & Pepper, J. M. (1998). *Conceptual bases of professional nursing* (4th ed.). Philadelphia: Lippincott.

Mason, D., & Leavitt, J. K. (1999). *Policy and politics in nursing and health care* (3rd ed.). Philadelphia: Saunders.

Milstead, J. A. (1999). *Health policy & politics: A nurse's guide.* Gaithersburg, MD: Aspen.

Mitchell, P. R., & Grippando, G. M. (1993). *Nursing perspectives and issues.* Clifton Park, NY: Delmar Learning.

Needleman, J., Buerhaus, P., Mattke, S., Stewart, M., & Zelevinsky, K. (2002). Nurse staffing levels or the quality of care in hospitals. *New England Journal of Medicine, 346*(22).

Seltzer, T. M. (2001). Collective bargaining: A wake-up call—part 2. *Nursing Management, 32*(4), 35–37, 48.

Shi, L., & Singh, D. A. (2001). *Delivering health care in America* (2nd ed.). Gaithersburg, MD: Aspen.

Wells, S. (1998). *Choosing the future: The power of strategic thinking.* Boston: Butterworth-Heinemann.

Williams, R. P. (1998). Nursing leaders' perceptions of quality nursing: An analysis from academe. *Nursing Outlook, 46*(6), 262–267.

Wiseman, R. (2003). *The luck factor 2003.* NY: Hyperion Miramax.

SUGGESTED READINGS

Baird, K. (2000). *Customer service in health care: A grassroots approach to creating a culture of service excellence.* San Francisco: Jossey-Bass.

Benner, P. E. (2000). *From novice to expert: Excellence and power in clinical nursing practice* (Commemorative edition). Upper Saddle River, NJ: Prentice Hall.

Birnbaum, G. (2001). Economic sequences of collective bargaining by physicians. *Journal of the American Medical Association, 15*, 1837–1839.

Bronder, E. (2001). Collective bargaining agreements. *American Journal of Nursing, 8*, 59–61.

Buerhaus, P. I., Staiger, D. O., & Auerbach, D. I. (2000). Implications of an aging registered nurse workforce. *Journal of the American Medical Association, 283*, 2948–2954.

Carson, W., & Franklin, P. (2001). Workplace advocacy. How can it help you? *American Journal of Nursing, 2*, 55–56.

Clifford, C. (2000). International politics and nursing education: Power and control. *Nursing Education Today, 1*, 4–9.

Disch, J. (2000, July-August). Nurse executive: Make the glue red. *Journal of Professional Nursing, 16*(4),189.

Dolan, B. (2001). *The power of nursing. Emergency Nurse, 10*, 1.

Fletcher, M. (2001). Advocacy 101. Nursing leadership: Unleashing the power. *Canadian Nurse, 4*, 14.

Foreman, S., Emmons, D., & Wozniak, G. (2001). Economic consequences of collective bargaining by physicians. *Journal of the American Medical Association, 15*, 1837–1839.

Government Technology (any recent issue). (Available free online at www.govtech.net or by writing to Government Technology at 100 Blue Ravine Road, Folsom, CA 95630.) Addresses the information age and the power of information.

Hanson, W. (2000). We shall be transformed. *e-gov: The Next Challenge*, available at www.govtech.net.

Jennings, C. P. (Ed.). (2000 to present). *Policy, Politics and Nursing Practice.* (Quarterly journal available through Sage Publications, Thousand Oaks, CA).

Jervis, L. L. (2002). Working in and around the 'chain of command': Power relations among nursing staff in an urban nursing home. *Nursing Inquiry, 1*, 12–23.

Kerfoot, K. (2000). On leadership—"Customerizing" in the new millennium. *MedSurg Nursing: The Journal of Adult Health, 9*(2), 97–99.

Kuokkanen, L., & Leino-Kilpi, H. (2002). Power and empowerment in nursing: Three theoretical approaches. *Journal of Advanced Nursing, 1*, 235–241.

Laschinger, H. K. S., & Wong, C. (1999). Staff nurse empowerment and collective accountability: Effect on perceived productivity and self-rated work effectiveness. *Nursing Economic$, 17*(6), 308–316.

McCullough, C., Tabone, S., & Brunell, M. L. (2000). Collective bargaining and workplace advocacy. Three states present their views. *Imprint, 1,* 29–33.

Ogren, K. E. (2001).The risk of not understanding nursing history. In E. C. Hein (Ed.), *Nursing issues in the 21st century: Perspectives from the literature* (pp. 3–9). Philadelphia: Lippincott.

O'Reilly, P. (2000). *Health care practitioners: An Ontario case study in policy making.* Toronto: University of Toronto Press.

Phan, C. (1999). Physician unionization: The impact on the medical profession. *Journal of Legal Medicine, 20*(1), 114–140.

Polston, M. D. (1999). Whistleblowing: Does the law protect you? *American Journal of Nursing, 99*(1, pt.1), 26–31.

Porter-O'Grady, T. (2001). Collective bargaining: The union as partner. *Nursing Management, 32*(6, pt. 1), 30–32.

Porter-O'Grady, T. (2001). Profound change: 21st century nursing. *Nursing Outlook, 4,* 182–186.

Rehtmeyer, C. M. (2000). Seeing change as an opportunity. In F. L. Bower (Ed.), *Nurses taking the lead: Personal qualities of effective leadership* (pp. 173–198). Philadelphia: Saunders.

Stafford, M. J., Taylor, J. W., Zimmerman, A., Henrick, A., Perry, K., & Lambke, M. R. (2000). Re: "A new version of collective bargaining." *Nursing Outlook, 2,* 92.

United American Nurses (UAN) mobilizes nurses on staffing crisis. (2001). *American Journal of Nursing, 101*(1), 65.

Young, S. W., Hayes, E., & Morin, K. (1995). Developing workplace advocacy behaviors. *Journal of Nursing Staff Development, 5,* 265–269.

CHAPTER 10

> Never doubt that a
> small group of
> thoughtful, commit-
> ted citizens can
> change the world;
> indeed, it's the only
> thing that ever has.
> (Margaret Mead)

Change and Conflict Resolution

OBJECTIVES

Upon completion of this chapter, the reader should be able to:

1. Discuss traditional theories of change.
2. Discuss chaos theory and the concept of the learning organization.
3. Apply strategies for implementation of change.
4. Identify common responses to change.
5. Discuss conflict.
6. Review conflict resolution.
7. Identify strategies to facilitate conflict resolution.

Mary has been a nursing assistant on a patient care unit for 2 years while completing her nursing degree. In that time, she has had two supervisors. In addition, she has had to work with three different methods of care delivery on her unit and has just experienced a corporate merger resulting in many changes in corporate culture and mission. Mary just completed her nursing degree and wonders whether she can make it through another change. She raises her head, looks in a mirror, and says to herself, "Of course I can. Change is inevitable and ever-present. The opportunities another change presents are exciting and pervasive." With that, Mary puts on a smile, walks out the office door, and greets her fellow workers.

What do you think Mary is feeling?

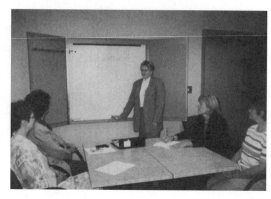

How can Mary begin to cope with another change?

In health care, is change always inevitable, pervasive, and exciting?

This chapter is designed to introduce the concepts of change and conflict resolutions. Change is an inevitable and frequent occurrence in health care and life. This chapter discusses change and conflict resolution. It will help the nurse gain understanding of these important concepts.

CHANGE

There are many definitions of change, and there are many types of change, for example, personal, professional, and organizational. For simplicity, change can be defined as "making something different from what it was" (Sullivan & Decker, 2001, p. 6). The outcome may be the same, but the actions performed to get to the outcome may be different.

Traditional Change Theories

The change theories illustrated here are Lewin's Force-Field Model (1951), Lippitt's Phases of Change (1958), Havelock's Six-Step Change Model (1973), and Rogers' Diffusion of Innovations Theory (1983). These are classic change theories and are based on Lewin's original model.

Lewin's model has three simple steps: unfreezing, moving to a new level, and refreezing. Unfreezing means that the current or old way of doing is thawed. People begin to be aware of the need for doing things differently, that change is needed for a specific reason. In the next step, the intervention or change is introduced and explained. The benefits and disadvantages are discussed, and the change—the move to a new level—is implemented. In the third step, refreezing occurs. This means that the new way of doing is incorporated into the routines or habits of the affected people. Although these steps sound simple, the process of change is, of course, more complicated (Lancaster, 1999).

The theories described in Table 10-1 are linear in nature, meaning they more or less proceed in an orderly manner from one step to the next. Unfortunately, health care organizations are not often this simple and often require more complex theories of change.

LITERATURE APPLICATION

Citation: Ingersoll, G. L., Kirsch, J. C., Merk, S. E., & Lightfoot, J. (2000, January). Relationship of organizational culture and readiness for change to employee commitment to the organization. *Journal of Nursing Administration, 30*(1), 11–20.

Discussion: This is a research article on employees' commitment to the organization and readiness for change. It discusses the relationship of organizational culture and readiness for change to employee commitment to the organization. The authors found that employee readiness for change often lagged behind the need for change within the organization.

Implications for Practice: Both employers and employees should recognize that change is inevitable. In these times of rapid health care change, employee readiness and commitment are important, but they cannot be the deciding factor in whether to change. The employer must change to keep up with the economic climate. The employee has a responsibility to change as necessary to help the employer maintain fiscal health.

Emerging Change Theories

There are some emerging theories of change that are much more complex in breadth and depth than the theories previously discussed. Some of these theories are chaos theory and learning organization theory.

Chaos Theory

Chaos theory (Gleick, 1987), often referred to as the science of complexity (Waldrop, 1992), states that the behavior of relatively simple physical systems is fundamentally unpredictable. Chaos theory's second insight is that patterns do lurk under the seemingly random behavior of these systems. These patterns enable scientists to determine within broad statistical parameters what a system is likely to do, not exactly what it is going to do. These systems are complex and self-organizing. These self-organizing complex adapting systems do not respond passively to events. They actively try to turn whatever happens to their advantage. These complex adaptive systems contain individual agents that network to (1) create self-managed highly organized behavior, (2) respond to feedback from the environment and fit their behavior accordingly, (3) learn from experience and incorporate that learning in the structure of the system, and (4) reap the advantages of specialization without being "stuck" in rigidity. Chaos theory suggests that the organism must be able to adapt quickly to change.

The Learning Organization

Peter Senge (1990) first described learning organization theory. Learning organizations demonstrate responsiveness and flexibility. Senge believes that because organizations are open systems, they could best respond to unpredictable changes in the environment by using a learning approach in their interactions and interdisciplinary workings with one another. The whole cannot function well without a part regardless of how small that part may seem. Senge, Kleiner, Roberts, Ross, and

TABLE 10-1
COMPARISON CHART OF TRADITIONAL CHANGE THEORIES

Theorist and Year	Lewin (1951)	Lippitt (1958)	Havelock (1973)	Rogers (1983)
Title of Model	Force-Field Model	Phases of Change	Six-Step Change Model	Diffusion of Innovations Theory
Steps in Model (The steps in the models are spaced to indicate their correlation to Lewin's model.)	1. Unfreeze	1. Diagnose problem 2. Assess motivation and capacity for change 3. Assess change agent's motivation and resources	1. Build relationship 2. Diagnose problem 3. Acquire resources	1. Awareness
	2. Move	4. Select progressive change objectives 5. Choose appropriate role of change agent	4. Choose solution 5. Gain acceptance	2. Interest 3. Evaluation 4. Trial
	3. Refreeze	6. Maintain change 7. Terminate helping relationship	6. Stabilization and self-renewal	5. Adoption

Adapted from *Introductory Management and Leadership for Nurses* (2nd ed., p. 327) by R. C. Swansburg and R. J. Swansburg (1998), Boston: Jones & Bartlett Publishers.

Smith (1994) emphasize that the core of the learning organization is based on five "learning disciplines"—lifelong programs of study and practice.

- Personal Mastery. Learning to expand our personal capacity to create the results we most desire, creating an organizational environment that encourages all members of the team to develop themselves toward the goals and purposes they choose.

- Mental Models. Reflecting on, continually clarifying, and improving our internal pictures of the world, and seeing how this vision shapes our actions and decisions.

- Shared Vision. Building a sense of commitment in a group by developing shared images of the future we seek to create, and developing the principles and guiding practices by which we hope to get there.
- Team Learning. Encouraging conversational and collective thinking skills, so groups of people can reliably develop intelligence and ability greater than the sum of individual members' talents.
- Systems Thinking. A way of thinking about and understanding the forces and interrelationships that shape the behavior of systems. Systems thinking highlights the fact that change in one area will affect other areas of the system. This discipline helps us to see how we can act more in tune with the larger processes of the natural and economic world.

In organizations, Senge believes the individuals who contribute the most to the enterprise are the ones who are committed to the practice of these disciplines for themselves. They are expanding their own capacity to improve and master their environment; seek, clarify, and share their vision; build team learning; and understand systems.

Implementation of Change

Bennis, Benne, and Chin (1969) identified three strategies to promote change in groups or organizations. Different strategies work in different situations. The power or authority of the change agent has an impact on the strategy selected. The change agent is one who is responsible for implementation of a change project. This person may be from within or outside an organization. Most change agents use a variety of strategies to promote successful change. See Table 10-2.

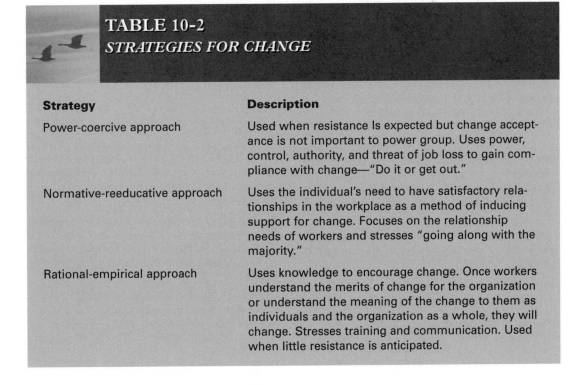

TABLE 10-2
STRATEGIES FOR CHANGE

Strategy	Description
Power-coercive approach	Used when resistance Is expected but change acceptance is not important to power group. Uses power, control, authority, and threat of job loss to gain compliance with change—"Do it or get out."
Normative-reeducative approach	Uses the individual's need to have satisfactory relationships in the workplace as a method of inducing support for change. Focuses on the relationship needs of workers and stresses "going along with the majority."
Rational-empirical approach	Uses knowledge to encourage change. Once workers understand the merits of change for the organization or understand the meaning of the change to them as individuals and the organization as a whole, they will change. Stresses training and communication. Used when little resistance is anticipated.

Response to Change

People have responses to change. A typical response to change is resistance. Humans like order and familiarity; they enjoy routine and the status quo.

There are several factors that affect resistance to change. The first is trust. The employee and employer must trust that each is doing the right thing and that each is capable of producing successful change. In addition to capability, predictability is important. The employee wants a predictable work environment and security. When change is introduced, then that predictability—and, therefore, capability—begins to come into question (Duck, 1993). Another factor is the individual's ability to cope with change. Silber (1993) points out four factors that affect an individual's ability to cope with change:

1. Flexibility for change; that is, the ability to adapt to change

2. Evaluation of the immediate situation; that is, if the current situation is unacceptable, then change will be more welcome

3. Anticipated consequences of change; that is, the impact change will have on one's current job

4. Individual's stake or what the individual has to win or lose in the change; that is, the more individuals perceive they have to lose, the more resistance they will offer.

Change can be a scary prospect if one has not had much experience with change or if one has had negative experiences with change. It is important to help individuals remember that change is inevitable and ever present.

Bushy (1992) has identified six behavioral responses to planned change. These behaviors are usually apparent in every health care facility and every nursing unit. These behavioral responses are as follows:

1. Innovators: Change embracers. Enjoy the challenge of change and often lead change.

2. Early adopters: Open and receptive to change but not obsessed with it.

3. Early majority: Enjoy and prefer the status quo but do not want to be left behind. They adopt change before the average person.

4. Late majority: Often known as the followers. They adopt change after expressing negative feelings and are often skeptics.

5. Laggards: Last group to adopt a change. They prefer tradition and stability to innovation. They are somewhat suspicious of change.

6. Rejectors: Openly oppose and reject change. May be surreptitious or covert in their opposition. They may hinder the change process to the point of sabotage.

Other responses to change have been identified. These include grieving, denial, anger, depression, and bargaining (Marquis & Huston, 2000). Regardless of the importance and necessity of change, the human response is very important and cannot be dismissed. So often, in one's zeal to respond to a need, the change agent forgets that the human side of change must be dealt with. People have a right to their feelings and a right to express them. The important point is the change agent works with people's response and help them move on to the goal of implementing the change. Table 10-3 summarizes the roles and characteristics of the change agent.

CONFLICT

An important part of the change process is the ability to resolve conflict. Conflict is a disagreement about something of importance to the people involved. Conflict resolution skills are leadership and management tools that all registered nurses should have in their repertoire. Conflict itself is not bad. Conflict can be healthy. It, like change, allows for creativity, innovation, new ideas, and new ways of doing things. It allows for the healthy discussion of different views and values and adds an important dimension to the provision of quality patient care. Without some conflict, groups or work teams

TABLE 10-3
ROLES AND CHARACTERISTICS OF THE CHANGE AGENT

- Leader of change process and sets time frame for completion
- Manages process and group dynamics. Seeks input from people involved
- Understands feelings of group experiencing the change. Works with conflict, as needed
- Maintains momentum and enthusiasm
- Maintains vision of change.
- Intuitive
- Facilitates, resources, and time for group change
- Communicates change, progress, and feelings constantly to key people in the group and organization
- Knowledgeable about the organization
- Trustworthy and innovative
- Respected and honest

REAL WORLD INTERVIEW

Change is all about growing and developing, but the change agent or nurse manager has to be honest and truthful. Once he or she lies to us, then trust is destroyed and the change will surely fail. It's okay to not have the answer or not to be able to give the answer, but don't lie about it.

Caron Martin, RN
Staff Nurse

STOP AND THINK

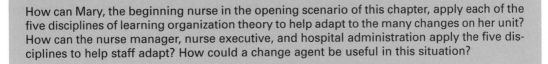

How can Mary, the beginning nurse in the opening scenario of this chapter, apply each of the five disciplines of learning organization theory to help adapt to the many changes on her unit? How can the nurse manager, nurse executive, and hospital administration apply the five disciplines to help staff adapt? How could a change agent be useful in this situation?

tend to become stagnant and routinized. Nothing new is allowed to penetrate the "way we have always done it" mentality. There are three broad types of conflict: intrapersonal, interpersonal, and organizational.

Conflict Resolution

In 1975, Filley suggested a process for conflict resolution that is widely accepted. In this process, there are five stages of conflict: (1) antecedent conditions, (2) perceived and/or felt conflict, (3) manifest behavior, (4) conflict resolution or suppression, and (5) resolution aftermath. In Filley's model, conflict and conflict resolution follow a specific course. The process begins with specific preexisting conditions called antecedent conditions. As the situation develops, conflict is perceived or felt by the involved parties. This triggers a response or manifest behavior. The conflict is either resolved or suppressed, leading to the development of new feelings and attitudes, and may create new conflicts. Conflict resolution is vital in change. The antecedent conditions that Filley suggests may or may not be the cause of the conflict, but they certainly move the disagreement to the conflict level. The sources of these conditions include disagreement in goals, values, or resource utilization. Other issues may also serve as antecedent conditions such as the dependency of one group on another. For instance, the nursing department is dependent on the pharmacy department to provide drugs for the nursing unit in a timely fashion. The goals and priorities of pharmacy and nursing may be different at the time the nurse requests the drugs and so a source of disagreement arises. If the circumstances for disagreement continue, a conflict will develop. According to Sullivan and Decker (1997), goal incompatibility is the most important antecedent condition to conflict.

Methods of Conflict Resolution

There are essentially seven methods of conflict resolution. These methods dictate the outcomes of the conflict process. Although some methods are more desirable or produce more successful outcomes than others, there may be a place in conflict resolution for all the methods, depending on the nature of the conflict and the desired outcomes. Table 10-4 is a summary of these methods, highlighting some of their advantages and disadvantages.

According to Lewicki, Hiam, and Olander (1996), there are five basic approaches to negotiating in conflict resolution; collaborative (win-win), competitive (win at all costs), avoiding (lose-lose), accommodating (lose to win), and compromise (split the difference). These five approaches to negotiation are influenced by the importance of maintaining the relationship relative to the importance of achieving one's desired outcomes (Figure 10-1). Note that as the relationship and the outcome's value increase, the amount of collaboration increases.

Strategies to Facilitate Conflict Resolution

Open, honest, clear communication is the key to successful conflict resolution. The nurse manager/leader and all parties to the conflict must agree to communicate with one another openly and honestly. Courtesy and active listening are encouraged.

The setting for the discussions for conflict resolution should be private, relaxed, and comfortable. If possible, external interruptions from phones, pagers, overhead speakers, and personnel should be avoided or kept to a minimum. The setting should be on neutral territory so that no one feels overpowered. The ground rules, such as not interrupting, who should go first, time limits, and so on, should be agreed upon in

TABLE 10-4
SUMMARY OF CONFLICT RESOLUTION TECHNIQUES

Conflict Resolution Technique	Advantages	Disadvantages
Accommodating— smoothing or cooperating. One side gives in to the other side	One side is more concerned with an issue than the other side; stakes not high enough for one group and that side is willing to give in	One side holds more power and can force the other side to give in; the importance of the stakes are not as apparent to one side as the other; can lead to parties feeling "used" if they are always pressured to give in
Avoiding—ignoring the conflict	Does not make a big deal out of nothing; conflict may be minor in comparison to other priorities; allows tempers to cool	Conflict can become bigger than anticipated; source of conflict might be more important to one person or group than others
Collaborating—both sides work together to develop optimal outcome	Best solution for the conflict and encompasses all important goals to each side	Takes a lot of time; requires commitment to success
Competing—forcing; the two or three sides are forced to compete for the goal	Produces a winner; good when time is short and stakes are high	Produces a loser; may leave anger and resentment on losing side
Compromising—each side gives up something and gains something	No one should win or lose but both should gain something; good for disagreements between individuals	May cause a return to the conflict if what is given up becomes more important the original goal
Confronting—immediate and obvious movement to stop conflict at the very start	Does not allow conflict to take root; very powerful	May leave impression that conflict is not tolerated; may make something big out of nothing
Negotiating—high-level discussion that seeks agreement but not necessarily consensus	Stakes are very high and solution is rather permanent; often involves powerful groups	Agreements are permanent, even though each side has gains and losses

STOP AND THINK

Review Table 10-4, Summary of Conflict Resolution Techniques. Think about a recent personal or professional time when you disagreed with someone. Which conflict resolution technique did you use? Did it help you achieve your goal?

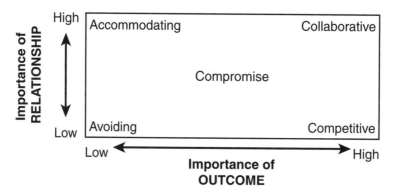

Figure 10-1 Negotiation Strategies

the beginning. Adherence to ground rules should be expected.

In the conflict resolution process, it is expected that both sides in the conflict will comply with the results. If one party cannot agree to comply with the decisions or outcomes, there is no point to the process. A tool for assessing conflict is identified in Figure 10-2. This tool can be used to determine interpersonal or intergroup conflict within an organization and whether a given conflict is functional or dysfunctional. Figure 10-3 provides a guide for assessment of the level of conflict. As noted earlier, a reasonable level of conflict can be healthy and stimulate creativity.

Interpersonal or intergroup?

1. Who?
   • Who are the primary individuals or groups involved? Characteristics (values; feelings; needs; perceptions; goals; hostility; strengths, past history of constructive conflict management; self-awareness)?
   • Who, if anyone, are the individuals or groups that have an indirect investment in the result of the conflict?
   • Who, if anyone, is assisting the parties to manage the conflict constructively?
   • What is the history of the individuals' or groups' involvement in the conflict?
   • What is the past and present interpersonal relationship between the parties involved in the conflict?
   • How is power distributed among the parties?
   • What are the major sources of power used?
   • Does the potential for coalition exist among the parties?
   • What is the nature of the current leadership affecting the conflicting parties?

2. What?
   • What is (are) the issues(s) in the conflict?
   • Are the issues based on facts? Based on values? Based on interests in resources?
   • Are the issues realistic?
   • What is the dominant issue in the conflict?
   • What are the goals of each conflicting party?
   • Is the current conflict functional? Dysfunctional?
   • What conflict management strategies, if any, have been used to manage the conflict to date?
   • What alternatives in managing the conflict exist?
   • What are you doing to keep the conflict going?
   • Is there a lack of stimulating work?

3. How?
   • What is the origin of the conflict? Sources? Precipitating events?
   • What are the major events in the evolution of the conflict?
   • How have the issues emerged? Been transformed? Proliferated?
   • What polarizations and coalitions have occurred?
   • How have parties tried to damage each other? What stereotyping exists?

4. When/Where?
   • When did the conflict originate?
   • Where is the conflict taking place?
   • What are the characteristics of the setting within which the conflict is occurring?
   • What are the geographic boundaries? Political structures? Decision-making patterns? Communication networks? Subsystem boundaries?
   • What environmental factors exist that influence the development of functional versus dysfunctional conflict?
   • What resource persons are available to assist in constructive conflict management?

Functional or dysfunctional?	**YES**	**NO**
Does the conflict support the goals of the organization?	[ ]	[ ]
Does the conflict contribute to the overall goals of the organization?	[ ]	[ ]
Does the conflict stimulate improved job performance?	[ ]	[ ]
Does the conflict increase productivity among work group members?	[ ]	[ ]
Does the conflict stimulate creativity and innovation?	[ ]	[ ]
Does the conflict bring about constructive change?	[ ]	[ ]
Does the conflict contribute to the survival of the organization?	[ ]	[ ]
Does the conflict improve initiative?	[ ]	[ ]
Does job satisfaction remain high?	[ ]	[ ]
Does the conflict improve the morale of the work group?	[ ]	[ ]

A yes response to the majority of the questions indicates that the conflict is probably functional. If the majority of responses are no, then the conflict is most likely a dysfunctional conflict.

Figure 10-2 Guide for the Assessment of Conflict (From *Nursing Leadership and Management*, by G. MacFarland, H. Leonard, and M. Morris, 1984, Clifton Park, NY: Delmar Learning).

Is conflict too low?	YES	NO
Is the work group consistently satisfied with the status quo?	[ ]	[ ]
Are no or few opposing views expressed by work-group members?	[ ]	[ ]
Is little concern expressed about doing things better?	[ ]	[ ]
Is little or no concern expressed about improving inadequacies?	[ ]	[ ]
Are the decisions made by the work group generally of low quality?	[ ]	[ ]
Are no or few innovative solutions or ideas expressed?	[ ]	[ ]
Are many work-group members "yes-men"?	[ ]	[ ]
Are work-group members reluctant to express ignorance or uncertainties?	[ ]	[ ]
Does the nurse manager seek to maintain peace and group cooperation regardless of whether this is the correct intervention?	[ ]	[ ]
Do the work-group members demonstrate an extremely high level of resistance to change?	[ ]	[ ]
Does the nurse manager base the distribution of rewards on "popularity" as opposed to competence and high job performance?	[ ]	[ ]
Is the nurse manager excessively concerned about not hurting the feelings of the nursing staff?	[ ]	[ ]
Is the nurse manager excessively concerned with obtaining a consensus of opinion and reaching a compromise when decisions must be made?	[ ]	[ ]

A yes response to the majority of these questions can be indicative of a too-low conflict level in a work group.

Is conflict too high?	YES	NO
Is there an upward and onward spiraling escalation of the conflict?	[ ]	[ ]
Are the conflicting parties stimulating the escalation of conflict without considering the consequences?	[ ]	[ ]
Is there a shift away from conciliation, minimizing differences, and enhancing goodwill?	[ ]	[ ]
Are the issues involved in the conflict being increasingly elaborated and expanded?	[ ]	[ ]
Are false issues being generated?	[ ]	[ ]
Are the issues vague or unclear?	[ ]	[ ]
Is job dissatisfaction increasing among work-group members?	[ ]	[ ]
Is the work-group productivity being adversely affected?	[ ]	[ ]
Is the energy being directed to activities that do not contribute to the achievement of organizational goals (e.g., destroying opposing party)?	[ ]	[ ]
Is the morale of the nursing staff being adversely affected?	[ ]	[ ]
Are extra parties getting dragged into the conflict?	[ ]	[ ]
Is a great deal of reliance on overt power manipulation noted (threats, coercion, deception)?	[ ]	[ ]
Is there a great deal of imbalance in power noted among the parties?	[ ]	[ ]
Are the individuals or groups involved in the conflict expressing dissatisfaction about the course of the conflict and feel that they are losing something?	[ ]	[ ]
Is absenteeism increasing among staff?	[ ]	[ ]
Is there a high rate of turnover among personnel?	[ ]	[ ]
Is communication dysfunctional, not open, mistrustful, and/or restrictive?	[ ]	[ ]
Is the focus being placed on nonconflict relevant sensitive areas of the other party?	[ ]	[ ]

A yes response to the majority of these questions can be indicative of a conflict level in a work group that is too high.

Figure 10-3 Guide for the Assessment of Level of Conflict (From *Nursing Leadership and Management,* by G. MacFarland, H. Leonard, and M. Morris, 1984, Clifton Park, NY: Delmar Learning).

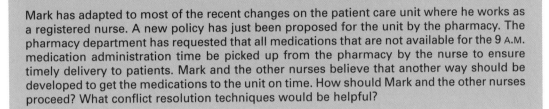

CASE STUDY 10-1

Mark has adapted to most of the recent changes on the patient care unit where he works as a registered nurse. A new policy has just been proposed for the unit by the pharmacy. The pharmacy department has requested that all medications that are not available for the 9 A.M. medication administration time be picked up from the pharmacy by the nurse to ensure timely delivery to patients. Mark and the other nurses believe that another way should be developed to get the medications to the unit on time. How should Mark and the other nurses proceed? What conflict resolution techniques would be helpful?

KEY CONCEPTS

- Change is defined as making something different from what it was.
- Major change theorists include Lewin, Lippitt, Havelock, and Rogers.
- Senge's model of five disciplines describes the learning organization. This model describes organizations undergoing continuous and unrelenting change.
- Strategies for change include the power-coercive approach, the normative-reeducative approach, and the rational-empirical approach.
- The techniques for conflict resolution include avoiding, accommodating, compromising, competing, negotiating, confronting, and collaborating.
- Chaos theory is often referred to as the science of complexity.
- Conflict can be healthy and stimulate creativity.

KEY TERMS

change
change agent
chaos theory

conflict
learning
  organization
  theory

REVIEW QUESTIONS

1. What is the most desirable conflict resolution technique?
   A. Avoiding
   B. Competing
   C. Negotiating
   D. Collaborating

REVIEW ACTIVITIES

1. Select a change project that either you have personally achieved or you have experienced in a clinical situation, and discuss with your classmates how you felt and how the change agent maintained momentum and enthusiasm for the project. If this is a personal change, how did you maintain enthusiasm?

2. Recall a conflict with which you have been involved in the clinical situation. Discuss each of the methods of conflict resolution identified in the chapter. Identify which ones would have worked. Did the conflict ever get resolved? How?

EXPLORING THE WEB

- Note this journal. Would it be useful to the new nurse? Anyone else in health care? Journal of Conflict Resolution: *http://www.ingenta.com*

REFERENCES

Bennis, W., Benne, K., & Chin, R. (Eds.). (1969). *The planning of change* (2nd ed.). New York: Holt, Rinehart, Winston.

Bushy, A. (1992). Managing change: Strategies for continuing education. *The Journal of Continuing Education in Nursing, 23,* 197–200.

Duck, J. D. (1993, November/December). Managing change: The art of balancing. *Harvard Business Review,* 109–118.

Filley, A. C. (1975). *Interpersonal conflict resolution.* Glenview, IL: Scott, Foresman.

Gleick, J. (1987). *Chaos: Making a new science.* New York: Viking.

Havelock, R. G. (1973). *The change agent's guide to innovation in education.* Englewood Cliffs, NJ: Educational Technology.

Ingersoll, G. L., Kirsch, J. C., Merk, S. E., & Lightfoot, J. (2000, January). Relationship of organizational culture and readiness for change to employee commitment to the organization. *Journal of Nursing Administration, 30*(1), 11–20.

Lancaster, J. (1999). *Nursing issues in leading and managing change.* St. Louis, MO: Mosby.

Lewicki, R. J., Hiam, A., & Olander, K. W. (1996). *Think before you speak.* New York: John Wiley & Sons.

Lewin, K. (1951). *Field theory in social science.* New York: Harper & Row.

Lippit, R., Watson, J., & Westley, B. (1958). *The dynamics of planned change.* New York: Harcourt, Brace.

MacFarland, G., Leonard, H., & Morris, M. (1984). *Nursing leadership and management.* Clifton Park, NY: Delmar Learning.

Marquis, B. L., & Huston, C. J. (2000). *Leadership roles and management functions in nursing: Theory applied* (3rd ed.). Philadelphia: Lippincott.

Mead, M. Retrieved October, 2002, from http://www.brainyquote.com.

Rogers, E. M. (1983). *Diffusion of innovations* (3rd ed.). New York: Free Press.

Senge, P. M. (1990). *The fifth discipline: The art and practice of the learning organization.* New York: Doubleday.

Senge, P., Kleiner, A., Roberts C., Ross, R. B., & Smith, B. (1994). *The fifth discipline fieldbook.* New York: Doubleday.

Silber, M. B. (1993, September). The "C"s in excellence: Choice and change. *Nursing Management, 24*(9), 60–62.

Sullivan, E. J., & Decker, P. J. (2001). *Effective leadership & management in nursing* (5th ed.). Menlo Park, CA: Addison-Wesley.

Waldrop, M. M. (1992) *Complexity: The emerging science at the edge of order and chaos.* New York: Simon & Schuster.

SUGGESTED READINGS

Bennis, W., & Nanus, B. (1985). *Leaders: The strategies for taking charge.* New York: Harper & Row.

Diggs, W. W. (1999). *Chaos theory! Journal of Nursing Administration, 29*(8), 7–8.

Docimo, A .B., Pronovost, P. J., Davis, R. O., Concordia, E. B., Gabrish, C. M., Adessa, M. S., & Bessman, E. (2000). Using the online and offline change model to improve efficiency for fast-track patients in an emergency department. *Joint Commission Journal on Quality Improvment, 9,* 503–514.

Donabedian, A. (1976). Foreword. In M. Phaneuf, *The nursing audit and self-regulation in nursing practice* (2nd ed.). New York: Appleton-Century-Crofts.

Haigh, C. (2002). Using chaos theory: The implications for nursing. *Journal of Advanced Nursing, 5,* 462–469

Johnson, S. (1998). *Who moved my cheese?* New York: G.P. Putnam.

Kotter, J. P. (1996). *Leading change.* Boston: Harvard Business School Press.

McDaniel, R. R. (1997). Strategic leadership: A view from quantum and chaos theories. *Health Care Management Review, 22*(1), 21–37.

Rolfe, G. (1999). The pleasure of the bottomless: Postmodernism, chaos and paradigm shifts. *Nurse Education Today, 8,* 668–672.

Rosswurm, M. A., & Larrabee, J. H. (1999). A model for change to evidence-based practice. *Image: Journal of Nursing Scholarship, 31*(4), 317–322.

Sebastian, J. G. (1999). Organizational change and the change process. In J. Lancaster, *Nursing issues in leading and managing change.* St. Louis, MO: Mosby.

Simms, L. M., Price, S. A., & Ervin, N. E. (2000). *The professional practice of nursing administration* (3rd ed.). Clifton Park, NY: Delmar Learning.

Tappen, R. M. (2001). *Nursing leadership and management: Concepts and practice* (4th ed.). Philadelphia: F. A. Davis.

Thietart, R. A., & Forgues, B. (1995). Chaos theory and organizations. *Organization Science, 6*(1), 19–31.

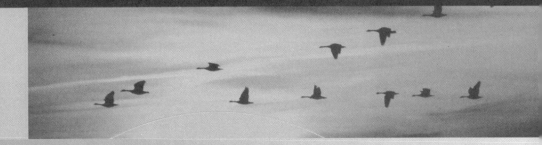

CHAPTER 11

Sound judgment, with discernment, is the best of seers. (Euripides)

Decision Making and Critical Thinking

OBJECTIVES

Upon completion of this chapter, the reader should be able to:

1. Review the concept of critical thinking.
2. Apply the decision making process to patient care using critical thinking.
3. Examine tools to improve decision making and build self-confidence.
4. Discuss individual vs. group decision making.
5. Identify how technology can help with decision making.
6. Identify how to determine if you are pleased with an Internet search for decision-making assistance.
7. Discuss evaluation of information found on the Internet.

You are a new nurse on a medical-surgical unit and have just come from a unit meeting. At the meeting, your nurse manager reported the results of the patient satisfaction survey from the previous year. Patient satisfaction has steadily declined, and for the past 3 months, only 20% of patients were satisfied. The manager selected a task force to investigate potential solutions to this problem and appointed you to the committee. The survey identified some reasons for the dissatisfaction: long waiting periods after pushing the nurse call light, not being informed about tests and procedures being performed, and being treated in an impersonal manner.

What should be the first step of the task force?

How can critical thinking and the decision-making process help the group solve the situation?

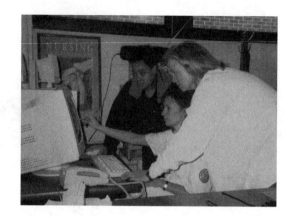

Rapid changes in the health care environment have expanded the decision-making role of the nurse. Critical thinking is essential when making these decisions. The Pew Health Professions Commission asserted that nurses must "demonstrate critical thinking, reflection, and problem solving skills" to thrive as effective practitioners in the 21st century (Bellack & O'Neil, 2000). This chapter explores the decision-making process and the critical thinking process. It also examines advantages and limitations to group decision making as well as the use of technology in decision making.

CRITICAL THINKING

What does it mean to be a critical thinker? Paul (1992) defines **critical thinking** as "thinking about your thinking while you're thinking in order to make your thinking better" (p. 7). Alfaro-Lefevre (1999) describes critical thinking as purposeful, outcome-directed thinking that aims to make judgments based on scientific evidence rather than tradition or conjecture (guesswork). Miller and Babcock (1996) state that critical thinking involves metacognition, which

means examining one's own reasoning or thought process while thinking—a process that helps to strengthen and refine thinking skills. A good critical thinker is able to examine situations from all sides and make decisions, taking into account research and the best evidence and various points of view. A good critical thinker does not say, "We've always done it this way," and refuse to consider alternate ways. The critical thinker thinks "out of the box" and generates new ideas and alternatives when making decisions. The critical thinker asks "why?" questions about a situation to arrive at the best decision. Four basic skills—critical reading, critical listening, critical writing, and critical speaking—are necessary for the development of critical thinking skills. These skills are part of the process of developing and using thinking for decision making. Ability in these four areas can be developed by using the universal intellectual standards illustrated in Table 11-1.

As you begin to apply critical thinking to nursing, use these universal intellectual standards when you are reading material from a textbook, listening to an oral presentation, writing a paper, answering test questions, or presenting ideas in oral form. Ask yourself whether the ideas are clear or unclear, precise or imprecise, specific or vague, accurate or inaccurate, and so forth. Critical thinking involves going beyond basic problem solving into a realm of inquisitive exploration, looking for all relevant factors that have an impact on the issue. It includes questioning all findings until a comprehensive picture emerges that explains the phenomenon, possible solutions, and creative methods for proceeding (Kennison & Brace, 1997). Development of critical thinking takes time and practice.

TABLE 11-1
THE SPECTRUM OF UNIVERSAL INTELLECTUAL STANDARDS

Clear	Unclear
Precise	Imprecise
Specific	Vague
Accurate	Inaccurate
Relevant	Irrelevant
Consistent	Inconsistent
Logical	Illogical
Deep	Superficial
Complete	Incomplete
Significant	Insignificant
Adequate	Inadequate
Fair	Unfair

Adapted from Foundation for Critical Thinking. Please see Web site: www.criticalthinking.org.

STOP AND THINK

Ask yourself the critical thinking questions inspired by Table 11-1 when you are making decisions at every step of the nursing process. Have I gathered the best, most up-to-date research and evidence to help with the decision? Is my assessment accurate and complete? Is the nursing diagnosis logical and clear? Is the plan of care relevant and complete? Is the implementation consistent? Is the evaluation adequate? Have I been fair in working with my patient? Have I avoided being vague, inaccurate, inconsistent, and illogical? Have I tried to think in new "out of the box" ways to solve my patient's problems? Continue to apply the critical thinking questions and to review the research and best evidence at each step.

Reflective Thinking

Pesut and Herman (1999) describe reflective thinking as watching or observing ourselves as we perform a task or make a decision about a particular situation. We have two selves, the active self and the reflective self. The reflective self watches the active self as it engages in activities. The reflective self acts as observer and offers suggestions about the activities. To be a good critical thinker, one must practice reflective thinking. Reflection upon a situation or problem after a decision is made allows the individual to evaluate the decision. Students can become better reflective thinkers through the use of clinical journals.

PROBLEM SOLVING AND DECISION MAKING

Problem solving is the process of identifying possible courses of action or alternatives that will alleviate a problem. This process may be applied to a problem of any type.

Decision Making

Huber (2000) defines decision making as a "behavior exhibited in making a selection and implementing a course of action from alternatives. It may or may not be the result of an immediate problem" (p. 378). Both decision making and problem solving use critical thinking. See Figure 11-1.

There are five steps to the decision-making process:

1. Identify the need for a decision.
2. Determine the goal or outcome.
3. Identify alternatives or actions, with benefits and consequences of each.
4. Choose an alternative.
5. Evaluate the alternative chosen. Did you meet your goal?

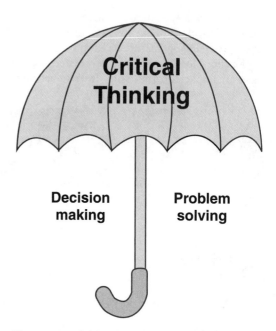

Figure 11-1 Critical Thinking Is Used in Both Problem Solving and Decision Making

Clinical Application

You are the night shift nurse caring for Mr. Cintas. In the morning, Mr. Cintas is scheduled for a permanent pacemaker insertion to replace his temporary pacemaker, which is still functioning. Hospital policy states that no visitor may stay all night with a patient unless that patient is very critically ill. Mr. and Mrs. Cintas are both requesting that Mrs. Cintas stay all night in a chair beside Mr. Cintas's bed because both are anxious about his upcoming procedure. Use your decision-making and problem-solving skills to help you decide what to do.

- Step 1: Identify the need for a decision. Should you let Mrs. Cintas spend the night? Consider all the information (hospital policy, the patient's wishes, anxiety level, and so on).
- Step 2: Determine the goal or outcome. Questions to consider include the following: Can an exception to hospital policy be

REAL WORLD INTERVIEW

I was in a situation where I just didn't think my patient looked good. I decided to go ahead and start two new IV sites, just in case. The patient arrested 2 hours later, and we really needed those IV sites. I felt good about my decision.

Cheryl Buntz, RN,

New Graduate

made? Is the goal to alleviate Mr. Cintas's anxiety? Will Mr. Cintas's level of anxiety adversely affect the outcome of the surgery? Will Mr. and Mrs. Cintas be satisfied? Are there other goals?

- Step 3: Identify all alternative actions and the benefits and consequences of each. If you enforce hospital policy, the benefits are that all patients are treated equally and the written policy supports the decision. The consequences are that Mr. Cintas's anxiety level increases, perhaps adversely affecting the outcome of his surgery, and Mr. and Mrs. Cintas will not be advocates for the health center. The other alternative is to allow Mrs. Cintas to stay all night. The benefits are that Mr. Cintas's level of anxiety will decrease, and Mr. and Mrs. Cintas will be satisfied customers. The consequence is that a precedent is set that may make it difficult to enforce the existing hospital policy.
- Step 4: Choose an alternative and arrive at the decision. Consider the two alternatives and the benefits and consequences of each. Then implement the decision.
- Step 5: Evaluate the alternative chosen. Was the goal achieved?

From the beginning of their careers, new graduate nurses are faced with the responsibility of making decisions regarding patient care. For the beginning nurse, it is common to have more questions than answers. When nurses are faced

with a difficult clinical decision, Huston and Marquis (1995) recommend consulting with others as early as possible. These may include other RNs on the unit or house supervisors.

Certain vs. Uncertain Decisions

Sometimes, when a decision is made, the outcome is certain. Other times, a nurse will need to make a decision without having all of the information needed to ensure a good outcome. Decision making in both certain and uncertain times can be improved by using various tools.

Decision-Making Tools

Nurses may use tools to clarify their decisions. Figure 11-2 shows a decision analysis tree for choosing whether to go back to school. See Figure 11-3 for a decision analysis tree for a patient who smokes.

A decision-making grid may help to separate the multiple factors that surround a situation. Figure 11-4 illustrates use of a decision-making grid by a unit that was told it had to reduce the workforce by two full-time equivalents (FTEs). This grid is useful in this example to visually separate the factors of cost savings, effect on job satisfaction of remaining staff, and effect on patient satisfaction.

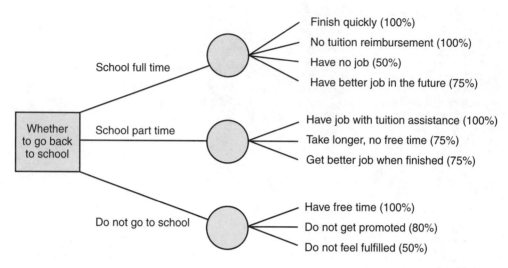

Key numbers represent percentage of possibility that event will occur

Figure 11-2 Decision Tree for Choosing Whether to Go Back to School

A decision-making grid is also useful when a nurse is trying to decide between two choices. Figure 11-5 is an example of a decision grid used by a nurse deciding between working at hospital A or hospital B.

The Program Evaluation and Review Technique (PERT) is useful in determining timing of decisions. The PERT flowchart provides a visual picture depicting the sequence of tasks that must take place to complete a project. Jones and Beck (1996) provide an example of a PERT flow diagram depicting a case management from beginning to end. See Figure 11-6. The chart shows the amount of time taken to complete the project and the sequence of events to complete the project. A Gantt chart can be useful for decision makers to illustrate a project from beginning to end. Figure 11-7 illustrates a Gantt chart.

Dos and Don'ts of Decision Making

A foundation for good decision making comes with experience and learning from those experiences. Table 11-2 gives the student some additional tips to consider when making decisions.

GROUP DECISION MAKING

Certain situations may call for group decision making. A group may offer innovative alternatives and decisions and afford some protection from mistakes because it uses the combined knowledge of all its members. Group decision making may increase the acceptance of the decision by all members. Vroom and Yetton (1973)

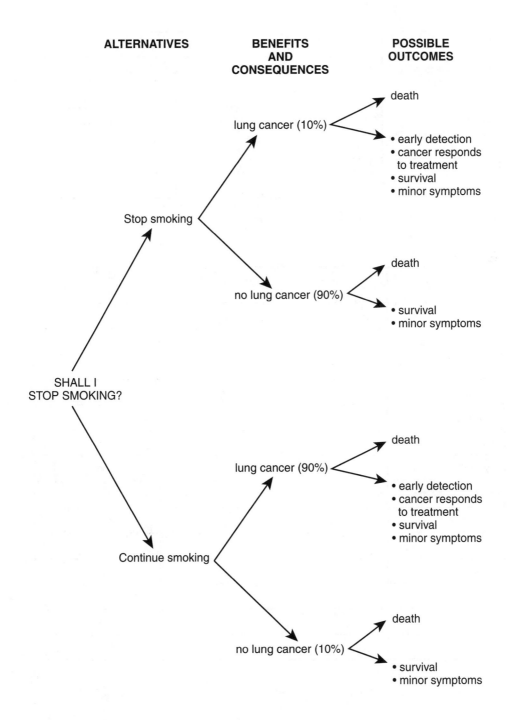

Figure 11-3 Decision Analysis Tree for a Patient Who Smokes

Methods of Reduction	Cost Savings	Effect on Job Satisfaction	Effect on Patient Satisfaction
Lay off the two most senior full-time employees	$93,500	Significant reduction	Significant reduction
Lay off the two most recently hired full-time employees	$63,200	Significant reduction	Moderate reduction
Reduce by staff attrition	$78,000	Minor reduction	Minor reduction

Figure 11-4 Sample Decision-Making Grid

Elements	Importance Score (out of 10)	Likelihood Score (out of 10)	Risk (multiply scores)
Work at hospital A			
Learning experience	10	10	100
Good mentor support	10	10	100
Financial reward	8	5	40
Growth potential	10	10	100
Good location	5	10	50
Total			390
Work at hospital B			
Learning experience	10	5	50
Good mentor support	10	5	50
Financial reward	8	10	80
Growth potential	10	5	50
Good location	5	5	25
Total			

Figure 11-5 Sample Decision-Making Grid

The vice president for nursing plans to change all units to include case managers. She believes that this can be accomplished within a year and one half. In order for this to be achieved, the following activities and events have to occur:

Activity Symbol	Activity Descriptions	Immediate Predecessor
A.	Form a multidisciplinary advisory group	None
B.	Agree upon definitions	A
C.	Notify members of subcommittees	B
D.	Write job descriptions	C
E.	Advertise for candidates for case manager	D
F.	Review qualifications of candidates	E
G.	Select candidates for case manager	F
H.	Review patient charts	None
I.	Write patient care maps	H
J.	Meet with case managers	None
K.	Orient case managers	J
L.	Orient unit and hospital staff	K
M.	Utilize case management process	L

Events

1.	Project begins
2.	Meeting of multidisciplinary committee
3.	Formation of subcommittees
4.	Subcommittee for job description meets
5.	Subcommittee for patient care maps meets
6.	Candidates for case managers are interviewed
7.	Candidates are hired
8.	Subcommittee for patient care maps meets to finalize maps
9.	Orientation begins
10.	Implementation begins
11.	Project is evaluated

Expected   Time Calculations

Activity	Duration
A	0.5 month
B	1 month
C	0.5 month
D	1 month
E	1 month
F	2 months
G	1 month
H	1 month
I	2 months
J	1 month
K&L	1 month
M	3 months

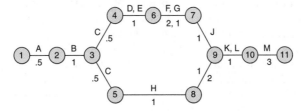

Figure 11-6 PERT Diagram with Critical Path for Implementation of Case Management

A nurse manager has agreed to have her unit pilot a new care delivery system within six months. The Gantt chart can be used to plan the progression of the project.

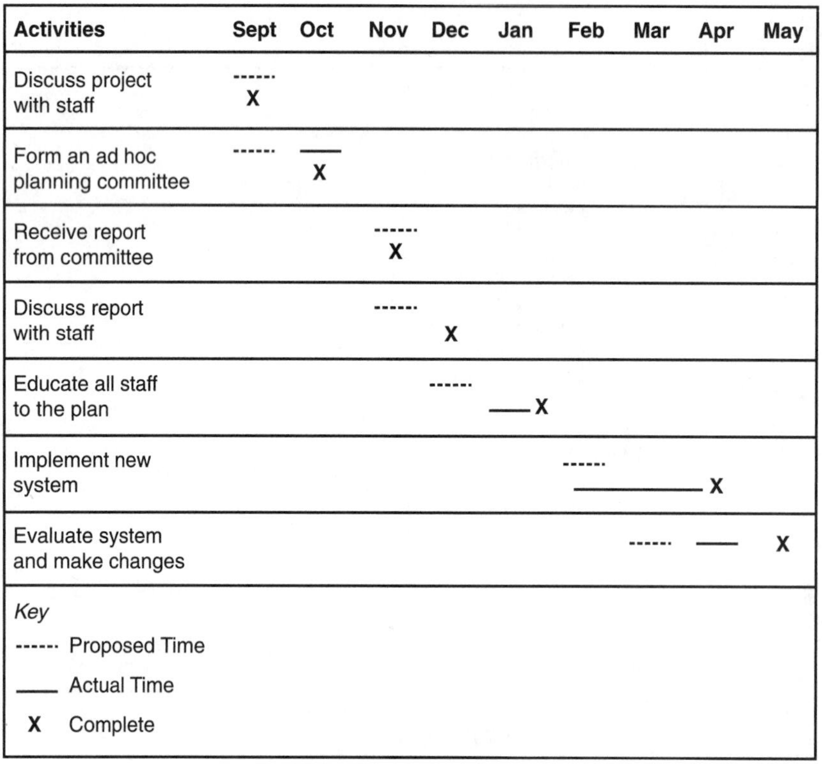

Activities	Sept	Oct	Nov	Dec	Jan	Feb	Mar	Apr	May
Discuss project with staff	------ X								
Form an ad hoc planning committee	------	— X							
Receive report from committee			------ X						
Discuss report with staff			------	X					
Educate all staff to the plan				------	— X				
Implement new system					------		— X		
Evaluate system and make changes						------	—	—	X
Key									
------ Proposed Time									
—— Actual Time									
X Complete									

Figure 11-7 Gantt Chart: Implementation of Care Delivery System

identified certain questions individuals should ask themselves before making a decision. See Table 11-3.

A major disadvantage of group decision making is the time involved. Without effective leadership, groups can waste time and be nonproductive. Group decision making can be more costly and can also lead to conflict. Groups can be dominated by one person or become the battleground for a power struggle among assertive members. Finally, groups will sometimes accept the first reasonable solution that occurs to them and disregard other solutions that might be better or less risky.

Groupthink Prevention

In groupthink, the goal is for everyone to be in 100% agreement on a decision. Groupthink discourages questioning and divergent thinking. It hinders creativity and usually leads to inferior decisions (Jarvis, 1997). The potential for groupthink increases as the cohesiveness of the group increases. An important responsibility of the group leader is to recognize symptoms of groupthink. Janis (as cited in Jarvis, 1997) described examples of these symptoms. One symptom is that group members develop an illusion of invulnerability, believing they can do no wrong. This

TABLE 11-2
DOS AND DON'TS OF DECISION MAKING

Do	Don't
Get good information before making a decision.	Make snap decisions.
Make notes and keep ideas visible about decisions to utilize all relevant Information.	Waste your time making decisions that do not have to be made.
Write down pros and cons of an issue to help clarify your thinking.	Consider decisions a choice between right and wrong. They are a choice among alternatives.
Make necessary decisions as you go along rather than letting them accumulate.	Prolong deliberation about decisions.
Consider those affected by your decision.	Regret a decision; it was the right thing to do at the time. Don't make decisions to justify earlier decisions.
Trust yourself. Delay or revise a decision as needed.	Always base decisions on the "way things have always been done."

Adapted from The Small Business Knowledge Base, 1999. Retrieved February 19, 2002, from http://www.bizmove.com.

CASE STUDY 11-1

You have been working on a medical-surgical unit. As you complete your nursing program, you are starting to interview at several hospitals. Set up a decision making grid to help you analyze your choices. What factors are most important to you as you begin to consider your decision? Use Figure 11-5.

problem has the greatest potential to develop when the group is powerful and group members view themselves as invincible. The second symptom of groupthink is stereotyping outsiders. This occurs when the group members rely on shared stereotypes—such as, all Democrats are liberal or all Republicans are conservative—to justify their positions. People who challenge or disagree with the decisions are also stereotyped. A third symptom is that group members reassure one another that their interpretation of data and their perspective on matters are correct regardless of the evidence showing otherwise. Old assumptions are never challenged, and members ignore

TABLE 11-3
INDIVIDUAL VS. GROUP DECISION MAKING

1. Does the nurse have all the information and resources needed to make the best decision?

2. Does the group have supplementary information needed to make the best decision?

3. Will individual personalities within the group work well together?

4. Is it absolutely critical that the group be involved in the decision and accept the decision prior to implementation?

5. Will the group accept a decision I make by myself?

6. Is there time for a group decision?

7. Does the course of action chosen make a difference to the organization?

8. Do the group and individual have the best interest of the organization foremost when considering the decision?

9. Will the decision cause undue conflict among the group?

Adapted from *Leadership and Decision-Making* (pp. 21–30), by V. Vroom and P. Yetton, 1973, Pittsburgh, PA: University of Pittsburgh Press.

what they do not know or what they do not want to know.

Strategies to avoid groupthink include appointing group members to roles that evaluate how group decision-making occurs. Group leaders should encourage all group members to think independently and verbalize their individual ideas. The leader should allow the group time to gather further data and reflect on data already collected. A primary responsibility of the group leader is to prevent groupthink from developing.

USE OF TECHNOLOGY IN DECISION MAKING

The best source of clinical decision making and judgment is the professional practitioner. However, computer technology has many uses to support information needs of nurses. Accessing current drug information, nursing and medical diagnostic information, and nursing intervention information in the clinical setting, as well as scheduling staff and making evidence-based changes in policy and procedure are but a few examples of how computers can assist nurses to make good decisions in patient care.

Computers have moved from the realm of a "nice to know" luxury item to a "need to know" essential resource for professional practice. Nurses are knowledge workers who require accurate and up-to-date information for their professional work. The explosion in information—some estimate that all information is replaced every 9 to 12 months—requires nurses to be on the cutting edge of knowledge to practice ethically and safely. Many nurses today are using personal digital assistants, such as the Palm Pilot, to assist with clinical decisions. See "Exploring the Web" in Chapter 12.

Using the Internet for Decision Making

There are a variety of strategies you can use for searching the Internet, including quick and dirty searching, links, and brute force. Keep in mind that you must be persistent: no one search strategy or search engine is going to work all the time.

The P-F-A Assessment

One strategy to develop your Internet search is to conduct a "purpose-focus-approach" (P-F-A) assessment. To determine your purpose, ask yourself why you are doing the search and why you need the information. Consider questions such as the following:

- Is it for personal interest?
- Do you want to obtain information to share with coworkers or a client?
- Are you verifying information given to you by someone else?
- Are you preparing a report or writing a paper for a class or project?

    Based on your purpose, your focus may be as follows:

- Broad and general (basic information for yourself)
- Lay oriented (to give information to a patient) or professionally oriented (for colleagues)
- Narrow and technical with a research orientation

Purpose combined with focus determines your approach. For example, information that is broad and general can be found using brute force methods or quick and dirty searching. Lay information can be quickly accessed at a few key sites, including MEDLINE*plus* (*http://www.medlineplus.gov*) and consumer health organizations. Similarly, professional associations and societies are a good starting point for professionally oriented information. Scientific and research information usually requires literature resources that can be found in databases such as MEDLINE *(http://www.ncbi.nlm.nih.gov)* or CINAHL (Cumulative Index to Nursing and Allied Health Literature).

Quick and Dirty Searching and Links

Quick and dirty searching is a very simple but surprisingly effective search strategy. First, start with a search engine, such as AltaVista (*http://www.altavista.com*) or Google (*http://www.google.com*). Next, type in the term of interest. At this point, do not worry about being overly broad or general. You will retrieve an enormous number of found references (called "hits"), but you are interested only in the first 10 to 20. Look at the universal resource locators (URLs), that is, the addresses of the sites that are returned by your search, and try to decipher what they mean. Pay attention to the domains: .com is commercial; .edu is an educational institution; .gov is the government. Quickly visit a few sites. Look for the information you need, or useful links. If a site is not relevant, use the back button on your browser to return to your search results and go to the next site. Once you find a site that appears to be useful, begin to explore the site. Many sites will connect you to other sites, using links, or hot buttons. If you click on a link, it will take you to a related site. If the site you are looking at has links (most do), use them to connect to other relevant sites. This process—quick search, quick review, clicking, and linking—can provide a starting point for finding useful information in a relatively short period of time. When you find a site of interest, "bookmark" it and add it to your list of favorites. See Table 11-4.

Brute Force

Brute force searching is another alternative. To do this, type in an address in the URL box (the address box at the top of the browser window) and see what happens. The worst outcome is an annoying error message, but you may land on a site that is exactly what you want. To be effective, think how URLs work: they usually start with www (for World Wide Web). Then there is the "thing in the middle" followed by a domain. Perhaps you are trying to find a school of nursing at a certain university. What is the common name for the university? *WWW.unh.edu* is the very logical URL for the

TABLE 11-4
LIST OF FAVORITE HEALTH CARE WEB SITES

http://www.allnursingschools.com

http://www.allHealth.com

http://www.aapcc.org

http://www.cancer.org

http://www.acb.org

http://www.acsh.org

http://www.diabetes.org

http://www.americanheart.org

http://www.lungusa.org

http://www.ama-assn.org

http://www.arthritis.org

http://www.bestdoctors.com

http://www.cochrane.org

http://www.cdc.gov

http://www.clinicaltrials.gov

http://www.health.discovery.com

http://www.drkoop.com

http://www.eMD.com

http://www.epilepsyfoundation.org

http://www.familydoctor.org

http://www.fda.gov

http://www.cms.hhs.gov

http://www.gon.ch

http://www.healthanswers.com

http://www.healthAtoZ.com

http://www.healthcentral.com

http://www.healthfinder.gov

http://www.healthgrades.com

http://www.healthhelper.com

http://www.healthy.net

http://www.intelihealth.com

http://www.kidshealth.com

http://www.mayoclinic.com

http://www.medlineplus.gov

http://www.medscape.com

http://www.ncsbn.org

http://www.netwellness.org

http://www.rarediseases.org

http://www.oncolink.org

http://www.pain.com

http://www.partnershipforcaring.org

http://www.pdr.net

http://www.personalMD.com

http://www.realage.com

http://www.rxlist.com

http://www.shapeup.org

http://www.oxygen.com

http://www.vh.org

http://www.webMD.com

http://www.nursingworld.org

http://www.ahrq.gov

http://www.nih.gov

http://www.ngc.gov

University of New Hampshire. Organizations are also quite logical in their URLs: *www.aorn.org* is the Association of periOperative Registered Nurses (AORN); *www.aone.org* is the American Organization of Nurse Executives (AONE).

Full Text Articles

The final element of searching for literature online is finding full-text articles. The databases so far discussed (MEDLINE and so on) do not contain full text—they include only literature citations. One option is to use a document delivery service such as the document delivery service at *http://www.ncbi.nih.gov*. Click on "literature database pubmed" and then on "pubmed medline." This resource allows you to conduct a search of the literature. It identifies articles which can be sent to you for a fee.

EVALUATION OF INFORMATION FOUND ON THE INTERNET

Traveling through the Internet, one must always use critical thinking skills to evaluate the information that is found. A simple mnemonic, "Are you PLEASED with the site?" is very helpful (Nicoll, 2003) (Table 11-5).

To determine whether you are PLEASED, consider the following:

- *P—Purpose.* What is the author's purpose in developing the site? Are the author's objectives clear? Many people will develop a Web site as a hobby or way of sharing information they have gathered. It should be immediately evident to you what the true purpose of the site is. At the same time, consider your purpose; that is, think back to your P-F-A assessment. There should be congruence between the author's purpose and yours.

- *L—Links.* Evaluate the links at the site. Are they working? Links that do not take you anywhere are called "dead links." Do they link to reliable sites? It is important to critically evaluate the links at sites hosted by organizations, businesses, or institutions because these entities are usually presenting themselves as authorities on the subject at hand. Some pages, such as those created by individuals, are really nothing more than a collection of links. These can be useful as a starting point for a search, but it is still important to evaluate the links that are provided at the site.

TABLE 11-5	
WEB SITE EVALUATION: ASK YOURSELF, "AM I PLEASED WITH THE SITE?"	
P	Purpose
L	Links
E	Editorial (site content)
A	Author
S	Site navigation
E	Ethical disclosure
D	Date site last updated

- *E—Editorial (site content)*. Is the information contained in the site accurate, comprehensive, and current? Is there a particular bias, or is the information presented in an objective way? Who is the consumer of the site: is it designed for health professionals, patients, consumers, or other audiences? Is the information presented in an appropriate format for the intended audience? Look at details, too. Are there misspellings and grammatical errors? "Under construction" banners that have been there forever? These types of errors can be very telling about the overall quality of the site.

- *A—Author*. Who is the author of the site? Does that person or group of people have the appropriate credentials? Is the author clearly identified by name and is contact information provided? One suggestion is to double-check an author's credentials by doing a literature search in MEDLINE. When people advertise themselves as "the leading worldwide authority" on such and such a topic, they should have a few publications to their credit that establish their reputations. It is surprising how many times this search brings up nothing.

  Be wary of how a person presents her credentials, too. Consider a site where "Dr. X" is touted as an expert. Upon further exploration, you may find that, in fact, Dr. X does have a PhD (or MD or EdD), but the discipline in which this degree was obtained has nothing to do with the subject matter of the site. Remember that there is no universal process of peer review on the WWW and anyone can present herself in any way that she wants. Be suspicious.

  Keep in mind that the webmaster and the author may be two (or more) different people. The webmaster is the person who designed the site and is responsible for its upkeep. The author is the person who is responsible for the content and is the expert in the subject matter provided. In your evaluation, make sure you determine who these people are.

- *S—Site*. Is the site easy to navigate? Is it attractive? Does it download quickly or have too many graphics and other features that make it inefficient? A site that is pleasing to the eye will invite you to return. Sites that cause your computer to crash should be viewed with a skeptical eye.

- *E—Ethical*. Is there contact information for the site developer and author? Is there full disclosure of who the author is and the purpose of the site? Is this information easy to find or is it buried deep in the Web site? There are many commercial services, particularly pharmaceutical companies, that have excellent Web sites with very useful information. But some of them exist only to sell their product, although this is not immediately evident on evaluation.

- *D—Date*. When was the site last updated? Is it current? Does the information need to be updated regularly? Generally, with health and nursing information, the answer to that last question is yes. You should be concerned with sites that have not been updated within 12 to 18 months. The date the site was last updated should be prominently displayed on the site. Keep in mind that different pages within the site may be updated at different times. Be sure to check the date on each of the pages that you visit.

As you become more proficient at evaluating Web sites, you may have additional criteria that you would add to this list or criteria that are important to you for a specific purpose, but, in general, this simple group of seven is surprisingly comprehensive. Test them for yourself. Do a quick search on a topic of interest, visit a number of sites, and determine just how PLEASED you are with what you find (Nicoll, 2003).

LITERATURE APPLICATION

Citation: Ward, B. O. (1999). "Internet-positive patients" driving you crazy? Find out how to get online and cope. *Internet Medicine: A Critical Guide, 4*(7), 1, 6.

Discussion: One of the major reasons that people go on-line is to search for health information on the Internet. In fact, since 1996, the number of people who use the Internet for health information climbed from 7.8 million to 31.1 million in the second quarter of 1999. Ready availability of electronic resources to patients is providing health care providers with unique challenges. Patients may arrive in an office or clinic with information that is more up to date and comprehensive than information the provider currently possesses.

What is the best approach to such Internet-positive patients? Keep in mind that your professional education has provided you with skills to critically analyze the information presented, something the patient may not be able to do. Use this as an opportunity to teach; empower the patient for taking the time to research and learn more about his health condition. In addition, you can take the following actions:

- React in a positive manner about information from the Internet, but remind the patient that its quality and reliability are unknown.
- Inform patients that time constraints will not permit you to read the information on the spot; ask them to send it to you (via e-mail, perhaps) before a scheduled appointment.
- Accept patients' contributions and acknowledge that they may have valuable information that you may not have come across yet.

Things you should *not* do include the following:

- Be dismissive or paternalistic
- Be derogatory about others' comments on the Internet
- Refuse Internet material
- Try to "one-up" the patient or family members regarding the information
- Break normal rules of patient confidentiality

Implications for Practice: Clinicians may improve their care delivery by incorporating Internet information gathered by patients, as appropriate, into their practice.

REAL WORLD INTERVIEW

Clinical care can no longer exist efficiently and effectively without electronic tools like the electronic patient record, decision support, and Internet access. Additionally, the external impetus to install electronic patient records is great. For example, the Leapfrog group set standards for hospitals to meet in order to obtain business from large corporations such as General Motors, Ford Motor Company, IBM, and 75 other companies. One of those standards is computerized physician order entry, which is projected to reduce prescribing errors by more than 50%. CFOs need to realize that their institutions will not be competitive in the health industry without electronic access for patients, computerized orders, and protections for patients like decision support. It is no longer a question of whether to install these computerized functions but when.

Nancy Staggers, PhD, RN, FAAN

Associate CIO

KEY CONCEPTS

- Critical thinking involves examining situations from every viewpoint when faced with any problem or situation. Use of the universal intellectual standards will improve a nurse's critical thinking.
- Practicing reflective thinking helps individuals become better critical thinkers.
- In the decision-making process, there are five levels: Level 1—identify the need for a decision; Level 2—determine the goal or outcome; Level 3—identify alternatives or actions, along with their benefits and consequences; Level 4—decide on the action and implement; Level 5—evaluate the action.
- Decision-making tools may be helpful when the nurse needs to separate multiple factors surrounding a situation during the decision-making process.
- The PERT model is useful for determining timing of decisions.
- There are situations in which the nurse makes an individual decision. Other situations call for group decision making.

- Groupthink occurs when individuals are not allowed to express creativity, question methods, or engage in divergent thinking. Managers must be able to identify the symptoms of groupthink.
- Effective searching for information on the Internet requires that you target your search. One technique is to conduct a P-F-A: a purpose-focus-approach assessment to determine what you are looking for and the best way to find it.
- PubMed is a search engine developed by the National Library of Medicine that allow you to search MEDLINE. It is free to anyone with an Internet connection.
- It is important to evaluate information found on the Internet. Ask yourself, "Am I PLEASED with the site?"

P-Purpose
L-Links
E-Editorial (site content)
A-Author
S-Site navigation
E-Ethical disclosure
D-Date site last updated

KEY TERMS

critical thinking   problem solving
decision making   reflective thinking

REVIEW QUESTIONS

1. Decision making is best described as
   A. the process one uses to solve a problem.
   B. the process one uses to choose between alternatives.
   C. the process one uses to reflect on a certain situation.
   D. the process one uses to generate ideas.

2. If a patient came to you asking for an Internet site where he could learn more about diabetes, which of the following would be appropriate for you to suggest?
   A. MEDLINE at the National Library of Medicine
   B. OncoLink
   C. MEDLINE*plus*
   D. All of the above

3. Decipher the following URL: *www.maine. edu*. This is the URL for which of the following Web sites?
   A. University of Maine
   B. Maine Visitors and Convention Bureau
   C. Maine State Government
   D. Maine State Nurses Association

4. Occasionally, making a decision is difficult because of the multiple factors that surround certain situations. To separate these factors, the nurse manager may utilize
   A. a decision grid.
   B. groupthink.
   C. brute force.
   D. links.

REVIEW ACTIVITIES

1. You are taking NCLEX in 10 weeks and need to prepare. Draw a PERT diagram to depict the sequence of things necessary for the successful completion of the NCLEX.

2. The education forms are not being filled out correctly on new admissions in your medical-surgical unit. Decide on your own the best action to take in this situation. Then, get into a group and attempt to decide on the best action to take. Compare the differences between individual and group decision making. What did you learn?

3. Identify a problem that you have been considering. Using the decision-making grid at the bottom of this page, rate the alternative solutions to the problem that you have been considering on a scale of 1 to 3 on the elements of cost, quality, importance, location, and any other elements that are important to you.

Did this exercise help you to clarify your thinking?

	Cost	Quality	Importance	Location	Other
Alternative A					
Alternative B					
Alternative C					

EXPLORING THE WEB

- Test your critical thinking in critical care with the scenarios on this Web site: *http://nursing.umaryland.edu*
- Note the universal intellectual standards at the Foundation for Critical Thinking: *http://criticalthinking.org*
- Visit these critical thinking sites: *http://www.criticalthinking.org* *http://www.insightassessment.com*
- Note the following site for clinical decision making—this site includes software for clinical decision making: *http://www.apache-msi.com*
- Review this site on applying artificial intelligence to clinical situations: *http://www.medg.lcs.mit.edu*
- The Nursing Information and Data Set Evaluation Center of the ANA was established "to review, evaluate against defined criteria, and recognize information systems from developers and manufacturers that support documentation of nursing care within automated Nursing Information Systems (NIS) or within computer-based Patient Record systems (CPR)." Visit the center at *http://www. nursingworld.org.* Search for "nidsec" to find answers to the following questions: How many nursing languages have been recognized by the ANA? Why have these languages been developed? What are they designed to do?
- Go to *http://www.criticalthinking.org* and click on standards and then on universal intellectual standards. How would you obtain more information on the approved languages?

REFERENCES

About Oncolink. (2001). University of Pennsylvania Cancer Center. Retrieved November 27, 2001, from http://www.oncolink.com

Alfaro-LeFevre, R. (1999). *Critical thinking in nursing: A practical approach.* (2nd ed.). Philadelphia: Saunders.

Bellack, J. P., & O'Neil, E. H. (2000). Re-creating nursing practice for a new century: Recommendations and implications of the Pew Health Professions Commission's final report. *Nursing and Health Care Perspectives, 21*(1), 14–21.

Huber, D. (2000). *Leadership and nursing care management.* Philadelphia: Saunders.

Huston, C. J., & Marquis, B. L. (1995, May). Seven steps to successful decision-making. *American Journal of Nursing,* 65–68.

Jarvis, C. (1997). *Groupthink.* Retrieved June 2, 1999, from Brunel University Web site: http://sol.brunel.ac.uk

Jones, R. A. P., & Beck, S. E. (1996). *Decision making in nursing.* Clifton Park, NY: Delmar Learning.

Kennison, M., & Brace, J. (1997). Critical thinking—digging deeper for creative solution. *Nursing, 27*(9), 52–54.

Miller, M. A., & Babcock D. E. (1996). *Critical thinking applied to nursing.* St. Louis, MO: Mosby.

Nicoll, L. H. (2003). Nursing and health care informatics. In P. L. Kelly-Heidenthal (Ed.), *Nursing leadership and management.* Clifton Park, NY: Delmar Learning.

Paul, R. (1992). *Critical thinking: What every person needs to survive in a rapidly changing world.* Santa Rosa, CA: Foundation for Critical Thinking.

Pesut, D. J., & Herman, J. (1999). *Clinical reasoning: The art & science of critical & creative thinking.* Clifton Park, NY: Delmar Learning.

The Small Business Knowledge Base. (1999). Retrieved January 19, 2002, from http://www.bizmove.com

Vroom, V. H., & Yetton, P. W. (1973). *Leadership and decision-making.* Pittsburgh, PA: University of Pittsburgh Press.

Ward, B. O. (1999). "Internet-positive patients" driving you crazy? Find out how to get online and cope. *Internet Medicine: A Critical Guide, 4*(7), 1, 6.

SUGGESTED READINGS

American Nurses Credentialing Center. (2001). *Informatics nurse certification. Basic eligibility requirements.* Retrieved July 19, 2001, from http://www.nursing world.org

Ball, M. J., Hannah, K. J., & Douglas, J. (2000). Nursing and informatics. In M. Ball, K. Hannah, S. Newbold, & J. Douglas (Eds.), *Nursing informatics: Where caring and technology meet* (3rd ed., pp. 6–14). New York: Springer-Verlag.

Bard, M. R. (2000). The future of e-health. *Cybercitizen Health, 1*(1), 1–13.

Jenkins, S. (2000). Nurses' responsibilities in the implementation of information systems. In M. J. Ball, K. J. Hannah, S. Newbold, & J. Douglas (Eds.), *Nursing informatics: Where caring and technology meet* (pp. 207–223). New York: Springer-Verlag.

LeStorti, A., Cullen, P., Hanzlik, E., Michiels, J. M., Piano, L., Ryan, P. L., et al. (1999). Creative thinking in nursing education: Preparing for tomorrow's challenges. *Nursing Outlook, 47*(2), 62–66.

Martinez de Castillo, S. L. (1999). *Strategies, techniques, and approaches to thinking: Case studies in clinical nursing.* Philadelphia: Saunders.

Parsons, L. (1999). Building RN confidence for delegation decision-making skills in practice. *Journal for Nurses in Staff Development, 15*(6), 263–269.

Schon, D. A. (1987). *Educating the reflective practitioner.* San Francisco: Jossey-Bass.

Simms, L. M., Price, S. A., & Ervin, N. E. (2000). *Professional practice of nursing administration* (3rd ed.). Clifton Park, NY: Delmar Learning.

Swansburg, R. C., & Swansburg, R. J. (2002). *Introductory management and leadership for nurse managers* (3rd ed.). Boston: Jones and Bartlett.

CHAPTER 12

Time Management and Setting Priorities

Autonomy means decision control over the kind and degree of service a client will receive. It involves a conscious decision about what will and what will not be done when there is more work than available time. Control over time use is a key aspect of professional nurse practice.

(Roxane Spitzer-Lehmann, 1996)

OBJECTIVES

Upon completion of this chapter, the reader should be able to:

1. Discuss concepts of time management.
2. Describe strategies for setting priorities.
3. Discuss shift report.
4. Apply time management strategies to enhance personal productivity.

Sharon has just completed her medical-surgical orientation as a new graduate registered nurse. This evening is her first solo shift. But she is not really alone. Sharon and Carole—the other RN—and one certified nursing assistant are responsible for 12 possible patients in this section of the unit. Currently there are 10 patients in this section, but a new admission is on the way, another patient is returning from surgery, the dinner trays are arriving, and Sharon has medications to pass. Just as the dinner trays arrive, a family member runs out to Sharon and states that her mom is confused and incontinent and has pulled out her IV.

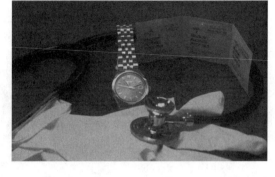

How would you react if you were Sharon? What would you do first?

M any nurses become nurses out of idealism. They want to help people by meeting all their needs. Unfortunately, most new graduates find it impossible to meet all or even most of their patients' needs. Needs tend to be unlimited, whereas time is limited. In addition to the direct patient care responsibilities, there are shift responsibilities, charting, doctors' orders to be transcribed or checked, medications to be given, and patient reports to be given.

New graduates often go home feeling totally inadequate. They wake up remembering what they did not accomplish. One young nurse shared with tears in her eyes that once, when she answered a call bell late in her shift, the patient requested a pain medication. She went to the narcotics cabinet to get the medication but was interrupted by an emergent situation. When she arrived home, she was so exhausted that she fell asleep rapidly, only to awaken with the realization that she had not returned with her patient's medication. Her guilt was tremendous. She had gone into nursing to relieve pain, not to ignore it.

Time management allows the novice nurse to prioritize care, decide on outcomes, and perform the most important interventions first. Time management skills are important not just for nurses on the job but for nurses in their personal lives as well. They allow nurses to make time for fun, friends, exercise, and professional development. This chapter discusses concepts of time management and strategies for setting priorities when delivering nursing care. Strategies to enhance personal productivity are also discussed.

TIME MANAGEMENT CONCEPTS

Time management has been defined as "a set of related common-sense skills that helps you use your time in the most effective and productive way possible" (Mind Tools, nd.-b). In other words, time management allows us to achieve more with available time. Time management requires self-examination of what pursuits are really important, analysis of how time is currently being used, and assessment of the distractions that have been siphoning time from more important pursuits.

There is a simple principle, the **Pareto principle**, which states that 20% of effort results in 80% of results, or conversely that 80% of unfocused effort results in 20% of results (Figure 12-1). The Pareto principle reminds us to focus our efforts on the most important activities to maximize the results we get.

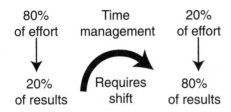

Figure 12-1 The Pareto Principle

The Pareto principle, formulated by Vilfredo Pareto in the late 1800s, was invoked by the total quality management (TQM) movement as a strategy for balancing life and work (Fryxell, 1997; Graham, 1998; Koch, 1999).

Analysis of Nursing Time

Analysis of nursing time use is the first step in developing a plan to effectively use time. Nurses often undervalue their time. Consider salary and benefits. Benefits are frequently forgotten, but they raise employer costs by 15% to 30% of salary. If a nurse is making $18 an hour, benefits add $2.70 to $5.40 to the hourly cost of a nurse's time. The value of nursing time in this example, excluding what the organization is paying in workers' compensation and payroll taxes, is $20.70 to $23.40 an hour. The organization has also invested in nurse recruitment, orientation, and development. Nursing time is a valuable commodity. Keeping this in mind will be invaluable when considering work that can be delegated to personnel who receive less compensation or when considering spending time on completing a task that does not support achieving an outcome.

Use of Time

Numerous studies have shown how nurses use their time. Most studies have been done on acute care nurses because they comprise the majority of nurses. Only 30% to 35% of nursing time is spent on direct patient care (Scharf, 1997). Twenty-five percent of a nurse's time is spent on charting and reporting, and the remainder of time is spent on admission and discharge procedures, professional communication, personal time, and providing care that could be provided by unlicensed personnel, such as transportation and housekeeping (Upenieks, 1998). Urden and Roode (1997) summarized various work sampling studies to show that RNs spend 28% to 33% of time on direct patient care, defined as activities performed in the presence of the patient or family; 42% to 45% of time on indirect care activities, which include all activities done for an individual patient but not in the patient's presence; 15% on unit-related activities, which include all unit general maintenance activities; and 13% to 20% on personal activities, which include activities that are not related to patient care or unit maintenance.

Given such a distribution of nurses' time, shifting the use of time could have a major impact on outcomes (Tappen, 2001). If nonnursing activities could be performed by nonnursing personnel instead of nurses, about 48 minutes per nurse per shift could be redirected toward essential nursing responsibilities (Prescott, Phillips, Ryan, & Thompson, 1991).

How do you use your time? Memory and self-reporting of time have been found to be unreliable. Nurses are often unaware of the time spent socializing with colleagues, making and drinking coffee, snacking, and other nonproductive time. Self-reporting of time is not recommended for estimating the total number of activities or the average time an activity takes to complete (Burke, Mckee, Wilson, Donahue, Batenhorst, & Pathak, 2000).

An **activity log** is a time management tool that can assist the nurse in determining how both personal and professional time is used. The activity log (Figure 12-2) should be used for several days. Behavior should not be modified while keeping the log. The nurse should record every activity, from the beginning of the day until the end. Review of this log will illuminate time use as well as time wasted. Analysis of the log will

Time	Name of Activity	Outcome Desired	Can You Delegate to Another? Who?
0500	Treadmill	Fitness	Keep for Self
0530	Shower and Breakfast	Cleanliness and Nutrition	Keep for Self
0600	Drive to Work	Arrive at Work	Keep for Self
0630			
0700	Shift Report	Identify Patients	Keep for Self
0730	Patient Rounds	Assess Patients	Keep for Self
0800	Give Report to UAP	Safe Patient Care	Keep for Self
0830	Bedmaking	Provide Clean Beds	Assign to UAP
0900	Pass Medications	Safe Medication Delivery	Keep for Self
0930	Dressing Change	Prevent Infection	Assign to LPN
1000			
1030			
1100			
1130			
1200			
1230			
1300			
1330			
1400			
1430			
1500			
1530			
1600			
1630			
1700			
1730			
1800			
1830			
1900			
1930			
2000			
2030			
2100			
2130			
2200			

Figure 12-2 Activity Log

allow the separation of essential activities from activities that can be performed by someone else (Grohar-Murray & DiCroce, 1997; Sullivan & Decker, 2001).

After completing the activity log for several days, a nurse needs to consider all activities that have been completed, how much time each activity took, what outcome was achieved by performing the activities, and whether the activities could have been done by someone else. When considering these questions, ask how would the Pareto principle apply? Has 80% of the effort resulted in 20% of the outcome achievement? If the activities have not achieved the desired outcomes, the nurse needs to change activities and focus on priorities. Start by noticing your most energetic time of day. Activities that take focus and creativity should be scheduled at high-energy times and dull, repetitive tasks at low-energy times. Scheduling time for proper rest, exercise, and nutrition allows for quality time.

Create More Time

There are three major ways to create time. One is to delegate work to others or hire someone else to do work. Another is to eliminate chores or tasks that add no value. The last way is to get up earlier in the day. When a person delegates a task, he or she cannot control when and how the task is completed. Initially, it may take more time to get others to do the chore than to just do it, but this investment of time should save the investor time and energy in the future. If a chore is boring and mundane, it makes more sense to work an hour more at a job one enjoys in order to pay for someone else to do unrewarding, boring work.

Getting up 1 hour earlier in the day for a year can free up 365 hours, or approximately nine weeks a year, extra time that can be used to enrich life. After several days of rising an hour earlier, an individual may feel tired and respond to the fatigue by going to bed a little earlier (Mind Tools, n.d.-a). This may be a good strategy for many people, especially those who are not productive in the evening and spend time doing activities that are minimally rewarding such as watching television. If a person does not try to get to bed earlier, though, and the end result of getting up early is fatigue, the strategy is not beneficial.

SETTING PRIORITIES

To plan effective use of time, nurses must understand the big picture, and decide on priority outcomes. Start by reviewing the big picture. No nurse works in isolation. Nurses should know

STOP AND THINK

The American public has become increasingly aware of and interested in health promotion (Leddy & Pepper, 1998). The relationship between personal lifestyle and the incidence of several diseases has been demonstrated through the mainstream media with public education campaigns. Many health promotion programs include the expectation that people invest in themselves. Do you invest in yourself with your daily activities to promote higher education, planned savings, healthy eating, regular exercise, deferred gratification, avoidance of smoking and excessive alcohol consumption, and regular physical checkups? Do you know people who seem to live only from one day to the next because their perspective of time is in the immediate and they do not seem to recognize the benefits of setting priorities and long-term planning?

what is expected of their coworkers, what is happening on the other shifts, and what is happening in this agency and the community. If the previous shift was stressed by a crisis, a shift may not get started as smoothly (Hansten & Washburn, 1998). If areas outside of the unit are overwhelmed, someone might be moved from a unit to assist on the overwhelmed unit elsewhere in the hospital. When nurses take the big picture into consideration, they are less likely to be frustrated when asked to assist others and more likely to avoid time wasters. See Table 12-1. They can also build into their time management plan the possibility of giving and receiving assistance.

TABLE 12-1
TIME WASTERS

Are you a time waster? We all sometimes behave in ways that sabotage the best of plans. Following are some examples of time wasters along with some strategies to help you reclaim those wasted hours.

1. Clutter: Wisdom holds that you can save 1 hour each day just by clearing your work area of clutter and keeping it clean. Organize your work area and take a few minutes at the end of your shift to prepare it for the next shift.

2. Interruptions: Intrusions into your work time (from either people or things) can be real time wasters. Try the following:
   • Learn to say "no." You do not have to agree to every request. Learn to pick your involvements carefully and pick those that are most important to reaching your goals.
   • Put your answering machine on at home and turn the telephone's ringer off. Delegate a time to listen and respond to messages.
   • Open your mail over the garbage can. Respond, delegate, or throw it out.
   • Organize your papers. Keep your notebooks, calendar, and telephone lists in one three-ring binder so you have your essentials together.

3. Procrastination: This refers to intentionally putting off or delaying something that should be done. Procrastination is a time waster because it does not afford effective use of time. Time management is not necessarily finishing everything at one sitting, but, rather, scheduling time to return to the task until you complete it; whereas procrastination is intentionally delaying the task without good cause or a plan to complete it in a time-efficient manner. Breaking the task down into manageable segments and rewards will encourage you to return to it again and again until it is complete.

4. Perfectionism: Very often we do not stick to a plan because it does not give us immediate results or the results we expected. Perfectionism affects your time-management plan by prohibiting you from accepting anything less than perfection; it also damages your positive attitude by setting unrealistic expectations of yourself. Focus on your positive accomplishments, look for ways to improve, accept your failures, and build on your experiences. Avoiding time wasters will help you achieve excellence. You want to achieve excellence, not perfection! (See Table 12-2.)

White, L. (2002). *Critical Thinking in Practical/Vocational Nursing.* Clifton Park, NY: Delmar Learning.

TABLE 12-2
BEHAVIORS OF PERFECTIONISTS AND PURSUERS OF EXCELLENCE

Perfectionists	Pursuers of Excellence
• Reach for impossible goals	• Enjoy meeting high standards within reach
• Value themselves for what they do	• Value themselves for who they are
• Get depressed and give up	• Experience disappointment but keep going
• Are devastated by failure	• Learn from failure
• Remember mistakes and dwell on them	• Correct mistakes, then learn from them
• Can only live with being number 1	• Are pleased with knowing they did their best
• Hate criticism	• Welcome criticism
• Have to win to maintain high self-esteem	• Do not have to win to maintain high self-esteem

White, L. (2002) *Critical Thinking in Practical/Vocational Nursing.* Clifton Park, NY: Delmar Learning.

Decide on Priority Outcomes

Nurses maximize their resources for safe patient care delivery by prioritizing their activities to achieve safe patient outcomes. Priority setting is one of the most critical skills a nurse must develop. Nurses determine priorities by applying the nursing process, assessing the patient, and making a nursing diagnosis then planning, implementing, and evaluating patient care. This is an ongoing process, calling for constant reassessment and reprioritization of patient care needs.

Differentiating between problems needing immediate attention and those that can wait requires great skill and judgment (Castledine, 2002). If the nurse does not prioritize care, a patient's problems may be missed and then the patient may become even more difficult to manage. Priorities should be set based on the patient's condition and responses to health care problems and treatments. Being flexible in prioritizing is a key to success because the patient's status may be continuously changing.

Vacarro (2001) states that prioritizing has several traps that nurses should avoid. See Table 12-3.

Frequently, nurses act on the "doing whatever hits first" trap. This means that a nurse may respond to things that happen first. For example, a nurse at the beginning of the day shift chooses to fill out the preoperative checklist for a patient going to surgery the next day rather than assess the rest of his or her patients first.

The second trap is "taking the path of least resistance." In this trap nurses may make a flawed assumption that it is easier to do a task rather than delegate it when they could be

TABLE 12-3
PRIORITIZING TRAPS TO AVOID

Doing whatever hits first

Taking the path of least resistance

Responding to the squeaky wheel

Completing tasks by default

Relying on misguided inspiration

Compiled with information from "Five Priority-Setting Traps," by P. J. Vaccaro, 2001, *Family Practice Management, 8*(4), p. 60. Adapted with permission.

completing another task that only nurses can complete. For example, a nurse who is admitting a patient needs to take the patient's vital signs and weight, complete the baseline assessment, and call the doctor for orders. The first two tasks can be delegated to a UAP so that the nurse may complete the baseline assessment of the patient and then call the doctor for orders.

The third trap is "responding to the squeaky wheel," wherein nurses feel compelled to respond to whatever need has been vocalized the loudest. In this case, the nurse may choose to respond to a family member who has come to the nursing station every half hour with some concern. To appease the family, the nurse may take time to focus on one of their many verbal concerns and overlook a more pressing patient need elsewhere.

The fourth trap is called "completing tasks by default." This trap occurs when nurses feel obligated to complete tasks that no one else will complete. A common example of this trap is emptying the garbage when it is full instead of asking housekeeping to do it.

The last trap is "relying on misguided inspiration." The classic example of this trap is when nurses feel "inspired" to document findings in the chart and avoid doing a higher priority responsibility. Unfortunately, some tasks will never become inspiring and need discipline, conscientiousness, and hard work to complete them.

Considerations in Setting Priorities

Priorities are established by nurses using Maslow's Hierarchy of Needs while considering the patients' immediate and short- and long-term goals and the importance and urgency of each patient care activity. Short-term goals are those that need to be met within 1 to 24 hours. Long-term goals are those that need to be met after 24 hours but usually prior to discharge. See Table 12-4.

Once nurses have decided on priority outcomes, they must consider what else can and should be achieved given less than optimal circumstances and limited resources. These circumstances could include a rough start to a busy shift; personnel who are late, absent, or uncooperative; and a patient crisis. If someone has called in sick and no replacement is available, it might be unreasonable for a nurse to plan to reinforce teaching or discuss the home environment with a patient scheduled to leave the next day. However, there would be no question that interventions that prevent life-threatening emergencies

TABLE 12-4
SETTING PRIORITIES FOR SAFE PATIENT OUTCOMES

- First Priority—Remember Maslow's (1970) Hierarchy of Human Needs. Assess physiological needs first. See high-priority unstable patients who have any threats to their ABCs first (i.e., airway, breathing, and circulation). These patients require nursing assessment, judgment, and evaluation until transfer or stabilization. Life-threatening conditions can occur at any time during the shift and may or may not be anticipated. Remember that all equipment and observations used to support and monitor the status of patients' ABCs are also a high monitoring priority (e.g., monitoring suicide threats, vital signs, level of consciousness, neurological status, skin color and temperature, pain, IV access, cardiac monitor, oxygen, suction, urine output, etc.).

- Second Priority—Next, assess Maslow's second level of human needs, (i.e., safety and security). Are there any threats to patient safety and security such as violence threats, need for fall prevention, infection control, and so on? See these patients next.

- Third Priority—Assess the patients' other needs and prioritize using Maslow's Hierarchy of Human Needs. These patient needs may include love and belonging, self-esteem, and self-actualization. What does the nursing and medical plan of care include (i.e., comfort, ambulation, positioning, etc.)? Stable patients who need standard, unchanging procedures and have predictable outcomes are seen last.

REAL WORLD INTERVIEW

I am sometimes assigned to work in the triage section where patients are seen when they first enter the Emergency Department (ED). It can really be nerve wracking at times, with everyone needing or wanting to be cared for immediately. The principles of setting priorities really come in handy in this situation. I decide which patient will be cared for in the ED based on priorities. If a patient has a life-threatening threat to their ABCs, such as an asthma attack, chest pain, significant alteration in vital signs, or significant bleeding, I arrange for this patient to be cared for immediately. My next priority is to assure safety for my patients. I constantly monitor all the patients in the triage area of the ED until they can be seen. I want to be sure that their condition remains stable and that they are safe while waiting to be seen. I also think it is important to keep the patients who are waiting informed as to how patients are seen and cared for in the ED. When patients see that we care for them based on how ill they are, they don't seem to mind waiting as much when someone who is sicker than them is cared for first. Of course, they all want to be cared for reasonably quickly. That is my goal also!

Patricia Kelly-Heidenthal, RN

CASE STUDY 12-1

The charge nurse on a 24-bed orthopedic unit assigned each nurse on the day shift four patients. Sylvia, R.N., had just finished her 5-month orientation period on the unit. The charge nurse asked Sylvia how she felt about coming off orientation today. Sylvia stated, "I am comfortable with the procedures, routines, and doctor interactions. I am still having trouble prioritizing what I should do first." The charge nurse assured her that her lack of experience probably had a lot to do with her difficulty prioritizing. The charge nurse went to her locker and gave Sylvia a handy little prioritizing chart that the charge nurse has had since she graduated from nursing school. She told Sylvia how this quick little reference chart helped her in situations when she was unsure of priorities. Sylvia was grateful for the chart and she used it that day. See Table 12-5.

Sylvia was assigned four patients. Patient 1 is a stable 34-year-old male, Jerry Dougherty, admitted 4 hours ago after a multivehicle accident. He is diagnosed with a fracture of the right tibia. The fracture was placed in a Thomas splint with a Pearson attachment. Mr. Dougherty has required frequent pain medication but is comfortable now.

The second patient is a 17-year-old young man, Frank Smith, who had a posttraumatic cervical spine fusion performed 3 days ago. He states that he will not wear the prescribed cervical brace after he leaves the hospital.

The third patient is a 63 year-old woman, Moira Hack, who had her left knee replaced 4 days ago and is supposed to be discharged today. The nursing assistant has reported that Ms. Hack had just fallen in the bathroom and is short of breath.

The last patient on Sylvia's team is a stable 76-year-old man, Frank Glowacki, who was admitted 1 day ago with a diagnosis of cancer of the spine. He is scheduled for a chemotherapy medication port to be inserted at 2 p.m. today. Using the priority chart in Table 12-5, determine who Sylvia will see first at the start of the shift.

(continues)

Case Study 12-1 *(continued)*

TABLE 12-5
PRIORITY CHART

Patient's Diagnosis	Maslow's Hierarchy of Needs:	Goals:	Priority:	Total:
	1 - physiological 2 - safety 3 - love and belonging, self-esteem, self-actualization	1 - immediate 2 - short term 3 - long term	1 - critical 2 - necessary 3 - not essential	The patient with the lowest total score is seen first by the nurse.
Mr. Dougherty: Fractured tibia, 4 hours post admit, pain controlled now	2	2	2	6
Mr. Smith: Cervical fusion, 3 days postop, refusing brace use at home	2	2	3	7
Ms. Hack: Knee replacement, 4 days postop, just fell, short of breath	1	1	1	3
Mr. Glowacki: Cancer of spine, port insertion today	2	2	3	7

Based on the total points, Moira Hack, the patient with the knee replacement who was short of breath and had fallen, needs to be assessed by Sylvia first. Based on the priority chart, Mr. Dougherty, the patient with the fractured tibia should be assessed next.

Were you torn between the patient who has had many pain management needs and the patient who was short of breath and fell on the floor? Was it because you thought the nursing assistant should help the patient back to bed? Remember that a nurse must assess the patient to determine any injury and why the patient fell. Perhaps the fall was caused by a slippery floor, or the patient may have experienced hypotension, weakness, disorientation, pulmonary embolism, hypoglycemia, brain attack, or a myocardial infarction. The nurse must therefore, assess this patient first and ensure patient safety.

or save a life when a life-threatening event occurs are priorities. They must be done no matter how short the staffing. It is high priority that nurses protect their patients and maintain both patient and staff safety as well as perform important nursing activities.

Covey, Merrill, and Merrill (1994) developed another way of setting priorities. Activities are classified as:

- Urgent or not urgent
- Important or not important

If an activity is neither important nor urgent, then it becomes the lowest priority.

Some activities that are often thought of as important may not be. Sometimes laboratory data, vital signs, and intake and output reports are ordered more frequently than the status of the patient indicates. Frequent monitoring of these parameters when a patient is stable may make no significant difference in patient outcomes. When nurses begin their shifts, they should question the activities that make no difference in outcomes (Hansten & Washburn, 1998). If a physician orders these activities, a nurse should work to get the order changed. If

there is a nursing policy and procedure or order that does not make a difference in patient care, the nurse should work to change it. Nurses should give priority to the activities that they know are going to make a difference in patient outcomes. Table 12-6 can be useful in setting priorities.

Shift Report as a Tool for Making Assignments

Before a plan is made for the shift, the shift report at best can lead to a smooth and effective start to the shift. At worst it can leave the oncoming shift members with inadequate or old data on which to base their plan. There are several ways to give the end of shift report—a face-to-face meeting, audiotaping, and walking rounds (Table 12-7).

Whether the report is conducted face to face, via audiotape, or through walking rounds, information has to be transmitted to allow for the effective and efficient implementation of

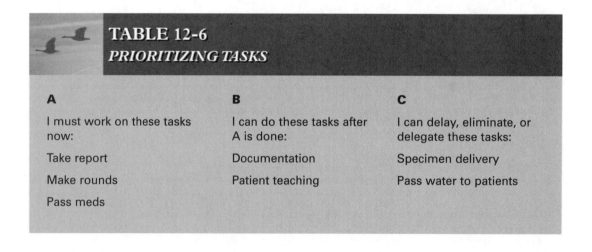

TABLE 12-6
PRIORITIZING TASKS

A	B	C
I must work on these tasks now:	I can do these tasks after A is done:	I can delay, eliminate, or delegate these tasks:
Take report	Documentation	Specimen delivery
Make rounds	Patient teaching	Pass water to patients
Pass meds		

TABLE 12-7
CHANGE OF SHIFT REPORTS: ADVANTAGES AND DISADVANTAGES

Method of Shift Report	Advantages	Disadvantages
Face-to-face report	• Nurses get clarification and can ask questions. • Nurse giving report has actual audience and tends to be less mechanical. • Nurses are more likely to give pertinent information than they would give to a tape recorder.	• It is time consuming. • It is easy to get sidetracked and gossip or discuss nonpatient-related business. • Both oncoming and departing nurses are in report. • Patients are not included in planning.
Audiotaped report	• Report is brief due to lack of interruptions by questions and comments. • Departing shift tapes report for oncoming shift prior to arrival of new shift workers. • Previous shift can provide care while oncoming shift gets report.	• Variables in the taping process such as the quality of tape and machine, the clarity and diction of the nurse who is recording, and the hearing of the oncoming shift can interfere with the communication. • It is difficult to get questions answered. The nurse must find the caregiver after report to ask questions. • Information is taped earlier in the shift and may no longer be accurate. • There is sometimes not enough information given due to the tendency of person talking into tape recorder to read from kardex instead of explaining about patient.

(continues)

Table 12-7 *(continued)*

Method of Shift Report	Advantages	Disadvantages
Walking rounds	• Provides the prior shift and oncoming shift staff the opportunity to observe the patient while receiving report. Staff can address any assessment or treatment questions. • Information is accurate and timely. • Patient is included in the planning and evaluation of care. • Accountability of outgoing care provider is promoted. • Patient views the continuity of care. • Oncoming shift makes initial nursing rounds with prior shift. • Departing nurse can show assessment and treatment data directly to oncoming nurse.	• It is time consuming. • There is a lack of privacy in discussing patient information.

care. If the outgoing nurse fails to cover all pertinent points, the oncoming shift must ask for the appropriate information. See Table 12-8 for a tool for taking and giving reports.

During or after report, the nurse can complete an assignment sheet or a written or computerized plan that sets the priorities for the shift and makes assignments to team members (Figure 12-3). Assignments should include specific reporting guidelines and deadlines for accomplishment of the tasks.

Make Patient Care Rounds

When nurses make patient care rounds, they perform rapid assessments of each patient. The information that is gathered on rounds may change the nurses' plans. They might get information that increases the need for patient monitoring. It is important to remember that plans are just that, plans, and have to be flexible based on ever-changing patient care needs.

STOP AND THINK

You are making rounds on your patients. Which types of patients have top-priority needs? Note the examples of top-priority patients below. What would your approach to these top-priority patients be?

Top-priority patient care groups

Respiratory	• Airway compromise
	• Severe respiratory distress, inadequate breathing
	• Critical asthma
	• Chest trauma with respiratory distress
Cardiovascular	• Cardiac arrest
	• Shock or hypotension
	• Exsanguinating hemorrhage
Neurological	• Major head injury
	• Unconscious or unresponsive
	• Active seizure state
Musculoskeletal (MSK)	• Major trauma
	• Traumatic amputation—extremity
	• Major cold injury—hypothermia
Skin	• Burn, >25% body surface area (BSA) or airway involvement
Gastrointestinal (GI)	• Difficulty swallowing, with airway or respiratory compromise
	• Abdominal trauma, penetrating or blunt
Gynecological (GYN)	• Vaginal bleeding, patient with abnormal vital signs
Hematologic/Immunologic (HEM/IMMUN)	• Anaphylaxis
Endocrine (ENDO)	• Diabetic—altered consciousness
Infection (INF)	• Septic shock
Child or elder abuse	• Unstable situation or conflict

Compiled with information from the Canadian Paediatric Triage and Acuity Scale: Implementation Guidelines for Emergency Departments. Retrieved from *http://www.caep.ca*

TABLE 12-8
TOOL FOR TAKING/GIVING REPORT

Patient room number Name Sex Physician Admit Date Surgery Date	
Primary and secondary diagnoses Nursing and medical	
Patient's current vital signs, lab work, diet, medications, IV fluids Oxygen saturation Pain score, intake and output Skin condition, fall risk, ambulation	
Signs/symptoms of potential complications Patient/family concerns New orders, or medications, or lab work, or changes in treatment/teaching plan	
Priority outcomes and interventions for priority nursing diagnoses Patient learning outcomes	
Expected date of discharge Referrals needed Progress toward outcomes and readiness for home	

Times for treatments and medications may have to be changed. Often nurses believe that the times for administering medication are inflexible, yet physicians usually write medication orders as daily, twice a day, three times a day, or four times a day. These kinds of orders give nurses flexibility in administration times. Although unit policy dictates when these medicines are given, unit policy is under nursing control.

Room Name	Patient Description	Special Needs and Outcomes	Assignment * All to report outcomes to Mary, RN at 8:30 P.M. -Report abnormals stat
1. Ms. J. D.	68-year-old female, Postop day 1 Post shoulder repair Confused Fall risk	Up in chair at 6 P.M. Vitals 4 P.M. and 8 P.M. Check distal pulse Posey, monitor LOC Check dressings 4 P.M. and 8 P.M Check voiding 6 P.M.	Mary, RN, charge nurse
2. Mr. D. B.	45-year-old male diabetic Postop day 1 Right below the knee amputee Insulin sliding scale c/o pain—restless	Accuchek stat and 9 P.M. Up in chair 6 P.M. Vitals 4 P.M. and 8 P.M. Pain medication as needed Monitor dressing	Cindy, LPN
3. Mr. J. K.	35-year-old male IV-5% Dextrose in water at 125 cc/hour Alert Hematemesis of coffee-ground fluid at 3 P.M. Hx of ETOH abuse c/o Abdominal pain	Vitals hourly Monitor hematemesis Monitor IV, LOC Monitor seizures Insert #16 IV catheter T&C Possible transfer to ICU	Jerry, RN

Figure 12-3 Assignment Sheet

REAL WORLD INTERVIEW

Ms. DuBose underwent elective surgery this summer. When asked about nurses and time management, she said, "The nurses that cared for me were always going back to the station to get something. It took three trips to get me my pain medication. If they had asked me when I requested the pain medication what I thought I needed, checked the order carefully, and brought the shot with an alcohol swab, they would have saved two extra trips and 30 minutes."

Ina DuBose

Patient

LITERATURE APPLICATION

Citation: Benner, P. (1984). *From novice to expert: Excellence and power in clinical nursing practice* (pp. 151–161). Menlo Park, CA: Addison-Wesley.

Discussion: Patricia Benner's work is a classic. It addresses issues faced by beginning nurses who struggle with time management issues and explains how expert nurses deal with time management using contingency planning.

Benner's study of how nurses cope with staffing shortages found that nurses who continuously respond to the challenge of each situation frequently end up feeling that they fail to meet their patients' needs in a timely manner. They lack two important sources of job satisfaction—interpersonal connection and a sense of accomplishment and competency that comes from meeting patients' needs when they need it. Nurses who work successfully and who consistently deal with a heavy workload develop a system of contingency planning that allows them to meet their patients' needs in a timely manner. This contingency planning includes rapidly assessing patient needs and setting and shifting priorities. They continuously evaluate routine standards and procedures. Standard priorities include attending to radically abnormal vital signs, signs and symptoms of respiratory or circulatory compromise, intravenous medications running dry, and intravenous medication administration. But even these priorities can be shifted when a patient on the unit actually is in a crisis. Expert nurses learn to anticipate and prevent periods of extreme workload within a shift.

Implications for Practice: This study emphasizes the importance of new nursing graduates learning to prioritize care and finding the human connection and a sense of competency and accomplishment in their work. Benner quotes a nurse who left nursing because of the lack of time to truly care for his patients. Often nurses leave practice before they develop time management skills that allow them to prioritize care and develop shift contingency plans.

Evaluate Outcome Achievement

At the end of the shift, the nurse reexamines the assignment sheet. Did the patient achieve the outcomes? If not, why? Were there staffing problems or patient crises? What was learned from this for future shifts?

FIND PERSONAL TIME FOR LIFELONG LEARNING

Finding time for lifelong learning and maintaining a balance with family, school, and work is a struggle for recent graduates and even more-seasoned nurses.

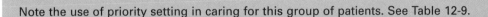

CASE STUDY 12-2

Note the use of priority setting in caring for this group of patients. See Table 12-9.

TABLE 12-9
PRIORITY SETTING IN CARING FOR PATIENTS, GROUP I

Patient	Priority Nursing Assessments
Ms. J. D. is a 68-year-old who is postop day 1 after a total shoulder replacement following a traumatic fall. She is confused and on multiple medications and has a history of hypertension and multiple falls. She is anxious and frightened by the "visiting spirits."	Vital signs, safety, distal pulse, incision/dressing check, breath sounds. See this patient third during rounds.
Mr. D. B. is a 55-year-old with insulin-dependent diabetes mellitus, juvenile onset at age 12. He is postop day 2 after a right below-the-knee amputation. He complains of severe right leg pain and is restless. Mr. D. B. has a history of noncompliance with diet and is on sliding scale insulin administration.	Glucoscan at 4 p.m. and 9 p.m., safety, incision/dressing check, pain, DB teaching. See this patient second during rounds.
Mr. J. K. is a 35-year-old patient with a history of alcohol abuse admitted for severe abdominal pain. He is throwing up coffee-ground-like emesis.	Level of consciousness, seizure and shock potential, hematemesis, DTs, safety, vital signs, CBC, hematocrit, type and cross-match, 16 gauge IV line for possible blood transfusion, oxygen, cardiac monitor. See this patient first during rounds.

(continues)

Case Study 12-1 *(continued)*

Now, identify the priority nursing assessments for this next group of patients. See Table 12-10.

TABLE 12-10
PRIORITY PATIENT ASSESSMENTS, GROUP II

Patient	Priority Nursing Assessments
Ms. H. M. is an 85-year-old patient who was transferred from a nursing home because of dehydration. She is vomiting and has abdominal pain of unknown etiology. Intravenous hydration continues and a workup is planned. Ms. H. M. is alert and oriented.	
Mr. A. B. is a 72-year-old patient who is status post cerebral vascular accident. He is to be transferred to rehabilitation. He needs his belongings gathered and a nursing summary written.	
Ms. V. G. is an 82-year-old patient who is postop five days after an open reduction of a femur fracture. She has a history of congestive heart failure, hypertension, and takes multiple medications. Her temperature is elevated. She is confused.	

There are many ways to achieve one's dreams, work, and have a personal life. Flaherty (1998) offers tips for balancing school, family, and work in Table 12-11.

TABLE 12-11
MAINTAINING BALANCE IN LIFE WHEN RETURNING TO SCHOOL

1. Let your employer know that you are interested in returning to school. Most employers are supportive of additional education and will be flexible with your schedule. But they will continue to expect a competent, dedicated employee.

2. Develop computer skills. By using a computer, you can e-mail professors and classmates at any time. You can do on-line research. You can easily incorporate constructive criticisms into papers and build on previous work. Technology is the working student's friend.

3. Discover a flexible, educational program. Many programs offer several classes in a row on a single day, weekend and night classes, or weeklong immersion classes. Some programs offer distance learning opportunities.

4. Do not be surprised by the demands of school. Courses will be difficult and demanding of time. Remember that you have faced difficult demands and challenges before. Use the same techniques that helped you in the past.

5. Solicit support from family and friends. They can offer emotional support as well as child care.

6. Use all available resources at the school and at work. Develop mentors and role models. Establish relationships with faculty. Discover and use academic support services such as writing centers and tutors. Read syllabi and course instructions carefully.

7. Focus on the outcome. Keep the end in sight and do not give up. Take it one course at a time. Reward yourself along the way. When a course is completed, celebrate.

8. Be careful of the sacrifices. You may replace some hobbies with school. But save some time for the things that are really meaningful to you and your family and friends.

9. Manage time. Ten minutes spent on planning saves time and energy later. Keep your sense of humor.

10. Take care of yourself and your responsibilities. Set aside a day to take care of personal chores and errands.

11. If you need a break, take one. Take time to reflect on what you are accomplishing. If you are feeling overwhelmed, take only one course or take a semester off.

12. Study on the run. Taping lectures and listening to them as you commute is a great way to study on the run.

Adapted from "The Juggling Act: 10 Tips for Balancing Work, School, and Family," by M. Flaherty, *Nurseweek*, retrieved July 15, 2000, from http://www.nurseweek.com

KEY CONCEPTS

- General time management strategies include having an outcomes orientation, analyzing time cost and use, focusing on priorities, and visualizing the big picture.
- Shift planning begins with developing priority outcomes.
- There are three alternatives for shift reports: face-to-face meetings, audiotaped reports, and walking rounds.
- Implementing an assignment sheet includes patient rounds and setting the times for monitoring, treatments, and outcome achievement.
- The assignment sheet is evaluated at the end of the shift by determining whether priority outcomes have been achieved.
- Time wasters that might interfere with outcome achievement include procrastination, inability to delegate, inability to say no, interruptions, perfectionism, and disorganization.
- Time management applies to one's personal life as well as one's job.
- Quality time can be achieved by analyzing time use and setting priorities.
- Delegating and getting up 1 hour earlier can create time for individuals.
- Efficient use can be made of travel and waiting time.
- Distractions can be controlled by making your environment less inviting, by using voice mail or an answering machine, by saying no, and by encouraging others to be independent.
- It is possible to balance work, family, and school.

 KEY TERMS

activity log   time management
Parento principle

 REVIEW QUESTIONS

1. All of the following are general time management techniques EXCEPT
   A. allowing distractions.
   B. outcomes orientation.
   C. time analysis.
   D. focus on priorities.

2. Today you get out of patient report late, your nursing assistant has not arrived, one of your patients is being transferred to the intensive care unit, and you are getting an admission into the bed that your transfer patient is vacating. What outcomes will you work toward for the shift?
   A. None. The situation is hopeless.
   B. Perfect outcomes. There is never an excuse not to do your best.
   C. Minimal outcomes. We can accomplish little today.
   D. Priority outcomes. We can be safe and effective.

3. Which of the following is the most efficient and effective way to give the shift report?
   A. Audiotaped report
   B. Walking rounds
   C. Face-to-face meeting
   D. Any of the above

4. Personal productivity can be enhanced by
   A. analyzing time, getting up an hour early, delegating unwanted tasks.
   B. getting up an hour early, answering your phone, and inviting a friend in to talk.
   C. analyzing use of time, getting up early, waiting patiently.
   D. limiting working and going to school at the same time.

REVIEW ACTIVITIES

1. For the next 3 days, complete an activity log for both your personal time and your work time. On what activities are you spending the majority of time? When is your energy level the highest? Is your energy level related to food intake or anythig else?

   - What are your biggest time wasters?

   - What are your distractions from outcome achievement?

2. Use Table 12-8 to organize your report.

3. Use Table 12-6 to prioritize your personal and work activities.

EXPLORING THE WEB

- If you would like to find a system for managing your time, the following Web sites offer electronic organizers (e.g., Personal Digital Assistant, Palm Pilot, Casio electronic organizer, Sharp electronic organizer):
  http://www.casio.com
  http://www.sharp-usa. com
  http://www.palm.com
- If you prefer a less technological time management system, the following Web sites offer non-electronic organizers and systems for time management (e.g., Day-Timer, Franklin Covey):
  http://www.daytimer.com
  http://www.covey.com
  http://www.franklin.com
- Want a free on-line calendar that you can access from anywhere?
  http://calendar. yahoo.com

- Look at all the hints and free tools on time management at the Mind Tools Web site. Can you put any of the ideas to use?
  http://www.mindtools.com
- If you find time management an impossible challenge, you can find professional assistance at the Professional Organizers Web site. *http://www.organizerswebring.com*

REFERENCES

Benner, P. (1984). *From novice to expert: Excellence and power in clinical nursing practice.* Menlo Park, CA: Addison-Wesley.

Burke, T. A., McKee, J. R., Wilson, H. C., Donahue, R. M., Batenhorst, A. S., & Pathak, D. S. (2000). A comparison of time-and-motion and self-reporting methods of work measurement. *Journal of Nursing Administration, 30*(3), 118–125.

Castledine, G. (2002). Prioritizing care is an essential nursing skill. *British Journal of Nursing, 11*(14), 987.

Covey, S. R., Merrill, A. R., & Merrill, R. R. (1994). *First things first: To love, to learn, to leave a legacy.* New York: Simon & Schuster.

Flaherty, M. (1998). The juggling act: 10 tips for balancing work, school, and family. *Nurseweek.* Retrieved July 15, 2000, from http://www.nurseweek.com

Fryxell, D. A. (1997). The 80% solution. *Writer's Digest, 77*(5), 57.

Graham, A. (1998). The vital few, the trivial many. *Internal Auditor, 55*(6), 6.

Grohar-Murray, M. E., & DiCroce, H. R. (1997). Managing Resources. In M. E. Grohar-Murray (Ed.), *Leadership and management in nursing* (2nd ed., pp. 291–315). Norwalk, CT: Appleton & Lange.

Hansten, R. I., & Washburn, M. J. (1998). *Clinical delegation skills: A handbook for professional practice.* Gaithersburg, MD: Aspen.

King, C. S. (1996). The politics of advanced practice: An interview with Roxanne Spitzer-Lehmann. *Advanced Practice Nursing Quarterly, 4*, 36–38.

Koch, R. (1999). *The 80/20 principle: The secret to success by achieving more with less.* New York: Doubleday.

Leddy, S., & Pepper, J. M. (1998). *Conceptual bases of professional nursing* (4th ed.). Philadelphia: Lippincott.

Maslow, A. H. (1970). *New knowledge in human values.* Washington, DC: Regency Publishing.

Mind Tools (n.d.-a). Creating extra hours—get up early! Retrieved September 5, 2000, from http://www. mindtools.com

Mind Tools (n.d.-b). How to achieve more with your time. Retrieved September 5, 2000, from http://www.mindtools.com

Prescott, P. A., Phillips, C. Y., Ryan, J. W., & Thompson, K. O. (1991). Changing how nurses spend their time. *Image: Journal of Nursing Scholarship, 23*(1), 23–28.

Scharf, L. (1997). Revising nursing documentation to meet patient outcomes. *Nursing Management, 28*(4), 38–39.

Sullivan, E. J., & Decker, P. J. (2001). *Effective leadership and management in nursing* (5th ed.). Menlo Park, CA: Addison-Wesley.

Tappen, R. M. (2001). *Nursing leadership and management: Concepts and practice* (4th ed.). Philadelphia: F. A. Davis.

Upenieks, V. B. (1998). Work sampling: Assessing nursing efficiency. *Nursing Management, 49*(4), 27–29.

Urden, L., & Roode, J. (1997). Work sampling: A decision-making tool for determining resources and work redesign. *Journal of Nursing Administration, 27*(9), 34–41.

Vacarro, P. J. (2001, April). Five priority-setting traps. *Family Practice Management, 8*(4), 60.

SUGGESTED READINGS

Anderson, L. A. (2001). Reality research: Project time management and recruitment. *Journal of Vascular Nursing, 4,* 137–138.

Bly, R. W. (1999). *101 ways to make every second count: Time management tips and techniques for more success with less stress.* New York: Career Press.

Brink, P. J. (2000). I'm too busy. *Western Journal of Nursing Research, 22*(4), 383.

Cericola, S. A. (2000). Time/stress management techniques. *Plastic Surgical Nursing, 20*(1), 48–49.

Dawes, B. S. (1999). Perspectives on priorities, time management, and patient care. *AORN Journal, 70*(3), 374–377.

Duffy, B. (1999). Organizing thoughts about time management. *Home Healthcare Nurse Manager, 6,* 14–17.

Folan, D. (1999). *Time management, world of Irish nursing by Irish Nurses Organization.* Retrieved September 10, 2000, from http://www.ino.ie.

Hemphill, B. (2000). 10 tips to beat post-travel clutter. *Nursing Management, 31*(6), 57.

Hindle, T. (1999). *Essential Managers: Manage Your Time.* London: DK.

Morgenstern, J. (2000). *Time management from the inside out: The foolproof system for taking control of your schedule—and your life.* New York: Henry Holt.

CHAPTER 13

Every act whatever of man that causes damage to another obliges him whose fault it happened to repair it. . . .(La. Civil Code art. 2315)

Legal Aspects of Patient Care

OBJECTIVES

Upon completion of this chapter, the reader should be able to:

1. Discuss the sources of law.

2. Name various federal administrative agencies and their areas of influence.

3. Name the most common areas of nursing practice cited in malpractice actions.

4. List some actions a nurse can take to minimize malpractice risk.

You are working on a geriatric nursing unit when you admit an 82-year-old female, Mrs. Perkins. She has a broken hip and many bruises and skin tears. The family with whom she is living tells you she is confused and falls often. While you are bathing Mrs. Perkins, she begins crying and tells you her grandson pushed her down the stairs and that he often hits her if she does not give him money. She says her daughter does not believe her if she says anything and she is afraid if she complains she will have no one to care for her.

Do you need any additional information to determine the validity of Mrs. Perkins's statement?

If abuse has occurred, what action should you take?

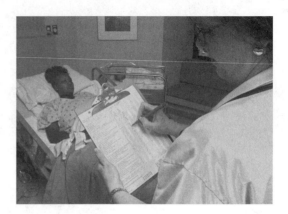

Do patient confidentiality concerns affect any actions you may take?

aw that affects the relationship between individuals is called civil law. Law that specifies the relationship between citizens and the state is called public law. This chapter reviews how various types of law affect nursing practice and actions a nurse can take to minimize risks to her professional practice.

SOURCES OF LAW

The authority to make, implement, and interpret laws is generally granted in a constitution. A **constitution** is a set of basic laws that specifies the powers of the various segments of the government and how these segments relate to each other.

Generally, it is the role of a legislative body, both on the federal and state levels, to enact laws. Agencies under the authority of the administrative branch of the government draft the rules that implement the law. Finally, the judicial branch interprets the law as it rules in court cases. Table 13-1 gives examples of these relationships.

Also, a judicial decision may set a precedent that is used by other courts and, over time, has the force of law. This type of law is referred to as **common law**.

Public Law

Public law consists of constitutional law, criminal law, and administrative law and defines a citizen's relationship with government.

Constitutional Law

Several categories of public law affect the practice of nursing. For example, the nurse accommodates patients' constitutional right to practice their religion every time the nurse calls a patient's clergy as requested, follows a specific religious custom for preparation of meals, or prepares a deceased person's remains for burial.

Controversial constitutional rights that may affect the nurse's practice include the recognized constitutional rights of a woman to have an abortion and an individual's right to die (see *Roe v. Wade* [1973] and *Cruzan v. Director* [1990]). Nurses may not believe in either of these rights personally and may refuse to work in areas where they would have to assist a patient in exercising these rights. Nurses may not, however, interfere with another person's right to have an abortion or to forgo lifesaving measures.

	Legislative Branch	Administrative Branch	Judicial Branch
TABLE 13-1 *THE THREE BRANCHES OF GOVERNMENT IN THE UNITED STATES*			
Example at federal level	Americans with Disabilities Act (ADA) (1990)	The Equal Employment Commission (EEOC) publishes rules specifying what employers must do to help a disabled employee.	In 1999, the U. S. Supreme Court interpreted the law to require that to be protected by this law, the individual must have an impairment that limits a major life activity and that is not corrected by medicine or appliances (glasses, blood pressure medicine) (*Sutton v. United Airlines* [1999]; *Murphy v. United Parcel Service, Inc.* [1999]).
Example at State Level	Nurse Practice Act	The state board of nursing develops rules specifying the duties of a registered nurse in that state.	Courts and juries determine whether a nurse's actions comply with the law governing the practice of nursing in a state.

Criminal Law

Criminal law focuses on the actions of individuals that can intentionally do harm to others. Often the victims of such abusive actions are the very young or the very old. These two categories of people generally cannot defend themselves against physical or emotional abuse. The nurse, in caring for patients, may notice that a vulnerable patient has unexplained bruises, fractures, or other injuries. Most states have mandatory statutes that require the nurse to report unexplained or suspicious injuries to the appropriate child or elderly protective agency. Generally, the institution where the nurse is employed will have clear guidelines to follow in such a situation. Failure to report the problem as required

by law can result in the nurse being fined for her inaction.

Another aspect of criminal law affecting nursing practice is the state and federal requirement that criminal background checks be performed on specified categories of prospective employees who will work with the very young or the elderly in institutions such as schools and nursing homes. Again, this is an attempt to protect the most vulnerable citizens from mistreatment or abuse. Failure to conduct the mandated background checks can result in the institution having to defend itself for any harm done by an employee with a past criminal conviction. A recent article related a case in which a hospital was found negligent for failing to conduct a criminal background check or investigate complaints against an employee who later sexually abused a patient (Fiesta, 1999c). However, in another case in which the hospital did investigate such complaints, the appellate court did not find it responsible for the sexual assault on a patient by an employee (Fiesta, 1999c). The rationale for this was that the hospital had done what it was required to do by law in investigating the employee's criminal background and was not liable for these unexpected actions.

The third area in which criminal law concerns affect nursing practice is the prohibition against substance abuse. Both federal and state law requires health care agencies to keep a strict accounting of the use and distribution of regulated drugs. Nurses routinely are expected to keep narcotic records accurate and current.

Nurses' behavior when off duty can also affect their employment status. Abusing alcohol or drugs on one's own time, if discovered, can result in nurses being terminated from employment and their license to practice nursing being restricted or revoked (Mantel, 1999). Frequently, boards of nursing have programs for the nurse with a drug problem, and completion of such a program may be required before the nurse can resume practice. Additionally, health care facilities may do random drug screens on their employees to identify those who may be using illegal substances.

Administrative Law

Both the federal government and state governments have administrative laws that affect nursing practice. The laws pertaining to Social Security and, more specifically, Medicare, are interpreted in the *Code of Federal Regulations*, which contains the administrative rules for the federal government. These rules have specific requirements that hospitals, nursing homes, and other health care providers must adhere to if they are to qualify for payment from federal funds. The Department of Health and Human Services is the federal agency that regulates hospitals and nursing homes. Likewise, state laws are interpreted in administrative rules that specify licensing requirements for health care providers in the state.

Federal Law. Administrative law deals with protection of the rights of citizens. It extends some rights and protections beyond those granted in the federal and state constitutions. An example of this type of law, at the federal level, is the Civil Rights Act of 1964, which prohibits many forms of discrimination in the workplace. This law may necessitate that the nurse manager make some scheduling accommodations for such things as an employee's religious practices.

STOP AND THINK

You work the afternoon shift in the ICU. You notice that when one particular nurse assigned to the afternoon shift is on duty, all of her patients receive narcotic pain medication at 4 P.M. This is true even when you have observed and documented that some of these patients have diminished responsiveness and no pain complaints when cared for by you or other nurses in the unit. Also, one of your patients complained to his doctor that the pain medication he received from this nurse "didn't work."

Given this scenario, what should you do as a nurse? What does your institution's policy and procedure manual say about this? How can you determine if your suspicions are accurate?

Another federal law that often affects employment in health care facilities is the Age Discrimination in Employment Act of 1967 (ADEA), which protects those 40 years of age and older by prohibiting employers from discriminating on the basis of age in all aspects of employment, including compensation, terms, conditions, and privileges. This law prohibits employers from using age as a factor in limiting or classifying people in any way that would deprive or tend to deprive them of employment opportunities or otherwise adversely affect their status (Nguyen, 2000b).

The Americans with Disabilities Act (ADA), another federal law, protects individuals with disabilities from discrimination-related employment practices. It protects people with a disability who otherwise meet the skill, experience, education, and other job-related requirements for a position of interest. If the applicant or worker is a qualified individual with a disability who can do the job in question, with or without a reasonable accommodation, then the individual has certain protected rights. These rights include the right to reasonable accommodation to perform the job; to be treated equally by the employer; and to be able to be promoted (Nguyen, 2000a).

Often, nurses must work with older people or people with disabilities who have different capabilities, judgments, and values, and they must be able to recognize and appreciate these differing perspectives and not be biased against the individuals because of these differences (Cofer, 1998). The Equal Employment Opportunity Commission is the federal agency that evaluates discrimination.

The Occupational Safety & Health Administration, an administrative agency, works to establish a safe workplace for employees. This includes enacting regulations concerning storage of hazardous substances; protection of employees from infection; and, recently, protection of employees from violence in the workplace. In a recent article, Sheehan noted that a physical attack may come from a coworker, a patient, or a family member and that the nurse must be alert for any warning that such a response is imminent. Some of the questions she suggests the nurse ask in evaluating the potential for violence in a patient include the following:

- Does the individual exhibit anger, irritation, or illogical thought processes?
- Does the patient exhibit confusion and agitation?
- Does the patient lack emotion or have a dull demeanor? (Sheehan, 2000)

These same observations would be valid for assessing the potential for violence in individuals other than patients.

State Law. An example of a state's administrative law is its nurse practice act. Under nurse practice acts, state boards of nursing are given the authority to define the practice of nursing within certain broad parameters specified by the legislature, mandate the requisite preparation for the practice of nursing, and discipline members of the profession who deviate from the rules governing the practice of nursing. Other professions such as medicine and dentistry have similar practice acts established in state law.

Currently, an issue that is affecting licensure of nursing is the multistate licensure compact, which affords mutual state recognition of nursing licenses.

Multistate Licensure Compact. The multistate licensure compact allows a nurse to have one license (in his or her state of residency) and to practice in other states (both physically and electronically), subject to each state's practice law and regulation. Under this mutual state licensure recognition, a nurse may practice across state lines unless otherwise restricted. Information about the multistate licensure compact is available at http://www.ncsbn.org. As of October 2002, 18 states had signed the compact.

Civil Law

Civil law governs how individuals relate to each other in everyday matters. It encompasses both contract and tort law. Most cases involving nurses fall into the category of civil tort law (Fiesta, 1999a).

Contract Law

Contract law regulates certain transactions between individuals and/or legal entities such as businesses. It also governs transactions between businesses. An agreement between two or more parties must contain the following elements to be recognized as a legal contract:

- Agreement between two or more legally competent individuals or parties stating what each must or must not do
- Mutual understanding of the terms and obligations that the contract imposes on each party to the contract
- Payment or consideration given for actions taken or not taken pursuant to the agreement

The terms of the contract may be oral or written; however, a written contract may not be legally modified by an oral agreement. Another way this is often expressed is by the phrase "all of the terms of the contract are contained within the four corners of the document"; that is, if it is not written, it is not part of the agreement or contract. A contract may be express or implied. In an express contract, the terms of the contract are specified, usually in writing. In an implied contract, a relationship between parties is recognized, although the terms of the agreement are not clearly defined, such as the expectations one has for services from the dry cleaner or the grocer.

The nurse is usually a party to an employment contract. The employed nurse agrees to do the following:

- Adhere to the policies and procedures of the employing entity
- Fulfill the agreed-upon duties of the employer
- Respect the rights and responsibilities of other health care providers in the workplace

In return, the employer agrees to provide the nurse with the following:

- A specified amount of pay for services rendered
- Adequate assistance in providing care
- The supplies and equipment needed to fulfill the nurse's responsibilities

- A safe environment in which to work
- Reasonable treatment and behavior from the other health care providers with whom the nurse must interact

This contract may be express or implied, depending on the practices of the employing entity. Sometimes, what is determined to be "reasonable" by the employer is not considered "reasonable" by the nurse. For instance, after 20 years of working as a nurse on the orthopedic unit, a nurse may not view it as reasonable to be pulled to the labor and delivery unit for duty as a nurse there. It would be prudent for this nurse to express any misgivings to the supervisor and then to cooperate but take only assignments that are in keeping with the responsibilities the nurse can safely complete. In this instance, it is reasonable to give nursing assistance on the labor and delivery unit that the nurse can competently deliver, although it may not be reasonable to assume total responsibility for these patients without additional education and experience.

Tort Law

Black's Law Dictionary (1996) defines tort as a private or civil wrong or injury, including action for bad faith breach of contract, for which the court will provide a remedy in the form of an action for damages. A tort can be any of the following:

- The denial of a person's legal right
- The failure to comply with a public duty
- The failure to perform a private duty that results in harm to another

A tort can be unintentional, as occurs in malpractice or neglect, or it can be the intentional infliction of harm such as assault and battery. In a tort suit, the nurse can be named as a defendant because of something the nurse did incorrectly or because the nurse failed to do something that was required. In either case, the suit is usually classified as a tort suit (Fiesta, 1999a). Other tort charges that a nurse may face include assault and battery, false imprisonment, invasion of privacy, defamation, and fraud.

Negligence and Malpractice. If a nurse fails to meet the legal expectations for care, usually defined by the state's nurse practice act, the patient, if harmed by this failure, can initiate an action against the nurse for damages. The term **malpractice** refers to a professional's wrongful conduct in the discharge of his or her professional duties or failure to meet standards of care for the profession, which results in harm to another individual entrusted to the professional's care (Zerwekh & Claborn, 2002). **Negligence** is the failure to provide the care a reasonable person would ordinarily provide in a similar situation.

Simply proving malpractice or negligence is not sufficient to recover damages. Proof of liability or fault requires the proof of the following four elements:

1. A duty or obligation created by law, contract, or standard practice that is owed to the complainant by the professional

2. A breach of this duty, either by omission or commission

3. Harm, which can be physical, emotional, or financial, to the complainant (patient)

4. Proof that the breach of duty caused the complained of harm

A Louisiana appellate court recently described the plaintiff's (patient's) specific burden of proof in a negligence or malpractice case against a nurse as follows:

[T]he three requirements which a plaintiff must satisfy to meet its burden of proving the negligence of a nurse are (1) the nurse must exercise the degree of skill ordinarily employed, under similar circumstances, by the members of the nursing or health care profession in good standing in the same community or locality; (2) the nurse either lacked this degree of knowledge or skill or failed to use reasonable care and diligence, along with her best judgment in the application of that skill; and (3) as a proximate result of this lack of knowledge or skill or the failure to exercise this degree of care, the plaintiff suffered injuries that would not otherwise have occurred. (*Odom v. State Dept. of Health & Hospitals* [1999])

Once a plaintiff presents his case, the defendant nurse must refute the claims either by showing that if a duty was owed, it was fulfilled or by demonstrating that the breach of that duty was not the cause of the plaintiff's harm.

Proving that a duty was owed is not difficult. The person need only show that the nurse was working on the day in question and was responsible for the plaintiff's care. This can usually be accomplished by producing staffing schedules and assignment sheets.

To demonstrate a breach of duty, the courts employ a *reasonable man* standard by asking what a reasonable nurse would do in a like situation. This is accomplished by reviewing the employing institution's policies and procedures and the state's nurse practice act and hearing testimony from nurses who are accepted as expert witnesses to the standard of nursing practice in the community.

The defendant nurse would employ the same methodology to refute the plaintiff's charges. The nurse would present evidence that the institution's policies and procedures were followed and that the care rendered adhered to accepted nursing standards. To present the nurse's case, the nurse's attorney would also use expert witnesses to document that the care given fulfilled the duty owed, was the kind that would be given by a reasonable nurse in such a circumstance, and that it was not the cause of the plaintiff's harm.

It is not sufficient for a patient plaintiff to show a breach of duty to prevail in a tort suit. He must also show that the breach of the duty caused him harm. Even if it is proved that a nurse made a medication error, if the error was not the cause of the plaintiff's harm, he will not win in recovering damages from the nurse. In a recent malpractice case, a patient with sickle cell anemia died after suffering a cardiopulmonary arrest, attributed to an aspiration that was witnessed by a visitor. The visitor immediately called for and obtained help. Although revived, the patient never regained consciousness and was eventually taken off life support. At trial, the plaintiff was able to prove that the nurse assigned to this patient did not follow the institution's policy of documenting frequent observations, which were mandated because the patient was receiving a blood transfusion at the time of the cardiac arrest. In reviewing the case on appeal, the appellate court noted the following:

[T]he record contains no evidence which suggests what could have been done even if the nurse had been seated at his bedside prior to the arrest. Plaintiff has failed to offer any proof that more immediate assistance would have prevented the catastrophic results of his aspiration. Based on the evidence in this record, we conclude that more frequent monitoring would have made no difference. (*Webb v. Tulane Medical Center Hospital* [1997])

Thus, even though the plaintiff successfully proved a breach of a duty, the breach was not found to be the cause of the patient's death, and the nurse was not found to be guilty of negligence. Table 13-2 reviews types of nursing actions involved in litigation reported in the *Professional Negligence Law Reporter*, July 2001 through July 2002 (Pozza, 2003). Table 13-3 identifies the clinical settings of these malpractice cases, and Table 13-4 identifies health care facility liabilities other than nursing actions identified in these cases.

When a nurse is listed as a party in a medical malpractice lawsuit, the nurse's liability is determined by state laws, such as the nurse practice act, the standards for the practice of nursing, and the institution's policies and procedures. Thus, if laws mandate that a nurse must have a doctor's order before doing something, then a

TABLE 13-2
TYPES OF NURSING ACTIONS INVOLVED IN LITIGATION

Treatment
- Failed to prevent and treat pressure ulcers and malnutrition, resulting in death
- Mishandled shoulder dystocia during delivery, resulting in brachial plexus injury
- Failed to perform intrauterine resuscitation, leading to infant's brain damage
- Failed to properly handle telephone triage calls, resulting in death
- Failed to incorporate patient's emergency room records into patient's hospital chart, resulting in death
- Failed to properly treat pediatric glaucoma, resulting in vision loss
- Burned patient with hair dryer, resulting in third-degree burns
- Failed to accurately count sponges after operation, resulting in retained sponge
- Failed to provide adequate nutrition and implement nursing plan of care, resulting in death
- Injected patient with used needle, leading to emotional distress from possible hepatitis infection
- Failed to properly treat patient's jaundice, resulting in infant's brain damage
- Failed to treat dehydration and pressure ulcers, resulting in death
- Removed internal pacemaker wires improperly, resulting in infection
- Administered suction tube improperly, leading to aspiration and death by suffocation
- Failed to detect arterial blockage after surgery, leading to leg amputation
- Failed to adequately hydrate patient prior to C section, resulting in maternal hypotension and infant's brain damage
- Failed to administer supplemental oxygen, resulting in vision loss and brain damage

(continues)

Table 13-2 *(continued)*

Communication

- Failed to notify physician of
  a. patient burns
  b. bleeding gastric ulcer, resulting in death
  c. increased heart rate, resulting in death
  d. fetal distress, resulting in death, or resulting in brain damage
  e. newborn jaundice, resulting in brain damage
  f. PT level
  g. pain and numbness after spinal surgery, resulting in cauda equina syndrome
  h. vision problems, resulting in vision loss
- Failed to report sexual abuse of patient/ resident to police and/or state department of human resources
- Failed to institute chain of command when physician refused to come to the hospital promptly

Medication

- Administered insufficient heparin, leading to death by pulmonary embolism
- Administered doses of Dilantin and insulin to a patient in excess of physician's order, leading to patient's disorientation and burns by bedside heater
- Administered excessive dose of IV antibiotics (nafcillin), leading to chemical burn
- Failed to send antibiotics home with patient with meningitis, leading to cerebral palsy
- Failed to recognize dosage error in doctor's order and thereby administered excessive dose of Dilaudid, leading to brain damage

Monitoring/ Observing/ Supervising

- Failed to monitor premature newborn, leading to death by cardiac arrest
- Failed to detect fetal distress, resulting in death, or resulting in brain damage
- Failed to monitor patient, leading to third-degree burns
- Failed to timely call a "code blue" in response to patient's respiratory arrest, resulting in death
- Failed to prevent patient falls, leading to death, or leading to quadriplegia, or leading to quadriparesis
- Failed to seek timely medical intervention, leading to death from bleeding ulcer
- Failed to properly monitor heart rate after surgery, resulting in death
- Misidentified and mixed up newborns in nursery
- Failed to monitor respiratory rate after surgery, resulting in death
- Failed to take vital signs of patient in waiting room, resulting in brain damage
- Failed to restrain demented patient, resulting in death
- Failed to properly insert Foley catheter during delivery, resulting in urinary sphincter trauma and incontinence
- Failed to monitor cornea in facial palsy, leading to corneal scarring and vision loss
- Failed to reattach cardiac monitor after x-rays, resulting in death
- Failed to detect brain swelling, resulting in vision loss and diminished IQ

Pozza, R., 2003

TABLE 13-3
CLINICAL SETTINGS OF NURSING MALPRACTICE CASES REPORTED IN PROFESSIONAL NEGLIGENCE LAW REPORTER (JULY 2001–JULY 2002)

Clinical Setting	No. of Cases
Hospital-Medical-Surgical	13
Maternity-Obstetrics	10
Nursing Home	9
Emergency Room	5
Pediatrics-Nursery	4
Recovery Room	2
Home Health Care	2
Clinic	1
Urgent Care Facility	1
Total	**47**

Pozza, R., 2003

doctor's order must be present. Problems arise when the orders are verbal, and later it is claimed that the nurse misunderstood and acted in error. Another pitfall is illegible writing, which is then misinterpreted and the result causes harm to the patient. Many nurses who have been in practice for a long time have encountered doctors who write orders that are contrary to accepted medical practice. In these situations, the nurse must exercise professional judgment and follow the policies and procedures of the institution. Usually these require the nurse to notify the nursing supervisor and the medical director for the area where the nurse works.

The institution's policies and procedures describe the performance expected of nurses in its employ, and a nurse deviating from them can be liable for negligence or malpractice. Occasionally, such failure to adhere to institutional protocol can result in the employer denying the nurse a defense in a lawsuit.

Practicing nurses must also adhere to the standards of practice for the nursing profession in the community. These standards include such things as checking the six "rights" in medication administration or repositioning the bed-bound patient at regular intervals. It is not uncommon for nurses to find conflicts between an employer's expectations and the nursing standards of care, resulting in problems such as having insufficient time or staffing to adhere to the standards taught in nursing school or receiving poor evaluations for taking too long to render care. In these situations, nurses must evaluate what standards they must follow to preserve their professional practice, protect patients, and protect themselves from liability, even if this requires a job change.

TABLE 13-4
HEALTH CARE FACILITY LIABILITIES OTHER THAN NURSING ACTIONS

- Failure to provide a safe environment
- Misrepresenting the level of care available at the nursing home
- Failure to adequately train personnel in fall prevention
- Failure to adequately supervise nursing home staff to ensure residents receive proper nutrition, custodial treatment, and medical care
- Failure to instruct and train personnel regarding the handling of jaundice in newborns
- Failure to adequately train staff on emergency procedures
- Failure to inform physician of patient burns
- Failure to properly supervise staff
- Failure to provide timely lab services
- Failure to appropriately dispose of used syringes
- Failure to enforce policies to adequately handle emergencies
- Failure to report abuse of nursing home resident
- Allowing unlicensed persons to administer IV medications

Pozza, R., 2003

Assault and Battery. Assault is a threat to touch another in an offensive manner without that person's permission. A battery is the touching of another person without that person's consent. In the health care arena, complaints of this nature usually pertain to whether the individual consented to the treatment administered by the health care professional. Most states have laws that require patients to make informed decisions about their treatment.

Fiesta (1999b) explained that informed consent laws protect the patient's right to practice self-determination. The patient has the right to receive sufficient information to make an informed decision about whether to consent or to refuse a procedure. The individual performing the procedure has the responsibility of explaining to the patient the nature of the procedure, benefits, alternatives, and the risks and complications. The signed consent form is used to document that this was done, and it creates a presumption that the patient had been advised of the appropriate risks.

Often the nurse is asked to witness a patient signing a consent form for treatment. When you witness a patient's signature, you are vouching for two things: that the patient signed the paper and that the patient knows he is signing a consent form (Olsen-Chavarriaga, 2000). For a consent form to be legal, a patient, in most states, must be at least 18 years old; be mentally competent; have the procedures, with their risks and benefits, explained in a manner he can understand; be aware of the available alternatives to the proposed treatment; and consent voluntarily. The nurse must also be familiar with which other people are allowed by state law to consent to medical treatment for another when that person cannot consent for himself. Frequently, these include the person possessing medical power of attorney; a spouse; adult children; or other relatives, if no one is available in one of the other categories listed.

A nurse may also face a charge of battery for failing to honor an advance directive, such as a medical power of attorney, durable power of attorney, or living will. Federal law requires that a hospital ask the patient, upon admission, whether she has a living will; if she does not, the hospital must ask the patient whether she would like to enact one. A living will is a written advance directive voluntarily signed by the patient that specifies the type of care she desires if and when she is in a terminal state and cannot sign a consent form or convey this information verbally. It can be a general statement such as "no life sustaining measures" or specific such as "no tube feedings or respirator." Often, the patient's family has difficulty allowing health care personnel to follow the wishes expressed in a living will and conflicts arise. These should be communicated to the hospital ethics committee, pastoral care department, risk management, or whichever hospital department is responsible for handling such issues. If the patient verbalizes her wishes regarding end-of-life care to the family, such difficult situations can sometimes be avoided, and the patient should be encouraged to do this, if possible.

Following Orders, Including Do Not Resuscitate (DNR).

The attending physician may write a do not resuscitate (DNR) order on an inpatient, which directs the staff not to perform the usual cardiopulmonary resuscitation (CPR) in the event of a sudden cardiopulmonary arrest. The doctor may write such an order without evidence of a living will on the medical record, and the nurse should be familiar with the institution's policies and state law regarding when and how a physician can write such an order in the absence of a living will. Often, a DNR order is considered a medical decision that the doctor can make, preferably in consultation with the family, even without a living will executed by the patient.

If the nurse feels that a DNR order or any order is contrary to the patient's good, the nurse should consult the policies and procedures of the institution. These may include going up the chain of command until the nurse is satisfied with the course of action. See the chain of command figure in the chapter on Delegation. This may entail notifying the nursing supervisor, the medical director, the institution's chief operating officer, the risk manager, the state regulators, or the Joint Commission on Accreditation of Healthcare Organizations (JCAHO). Often an institution has an ethics committee that examines such issues and makes a determination of the appropriateness of the order. Because of the opportunity for misunderstanding, verbal orders are not encouraged. When a nurse has a problem with a medical order, it is often prudent to discuss it first with the physician involved before reporting the problem up the chain of command. Often, problems can be resolved at this first step. However, if the problem is not resolved by discussing it with the physician, the nurse should report the problem to her supervisor and follow the state law and the agency's policies.

False Imprisonment.

False imprisonment occurs when individuals are incorrectly led to believe they cannot leave a place. This often occurs because the nurse misinterprets the rights granted to others by legal documents such as powers of attorney and does not allow a patient to leave a facility because the person with the power of attorney (agent) says the patient cannot leave. A power of attorney is a legal document executed by an individual (principal) granting another person (agent) the right to perform certain activities in the principal's name. It can be specific, such as "sell my house," or general, such as "make all decisions for me, including health care decisions." In most states, a power of attorney is voluntarily granted by the individual and does not take away the individual's right to exercise his own choices. Thus, if the principal (patient) disagrees with his agent's decisions, the patient's wishes are the ones that prevail. If a situation occurs in which an agent, acting on a power of attorney, disagrees with your patient regarding discharge plans, contact your supervisor for further assistance in deciding an action consistent with your patient's wishes and best interests.

The authority to make medical decisions for another may be granted in a general power of attorney document or in a specific document limited to medical decisions only such as a medical power of attorney. The requirements for a medical power of attorney vary from state to state, as do most legal documents.

A claim of false imprisonment may be based on the inappropriate use of physical or chemical restraints. Federal law mandates that health care institutions employ the least restrictive method of ensuring patient safety. Physical or chemical restraints are to be used only if necessary to protect the patient from harm when all other methods have failed. If the nurse uses restraints on a competent person who is refusing to follow the doctor's orders, the nurse can be charged with false imprisonment or battery. If restraints are used in an emergency situation, the nurse is to contact the doctor immediately after application to secure an order for the restraints. Also, the nurse must check the institution's policies regarding the type and frequency of assessments required for a patient in restraints and how often it is necessary to secure a reorder for the restraints. These policies ensure the patient's safety and must be consistent with state law.

Invasion of Privacy and Confidentiality. The nurse is required to respect the privacy of all patients. As a health care practitioner, the nurse may be privy to very personal information and must make every effort to keep it confidential. Only authorized individuals can access patient information, although patients have the right to access their own records. Only by obtaining the patient's permission can information be given to others. See the discussion of HIPAA in an earlier chapter. It is often necessary to police conversations with coworkers that have

the potential for being overheard by others so that no patient information is accidentally revealed. Sometimes the protection of a patient's privacy conflicts with the state's mandatory reporting laws for the occurrence of specified infectious diseases such as syphilis or human immunodeficiency virus (HIV). The need to protect an individual's privacy may also conflict with the state's mandatory reporting laws on suspected patient abuse, discussed previously. Other information that state or federal law may require to be revealed include a patient's blood alcohol level, incidences of rape, gunshot wounds, and adverse reactions to certain drugs. Failing to strictly follow reporting laws could lead to criminal, civil, or disciplinary action, termination of employment, or all of these; nurses must consult the institution's policies and confer with its risk management department to ascertain their responsibilities and course of action. The American Nurses Association (ANA) Code for Nurses states that nurses must protect the patient and the public when incompetence or unethical or illegal practice compromise health care and safety. Many states have adopted this concept in their nurse practice acts, thereby creating a legal obligation to report (Sloan, 1999). If a nurse were to observe unethical behavior in a hospital, the nurse should report this as directed in the institution's policies and procedures manual or by the laws of the state.

Defamation. Defamation is defined as an intentionally false communication/publication (*Black's Law Dictionary*, 1996). Other similar terms used for this tort are *slander*, which is verbal communication. *Libel* is the term for written

CASE STUDY 13-1

You are working the night shift. One of your patients' physicians has ordered a dose of a medication to be given to a patient that you know is too high for this patient. You are unable to locate the doctor to check the order. What would you do to ensure safe care for your patient?

communication. From its definition, one can see that two essential elements must be proved in a charge of defamation:

1. The information conveyed must be untrue.

2. The false information must be published or communicated to another party.

Note that publication or communication may mean simply telling one other person or writing a friend a letter containing the false information. The nurse may face such an accusation if the nurse communicates inaccurate information to another or if it is claimed that the information charted was untrue. However, several courts have ruled that charting information in a medical record, whether accurate or not, does not constitute publication as required for a charge of defamation.

PROTECTIONS IN NURSING PRACTICE

As discussed earlier in this chapter, nursing practice is guided by state nurse practice acts and agency policies and procedures. Other resources for the nurse include Good Samaritan laws, skillful communication, patient advocacy, and professional liability insurance.

Good Samaritan Laws

Good Samaritan laws are laws that have been enacted to protect the health care professional from legal liability. The essential elements of commonly enacted Good Samaritan law are as follows:

- The care is rendered in an emergency situation.
- The health care worker is rendering care without pay.
- The care provided did not recklessly or intentionally cause injury or harm to the injured party.

Note that these laws are intended to protect the volunteer who stops to render care at the scene of an accident. They would not protect a nurse, emergency medical technician (EMT), or other health care professionals rendering care at the scene of an accident as part of their assigned duties and for which they receive pay. In doing their duties, these paid emergency personnel would be evaluated according to the standards of their professions.

Skillful Communication

The nurse must communicate accurately and completely both verbally and in writing. Often a case involving patient care takes several years to come to trial; by that time, the nurse may have no memory of the incident in question and must rely on the written record done at the time of the incident. This record is frequently in the courtroom, blown up to billboard size for all to see. All errors are apparent and omissions stand out by their absence, especially if it is data that should have been recorded per institutional policy. The old adage that "if it isn't written, it wasn't done" will be repeated to the jury numerous times.

To protect themselves when charting, nurses should use the FLAT charting acronym: F—factual, L—legible, A—accurate, T—timely

F: Charting should be *factual*—what you see, not what you think happened.

L: Charting should be *legible*, with no erasures. Corrections should be made as you have been taught, with a single line drawn through the error and initialed.

A: Charting should be *accurate* and complete. What color was the drainage and how much was present? How many times, and at what times, was the doctor notified of changes? Was the supervisor notified?

T: Charting should be *timely*, completed as soon after the occurrence as possible. "Late entries" should be avoided or kept to a minimum.

Patient Advocacy

Nursing's role as a patient advocate can help nurses avoid being named in a lawsuit. Nurses often assist patients with health care needs in areas such as scheduling treatments, obtaining

REAL WORLD INTERVIEW

Most nurses are familiar with the phrase, "If it was not documented, it was not done." Insofar as this phrase is used to encourage thorough documentation, it reflects good nursing practice. Timely, accurate, and complete documentation is an excellent way to protect oneself from litigation. However, lawyers who represent plaintiffs in medical malpractice cases are aware of this "rule" and often attempt to use it against nurses in health care liability claims.

Imagine the following scenario: A patient is admitted to the hospital and Nurse A performs an initial assessment of the patient. Nurse A notes in the patient's chart that the patient has good capillary refill. Nurse A proceeds to take the patient's vital signs, including capillary refill, hourly throughout Nurse A's 8-hour shift. The patient's capillary refill remains reassuring and the nurse makes no further documentation in the chart relating to the patient's capillary refill. After Nurse A's shift, Nurse B takes over the patient's care. One hour into Nurse B's shift, the patient codes and expires. The patient's family sues Nurse A. The plaintiffs' lawyer is cross-examining Nurse A.

Lawyer: "Nurse A, are you familiar with the phrase, 'If it wasn't charted, it wasn't done'?"

Nurse A: "Yes."

Lawyer: "That's a common rule in nursing practice, isn't it?"

Nurse A: "Yes."

Lawyer: "You were taught that in nursing school, weren't you?"

Nurse A: "Yes, I was."

Lawyer: "And after you documented that the patient had good capillary refill upon admission, you did not document anything relating to the patient's capillary refill for the next 8 hours, did you?"

Nurse A: "Well, no."

Lawyer: "So if we use your rule, 'If it wasn't documented, it wasn't done' we can assume you never checked the patient's capillary refills during your shift after the initial assessment, right?"

Nurse A: "No. I checked, but they hadn't changed, so I didn't chart anything."

Do you see what just happened? Nurse A provided competent nursing care, but the lawyer made it appear as if Nurse A was negligent. A nurse involved in litigation should not blanketly agree with this documentation rule. The rule ignores the concept of charting by exception. You simply cannot document everything noted in an assessment of a patient. Moreover, most nurses would agree that patient care takes priority over charting. This rule ignores that. Bad charting looks bad. Good charting protects you. However, charting by exception does not correlate with providing bad nursing care. Even lapses in charting do not correlate with bad nursing care. Nurses should not lose sight of that when faced with litigation.

Robyn D. Pozza, JD

Austin, Texas

REAL WORLD INTERVIEW

The role of risk management in the health care environment is that of recognition, evaluation, and treatment of risks inherent in the organization. The goal of risk management is improving the quality of care provided by the organization while at the same time protecting its financial integrity. Risk management, while coordinated at a certain level of the organization, is not simply a one-department responsibility, but rather is the responsibility of each employee of the organization.

New graduates in nursing need to understand that in today's competitive health care environment, it is important that each practitioner look for ways to reduce the risks inherent in the delivery of health care. At a time when hospitals are receiving less and less reimbursement, our patients and consumers are demanding higher and higher quality of care.

Health care is at a crossroads, similar to the one that faced private industry during the 1970s. Our customers are demanding that we provide a safe environment and that we consistently strive for continuous quality improvement.

An incident report is a commonly used form that documents a variance from normal protocol or hospital procedures. It is not meant to place blame on an individual practitioner or department. It is used strictly to document the facts surrounding an event so the health care processes can be improved. Thus, the nurse should complete an incident report when any variance from a policy or a procedure is noticed.

When risk management receives the incident reports, they are logged into our database, and monthly reports are forwarded to nurse managers for follow-up and education with their staff.

Incident reports and the subsequent risk management department actions are generally reactive but we also do proactive/preventive interventions in the health care setting. These include the following:

1. Education of students completing their senior year of study in nursing

2. Participation on patient safety, environment of care, pharmacy, nursing, and other hospital committees, which work on proactive programs to reduce risks

3. Facilitation of the slips and falls task force to reduce our patients' fall risk

4. Education of new nurses and physicians on principles of risk management

Harriet Percy, RN
Risk Manager

appropriate referrals, explaining how the system works, assisting with follow-up activities, reinforcement of health teaching, coordination of care, and notification of appropriate individuals. The nurse, therefore, can play a unique role in the delivery of health care in acting as an advocate for the patient within the health care system. The nurse is often the key person involved in ensuring patient access to quality health care. Nurses who maintain good communication with their patients and fulfill these roles well have little problem with malpractice (Mitchell & Grippando, 1993).

TABLE 13-5
ACTIONS TO DECREASE THE RISK OF NURSING LIABILITY

- Treat all patients and their families with kindness and respect.
- Communicate with your patients by keeping them informed and listening to what they say.
- Acknowledge unfortunate incidents and express concern about these events without either taking the blame, blaming others, or reacting defensively.
- Chart and time your observations immediately, while facts are still fresh in your mind.
- Take appropriate actions to meet the patient's nursing needs.
- Follow the facility's policies and procedures for administering care and reporting incidents.
- Acknowledge and document the reason for any omission or deviation from agency policy, procedure, or standard.
- Complete incident reports immediately after they occur. Discuss critical factors with the risk manager to increase your retention of the facts.
- Maintain clinical competency and acknowledge your limitations. If you do not know how to do something, ask for help.
- Promptly report any concern regarding the quality of care, including the lack of resources with which to provide care, faulty equipment, staffing concerns, orientation or education concerns, and any complaints of discrimination or harassment and patient or family complaints to a nursing administration representative.
- Use appropriate standards of care.
- Document the time of changes in conditions requiring notification of the physician and include the response of the physician.
- Delegate patient care based on the documented education and experience of licensed and unlicensed personnel.
- Avoid taking verbal orders. If unavoidable, repeat them back to the practitioner.

Malpractice/ Professional Liability Insurance

Nurses may need to carry their own malpractice insurance. Nurses often think their actions are adequately covered by the employer's liability insurance, but this is not necessarily so. Although the hospital's insurance company almost always pays malpractice awards, insurance contracts often have provisions that allow them to refuse repayment if the insured intentionally injures another party (Pozza, 2003). Also, if in giving care, the nurse fails to comply with the institution's policies and procedures, the institution may deny the nurse a defense, claiming that

because of the nurse's failure to follow institutional policy, or because of the nurse working outside the scope of nursing employment, the nurse was not acting as an employee at that time. Also, nurses are being named individually as defendants in malpractice suits more frequently than in the past. More frequently, though, hospitals are often a plaintiff's primary target because they typically have deeper pockets than individual practitioners (Pozza, 2003).

It is advantageous for nurses to be assured of a defense independent of that of their employer. Professional liability insurance provides that assurance and pays for an attorney to defend nurses in a malpractice lawsuit. When purchasing malpractice insurance, nurses should clarify whether the insurance covers liability just as long as the premiums are being paid or if the insurance covers a prescribed time period.

Note that in the event that unaffiliated nurses, like agency per diem nurses, are held individually liable for a judgment, their personal insurance carrier will be responsible for paying the verdict rendered against them. Unaffiliated, uninsured nurses could be forced to pay for their own defense and be financially responsible for any judgments rendered against them.

In making the decision of whether to obtain separate insurance, nurses should consider the value of their personal assets. Nurses should also consider the laws of the state where they practice regarding those assets that are exempt from being seized to satisfy civil monetary judgments. Generally, one home and one automobile are exempt from seizure (Pozza, 2003). See Table 13-5.

Nurses Involved in Litigation

Nurses may be sued individually for damages resulting from their negligent acts. However, a plaintiff will often name the nurse's employer as a defendant instead of or in addition to suing the nurse individually. It is a well-established law throughout the United States that "a master is subject to liability for the torts of his servants committed while acting in the scope of employment" (Restatement (second) of the Law of Agency §219 [1958]). This law is called Respondeat Superior. In other words, a hospital, nursing home, clinic, and so on is legally responsible for the damages caused by the negligence of its nurses.

Customarily, plaintiffs in medical malpractice cases name a combination of health care providers as defendants. It is common for some or all of the defendants to settle the cases before they reach the trial phase. However, in the event that a case proceeds to trial, a jury may find that none, some, or all of the defendants were negligent in their care and treatment of the plaintiff. A jury may determine that the nursing care was appropriate but that the medical treat-

ment was substandard. Likewise, a jury could hold that the physician rendered appropriate care but that the nurses' conduct fell below the standard of care. Additionally, a new trend in medical malpractice litigation is to name the health maintenance organization (HMO) as a defendant as well. For example, the Illinois Supreme Court recently held that an HMO could be liable under theories of apparent authority, respondeat superior, direct corporate negligence, breach of contract, and breach of warranty (*Jones v. Chicago HMO Ltd. of Ill.* [2000]; Pozza [2003]).

Common Monetary Awards

Many malpractice cases are dismissed or settled prior to trial. In those cases that do reach the trial stage, jury verdicts are unpredictable and awards can vary dramatically. For instance, juries awarded the following for the listed injuries:

- Brachial plexus injury ($13.3 million) (Stonieczny v. Gardner, Ill. [2001])
- Wrongful death—pulmonary embolism ($5 million) (*Martinelli v. Lifemark Hospitals of Fla., Inc.* [2001])
- Microcephaly in newborn ($17 million) (*Diver v. Gingo* [2001])
- Vision loss ($8 million) (*Schwab v. Kamat* [2001])
- Arterial impairment ($260,000) (*In re Triss* [2002])

A jury may award the plaintiff both compensatory and punitive damages. Compensatory damages are awarded to compensate the plaintiff for injuries. Compensatory damages include damages for both economic losses (medical expenses, lost wages, lost earning capacity) and noneconomic losses (pain and suffering). Punitive damages are not intended to compensate the plaintiff for any loss. Rather, punitive damages are intended to punish the defendant for acting with "recklessness, malice or deceit" (*Black's Law Dictionary*, 1999). Punitive damage awards are particularly common in cases involving nursing homes. For example, a Texas jury awarded the family of a nursing home resident $90 million in punitive damages for gross negligence that caused the resident to develop pressure ulcers and contractures (*Horizon/CMS Healthcare Corp. V. Auld* [2000]; Pozza [2003]).

Monetary Liability Limits in Some States.

Since 1970, at least 30 states have enacted legislation capping the damages plaintiffs can recover in a lawsuit (Babcock & Pogarsky, 1999). Currently, there exist as many different cap schemes as states that employ them. Some states cap the amount that a plaintiff may receive for punitive damages. See Table 13-6.

Other states employ a flat dollar cap. These states limit the total amount the plaintiff may recover in both compensatory and punitive damages in any medical malpractice action. For example:

State	Total verdict limited to:
Colorado	$1 million per patient
Nebraska	$1.25 million per patient

Other states, like Texas, cap compensatory damages. Texas starts with a $500,000 cap per defendant and adjusts the cap for inflation by using the Consumer Price Index as a multiplier. However, in Texas the cap does not include punitive damages.

A plaintiff may claim that he or she is entitled to damages in excess of the applicable cap. Jurors are customarily not informed of the caps applicable in their states. Therefore, it is common for a jury's award to exceed the state's cap on damages. In the event that a jury awards a plaintiff damages in excess of a statutory cap, the judge will reduce the jury's award to the cap (Pozza, 2003).

TABLE 13-6
SELECTED STATES PUNITIVE DAMAGE LIMITS

State	Punitive Damages Limits
Alabama	$250,000
Alaska	Three times compensatory damages or $500,000, whichever is greater
California	$500,000
Georgia	$250,000
Illinois	$5 million or the highest annual gross income earned by the defendant within the past 5 years, whichever is less
Kansas	$5 million or the highest annual gross income earned by the defendant within the past 5 years, whichever is less
Nevada	$300,000 (when compensatory damages are less than $100,000)
North Dakota	Twice the compensatory damages or $250,000, whichever is greater
Virginia	$350,000

(Pozza, R., 2003)

Other Legal Risks for the Nurse, Doctor, or Hospital

Other than increased insurance premiums, health care providers have plenty at stake when named as defendants in medical malpractice cases. Physicians are required to report adverse verdicts and settlements to the National Practitioner's Data Bank. The National Practitioner's Data Bank was established through the Health Care Quality Improvement Act of 1986. The federal regulations regarding the data bank can be found in 45 CFR Part 60. Significant awards against a physician or numerous malpractice payments by a physician can affect the physician's licensure or ability to gain privileges to practice at certain hospitals and health care entities. Failure to report malpractice payments to the data bank can result in civil monetary penalties. The U.S. Department of Health and Human Services, Office of the Inspector General, may impose a civil money penalty of up to $11,000 for each violation.

Federal and state statutes and regulations prescribe nursing standards of care. See the Code of Federal Regulations Title 42—Public Health and Title 45—Public Welfare. Also see the U.S. Code Title 42—Public Health and Welfare. Every jurisdiction that licenses nurses has a Nurse Practice Act (Cavico & Cavico, 1995). In addition to instructing nurses on the definition of the standard of care for that jurisdiction, the Nurse Practice Act mandates strict rules for reporting and disciplining nurses who violate the standard. Likewise, state boards of nursing and administrative agencies may take action to suspend or revoke the licenses of nurses that it determines have violated the standard of care. Private entities, such as the Joint Commission on Accreditation of Healthcare Organizations (JCAHO), and nursing organizations, such as the American Nurses Association, promulgate their own rules of conduct that serve as guidelines for acceptable nursing care (Pozza, 2003).

Nurse/Attorney Relationship

Despite the nurse's best intentions, a nurse may be named as a defendant in a lawsuit and need to retain the services of an attorney. LaDuke (2000) made the following suggestions for consulting and collaborating with an attorney:

1. Retain a specialist. Generalists are competent to handle many matters, but professional malpractice, professional disciplinary proceedings, and employment disputes are best handled by specialists in those areas.

2. Be attentive. Read the documents the attorney produces and travel to court proceedings to observe the attorney's performance.

3. Notify your insurance carrier as soon as you are aware of any real or potential liability issue. Inform your agent about the status of your case every few months, even if it is unchanged.

4. Keep costs sensible. Your attorney should explain initially how the fee will be computed and how you will be billed. The attorney may require you to pay a retainer fee.

5. Keep informed. The attorney should address your questions and concerns promptly. You are entitled to be kept informed about the status of your case. You are entitled to copies of all correspondence, legal briefs, and other documents.

6. Weed through writing. Your attorney needs to explain all facts and options. Examine all relevant documents and do not hesitate to make corrections in the same way you would correct a medical record by drawing a line through the incorrect or misleading information, writing in the correction, and signing your initials after it.

7. Set your own course. Insist on a collaborative relationship with your attorney for the duration of your case.

KEY CONCEPTS

- Nursing practice is governed by civil, public, and administrative laws.
- Nurses are responsible for providing a safe environment for patients entrusted to their care.
- Nurses need to be familiar with their institution's policies and procedures in giving care and in reporting variances, illegal activities, or unexpected events.
- Nurses must have good oral and written communication skills.
- Common torts include negligence and malpractice, assault and battery, false imprisonment, invasion of privacy, and defamation.
- Nurses need to be familiar with their state nurse practice act.
- Good Samaritan laws exist in many states.
- Risk management programs improve the quality of care and protect the financial integrity of institutions.
- The Multistate Licensure Compact allows nurses to practice in more than one state.

KEY TERMS

administrative law	false imprisonment
assault	Good Samaritan laws
battery	living will
civil law	malpractice
common law	negligence
constitution	power of attorney
contract law	public law
criminal law	tort
defamation	

REVIEW QUESTIONS

1. Which of the following is the agency that evaluates complaints of discrimination?
   A. Occupational Safety & Health Administration
   B. Equal Employment Opportunity Commission
   C. Health and Human Services
   D. National Labor Relations Board

2. Which type of law authorizes state boards of nursing to enact rules that govern the practice of nursing?
   A. State law
   B. Federal law
   C. Common law
   D. Criminal law

3. An intentionally false communication, either published or spoken, is which of the following?
   A. Assault
   B. Defamation
   C. Malpractice
   D. False imprisonment

4. Invasion of privacy is an example of which of the following?
   A. Tort
   B. Administrative law violation
   C. Good Samaritan law violation
   D. Criminal law violation

5. A body of law that develops through precedents over time and has the force of law is called which of the following?
   A. Contract law
   B. Common law
   C. Public law
   D. Civil law

REVIEW ACTIVITIES

1. Talk to the risk manager at a hospital where you have your clinical assignments. Ask the risk manager how they handle an incident report. Is it used for improving the hospital's care in the future? How?

2. Review the living will policy at a hospital where you have your clinical assignments. Notice the forms that patients can sign. Do all patients sign them?

3. Discuss how nurses' off-duty behaviors can affect their nursing practice. Note if your state lists any actions in its nurse practice act that you might take outside of work that might cause your license to practice nursing to be revoked by your state nursing licensure board (e.g., a driving while intoxicated conviction).

EXPLORING THE WEB

- Where can you find state and federal laws regulating hospitals? *http://www.findlaw.com*
- You have a patient who is to be transferred to a nursing home for recuperation. Where can you tell the family to look to evaluate the local nursing homes regarding their adherence to the federal regulations for nursing homes? *http://www.medicare.gov*. Click on "long term care" and "nursing homes compare."
- Where can you find a copy of the ANA Code of Ethics? *http://www.ana.org*. Search for "code of ethics."
- Check these Internet resources for legal information:

  http://web2.westlaw.com

  http://www.lexis.com

  http://www.aslme.com (American Society of Law, Medicine and Ethics)

  http://www.lpig.org (Law and Policy Institutions Guide)

  http://www.law.cornell.edu

  http://www.jcaho.org

  http://cms.hhs.gov

  http://www.nursefriendly.com

REFERENCES

Babcock, L., & Pogarsky, G. (1999) Damages caps and settlement: A behavioral approach. *Journal of Legal Studies, 28,* 341.

Black's law dictionary (6th ed.). (1996). St. Paul, MN: West.

Black's law dictionary (7th ed.). (1999). St. Paul, MN: West.

Boze v. Universal Nursing Services. Ltd., Florida, No. H-27-CA-2001-1706, Hernando County Cir. Mar. 21, 2002 (17 PNLR 104, July 2002).

Cavico, F. J. and Cavico, N. M. (1995). The nursing profession in the 1990s: Negligence and malpractice liability. 43 Clev. St. L. Rev. 557.

Cofer, M. J. (1998). How to avoid age bias. *Nursing Management, 29*(11), 34–36.

Cruzan v. Director, Missouri Department of Health, 110 S. Ct. 2841 (1990).

Diver v. Gingo, Ohio, No. 305538, Cuyahoga County C.P., Jan. 2001 (16 PNLR 152, Oct. 2001).

Fiesta, J. (1999a). Do no harm: When caregivers violate our golden rule, part 1. *Nursing Management, 30*(8), 10–11.

Fiesta, J. (1999b). Informed consent: What health care professionals need to know, part 2. *Nursing Management, 30*(7), 6–7.

Fiesta, J. (1999c). Know your boundaries in sexual assault litigation. *Nursing Management, 30*(10), 10.

Horizon/CMS Healthcare Corp. v. Auld, 34 S.W.3d 887 (Tex. 2000).

Huckaby v. Lake Pointe Partners, Ltd., Texas, No. 1-00-592, Rockwall County 382d Jud. Dist. Ct. Dec. 14, 2001 (17 PNLR 67, May 2002).

In re Triss, 2002 WL 1271492 (La.App. 4 Cir., 2002).

Jones v. Chicago HMO Ltd. of Illinois, 730 N.E.2d 1119 (Ill. 2000).

LaDuke, S. (2000). What should you expect from your attorney? *Nursing Management, 31*(1), 10.

Lavalis v. Copperas Cove L.L.C., Texas, No. 183,293-B, Bell County 146th Jud. Dist. Dec. 27, 2001 (17 PNLR 32, Mar. 2002).

Lewis v. Physicians Ins. Co. of Wisconsin, 627 N.W.2d 484 (Wis. 2001) (16 PNLR 175, Nov. 2001).

Mantel, D. L. (1999). Legally speaking: Off-duty doesn't mean off the hook. *RN, 62*(10), 71–74.

Marshal v. Methodist Healthcare Jackson Hospital, Mississippi, No. 251-99-000984CIV, Hinds County Cir. Jan. 23, 2001 (16 PNLR 174, Nov. 2001).

Martinelli v. Lifemark Hospitals of Florida, Inc., Fla., No. 99-14491 CA 05, Dade County Cir. Mar. 1, 2001 (16 ATLA PNLR 111, July 2001).

Mitchell & Grippando (1993) *Nursing Perspective & Issues.* Clifton Park, NY: Delmar Learning.

Murphy v. United Parcel Service, 527 U.S. 516 (1999).

Nguyen, B. Q. (2000a). ADA coverage: Defining who is a "qualified individual with a disability." *American Journal of Nursing, 100*(1), 87.

Nguyen, B. Q. (2000b). If you're replaced by a younger nurse. *American Journal of Nursing, 100*(3), 82.

Odom v. State Department of Health & Hospitals, 322 So. 2d 91 (La. 1999).

Olsen-Chavarriaga, D. (2000). Informed consent: Do you know your role? *Nursing2000, 30*(5), 60–61.

Pozza, R. (2003). *Nursing malpractice cases.* Unpublished manuscript.

Restatement (Second) of the Law of Agency § 219 (1958).

Roe v. Wade, 410 U.S. 133 (1973).

Schwab v. Kamat, New York, No. 97-887, Onondaga County Sup. Ct., June 8, 2001 (16 PNLR 154, Oct. 2001).

Sheehan, J. P. (2000). Protect your staff from workplace violence. *Nursing Management, 31*(3), 24–25.

Sloan, A. J. (1999). Legally speaking: Whistle-blowing: There are risks! *RN, 62*(7), 65–68.

Stonieczny v. Gardner, Illinois, No. 98 L 04578, Cook County Cir. May 29, 2001 (16 PNLR 131, Sept. 2001).

Sutton v. United Airlines, 527 U.S. 471 (1999).

Urgent v. Government of the Virgin Islands, U.S.V.I., No. 607/1998, V.I. Territorial Ct. St. Croix Div. Sept. 13, 2001 (17 PNLR 8, Feb. 2002).

Ventura, M. J. (1999). The great multistate licensure debate. *RN, 62*(5), 58–62.

Webb v. Tulane Medical Center Hospital, 700 So. 2d 1142 (La. 1997).

Zerwekh, J., & Claborn, J. C. (2002). *Nursing today: Transition and trends* (4th ed.). Philadelphia: Saunders.

SUGGESTED READINGS

Brown, S. M. (1999). Good Samaritan laws: Protection and limits. *RN, 62*(11), 65–68.

Court case: Defending against sexual assault charges. (1999). *Nursing99, 29*(6), 71.

DeLaune, S., & Ladner, P. K. (2002). *Fundamentals of nursing* (2nd ed.). Clifton Park, NY: Delmar Learning.

Fiesta, J. (1999). Greater need for background checks. *Nursing Management, 30*(11), 26.

Fiesta, J. (1999). When sexual harassment hits home. *Nursing Management, 30*(5), 16–18.

McKee, R. (1999). Clarifying advance directives. *Nursing99, 29*(5), 52–53.

Simpson, R. (1999). Tech talk on multistate licensure. *Nursing Management, 30*(1), 12–13.

Staten, P. A. (1999). How to cover all the bases on informed consent. *Nursing Management, 30*(9), 14.

Sullivan, G. H. (1999). Legally speaking: Minimizing your risk in patient falls. *RN, 62*(4), 69–70.

Sullivan, G. H. (2000). Legally speaking: Keep your charting on course. *RN, 63*(4), 75–79.

Ventura, M. J. (1999). The great multistate licensure debate. *RN, 62*(5), 58–62.

Ventura, M. J. (1999). Legally speaking: When information must be revealed. *RN, 62*(2), 61–62, 64.

CHAPTER 14

Peace requires that you do what in your heart you know— that your chosen values guide your actions. (Chinn, 1995)

Ethical Dimensions of Patient Care

OBJECTIVES

Upon completion of this chapter, the reader should be able to:

1. Discuss values and values clarification.
2. Identify philosophical influences on professional nursing practice.
3. Review the use of ethical theories and principles in professional nursing practice.
4. Identify a model for ethical decision making.
5. Promote ethical leadership and management in health care organizations.
6. Review the International Council of Nurses Code for Nurses.

In a large teaching hospital, a patient you are caring for says he does not want to go on living. He has had cancer for several years and states he is tired of being sick. When you ask him whether he has shared these feelings with his family, he says that he does not want them to think he is giving up. You report the patient's statements to the next shift and explain how you encouraged him to talk with his family and his doctor. That evening, the patient suddenly arrests and a code is called. The patient ends up on a ventilator, receives 5 units of blood, and is comatose.

What are your thoughts about maintaining the patient's life in this situation?

Who should make the decision about the patient's situation since he is comatose?

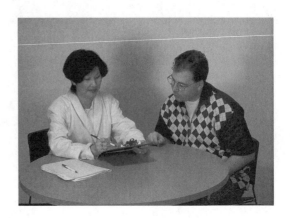

Nurses are confronted with ethical dilemmas in all types of practice settings. This chapter identifies selected virtues and explores the importance of clarifying personal values as a baseline for developing professional values. Personal and professional values contribute to the development of one's philosophy of nursing. This chapter provides a definition of ethics and reviews ethical theories and principles. It discusses the Patient's Bill of Rights and the International Council of Nurses Code for Nurses. It also identifies a model for ethical decision making and discusses how to promote ethical leadership and management in health care organizations.

VALUES AND VIRTUES

Values are personal beliefs about the truth of ideals, standards, principles, objects, and behaviors that give meaning and direction to life. If you were told that you must pack a bag for a special trip but you may bring only three items from your belongings, what items would you choose? The ones selected are what you value.

It is important to clarify your personal values. Personal values provide a baseline for identifying your professional nursing values.

Together, these personal and professional values contribute to your philosophy of nursing and guide your professional practice.

Virtue

Burkhardt and Nathaniel (2002) list four virtues that are more significant than others and that are illustrative of a virtuous person: compassion, discernment, trustworthiness, and integrity. **Compassion** is a trait nurses have, as perceived by society. It refers to the desire to alleviate suffering. **Discernment** is possession of acuteness of judgment. Trustworthiness and integrity are traits expected in all people but are especially necessary for professional nurses. These virtues form the foundation for an ethically principled discipline and have been endorsed throughout the profession's history (Burkhardt & Nathaniel, 2002). Nurses who subscribe to these four virtues are inclined to recall and value that patients also have their own personal values.

Values Clarification

Values clarification is the process of analyzing one's own values to better understand what is truly important. In their classic work *Values and Teaching*, Raths, Harmin, and Simon (1978, p. 47) formulated a theory of values clarification and proposed a three-step process of valuing, as follows:

1. *Choosing*: Beliefs are chosen freely (that is, without coercion) from among alternatives. The choosing step involves analysis of the consequences of various alternatives.

2. *Prizing*: The beliefs that are selected are cherished (that is, prized).

3. *Acting*: The selected beliefs are demonstrated consistently through behavior.

Nurses must understand that values are individual rather than universal. Professional nurses honor patients' rights to their own values. Nurses realize that it is common for patients and their nurses and other caregivers to hold different values.

Philosophical Influences on Nursing Practice

Philosophy is the rational investigation of the truths and principles of knowledge, reality, and human conduct. Personal philosophies stem from an individual's beliefs and values. These beliefs and values, in turn, develop based upon a person's experiences in life, cultural influences, and education.

Philosophy of Nursing

A professional nurse's personal philosophy affects her philosophy of nursing. Throughout the nursing educational process, students begin forming their philosophy of nursing. This philosophy is influenced significantly by a student's personal philosophy and experiences. One's personal philosophy should be compatible with the philosophy of the nursing department where she works. This helps the nurse to be an effective leader and practitioner. See Figure 14-1 for a nursing department's philosophy statement. An example of a personal nursing philosophy is:

I believe professional nursing care promotes an optimal level of wellness in body, mind, and spirit to those being served. I believe professional nurses must hold themselves to the highest standards of the profession and honor the profession's code of ethics in all aspects of practice.

DEFINITION OF ETHICS AND MORALITY

Ethics is the branch of philosophy that concerns the distinction of right from wrong on the basis of a body of knowledge, not just on the basis of opinions. Morality is behavior in accordance with custom or tradition and usually reflects personal or religious beliefs (DeLaune & Ladner, 2002). Ethics governs professional groups and provides a framework for determining the right course of action in a particular situation. For nurses, the actions they take in practice are primarily governed by the ethical principles of the profession. These principles influence practice, conduct, and relationships that nurses are held accountable for in the delivery of care. Health care ethics, also called bioethics, are ethics specific to health care and serve as a framework to guide behavior in ethical dilemmas. An ethical dilemma occurs when there is a conflict between two or more ethical principles; there is no "correct" decision.

Laws, in contrast, are state and federal government rules that govern all of society. Laws mandate behavior. In some situations in health care, the distinctions between law and ethics are not clear. There may be cases in which ethics and law are congruent; in others, ethics and law may be in conflict (Sullivan & Decker, 2001).

Ethical Theories

A standard way of making ethical decisions is to know the philosophical basis for making these decisions. When attempting to decide what is right and wrong, nurses find it useful to refer to ethical theories. Some of these theories are identified in Table 14-1.

Memorial's Professional Practice Model
Design for Excellence

Mission–
Professional nurses and Nursing teams exist to optimize the health of our patients and communities.

We believe many conditions must work together in order to nurture a professional environment. More specifically, the manner in which Beliefs, Practice, Structure, Relationships, and Operations interact will determine the quality of outcomes for us as well as for those we serve.

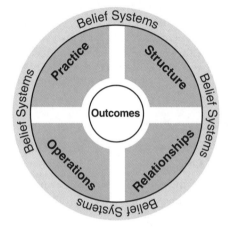

Figure 14-1 Nursing Philosophy (Adapted with permission from Memorial Health System's Professional Practice Philosophy, Springfield, IL)

STOP AND THINK

New graduates should formulate a philosophy of nursing based on personal beliefs and values. Reflections on the following questions can assist in the development of a philosophy:

What do I believe about nursing practice? Should nurses be patient advocates? How should professionals conduct themselves? How can I influence patient care based on my nursing philosophy? Are compassion, discernment, trustworthiness, and integrity essential both personally and professionally?

TABLE 14-1
SELECTED ETHICAL THEORIES

Ethical Theory	Interpretation
Deontology	Actions are based on moral rules and unchanging principles, such as "do unto others as you would have them do unto you." An ethical person must always follow the rules, even if doing so causes a less desirable outcome.
Teleology	A person must take those actions that lead to good outcomes. Achievement of a good outcome justifies using a less desirable means to attain the end.
Virtue Ethics	Virtues such as truthfulness and trustworthiness are developed over time. A person's character must be developed so that by nature and habit, the person will be predisposed to behave virtuously. Living a virtuous life contributes both to one's own well-being and to the well-being of society.
Social Justice and Equity	A "veil of ignorance" regarding who is affected by a decision allows for unbiased decision making. An ethical person chooses the action that is fair to all, including those persons who are most disadvantaged.
Relativism	There are no universal moral standards, such as "murder is always wrong." Moral standards are relative to person, place, time, and culture. Whatever a person thinks is right, is right. Theory has been largely rejected.

ETHICAL PRINCIPLES AND RULES

In addition to theories, ethical principles and rules provide a basis for nurses to determine the appropriate action when faced with an ethical dilemma in the practice setting. See Table 14-2 for a summary of the major ethical principles and rules.

A GUIDE FOR ETHICAL DECISION MAKING

Burkhardt and Nathaniel (2002) developed a guide for decision making, which nurses may use

when confronted with an ethical decision. See Figure 14-2.

An Ethics Test

A practical way of improving ethical decision making is to run decisions that you are considering through an ethics test when any doubt exists. The ethics test presented here was used at the Center for Business Ethics at Bentley College (Bowditch & Buono, 1997) as part of ethical corporate training programs. Decision makers are taught to ask themselves:

- Is it right?
- Is it fair?
- Who gets hurt?

TABLE 14-2
ETHICAL PRINCIPLES AND RULES

Ethical Principle/Rule	Definition	Example
Beneficence	The duty to do good to others and to maintain a balance between benefits and harms.	• Provide all patients, including the terminally ill, with caring attention and information. • Become familiar with your state laws regarding organ donations. • Treat every patient with respect and courtesy.
Nonmaleficence	The principle of doing no harm.	• Always work within your scope of practice. • Never give information or perform duties you are not qualified to do. • Observe all safety rules and precautions. • Keep areas safe from hazards. • Perform procedures according to facility protocols. Never take shortcuts. • Ask an appropriate person about anything you are unsure of. • Keep your skills and education up to date.
Justice	The principle of fairness that is served when an individual is given that which he or she is due, owed, deserves, or can legitimately claim.	• Treat all patients equally, regardless of economic or social background. • Learn the local, state, and national laws and your facility's policies and procedures for handling and reporting suspected abuse.
Autonomy and Confidentiality	Respect for an individual's right to self-determination; respect for individual liberty and privacy.	• Be sure that patients have consented to all treatments and procedures. • Become familiar with federal and state laws and facility policies dealing with privacy, e.g., HIPPA legislation. • Never release patient information of any kind unless there is a signed patient release.

(continues)

Table 14-2 *(continued)*

Ethical Principle/Rule	Definition	Example
		• Do not discuss patients with anyone who is not professionally involved in their care. • Protect the physical privacy of patients.
Fidelity	The principle of promise keeping; the duty to keep one's promise or word.	• Be sure that contracts have been completed. • Be very careful about what you say to patients. They may only hear the "good news."
Respect for others	The right of people to make their own decision	• Provide all persons with information for decision making. • Avoid making paternalistic decisions for others.
Veracity	The obligation to tell the truth.	• Admit mistakes promptly. Offer to do whatever is necessary to correct them. • Refuse to participate in any form of fraud. • Give an "honest day's work" every day.
Advocacy	The obligation to look out or speak up for the rights of others.	• Provide patients with high quality, evidence-based care.

- Would you tell your child or young relative to do it?
- How does it smell? This question is based on a person's intuition and common sense.
- Would you be comfortable if the details of your decision were reported on the front page of your local newspaper or through your hospital's e-mail system?

PATIENT RIGHTS

The American Hospital Association (1992) developed a Patient's Bill of Rights with the expectation that when patients and families par-ticipate in treatment decisions, the outcome will be more effective care. See the "Exploring the Web" section at the end of this chapter to view this document on-line.

ETHICAL LEADERSHIP AND MANAGEMENT OF HEALTH CARE ORGANIZATIONS

Health care leaders are charged with the responsibility of creating an environment that is

Gather Data and Identify Conflicting Moral Claims
- What makes this situation an ethical problem? Are there conflicting obligations, duties, principles, rights, loyalties, values, or beliefs?
- What are the issues?
- What facts seem most important?
- What emotions have an impact?
- What are the gaps in information at this time?

Identify Key Participants
- Who is legitimately empowered to make this decision?
- Who is affected and how?
- What is the level of competence of the person most affected in relation to the decision to be made?
- What are the rights, duties, authority, context, and capabilities of participants?

Determine Moral Perspective and Phase of Moral Development of Key Participants
- Do participants think in terms of duties or rights?
- Do the parties involved exhibit similar or different moral perspectives?
- Where is the common ground? The differences?
- What principles are important to each person involved?
- What emotions are evident within the interaction and with each person involved?
- What is the level of moral development of the participants?

Determine Desired Outcomes
- How does each party describe the circumstances of the outcome?
- What are the consequences of the desired outcomes?
- What outcomes are unacceptable to one or all involved?

Identify Options
- What options emerge through the assessment process?
- How do the alternatives fit the lifestyle and values of the person(s) affected?
- What are legal considerations of the various options?
- What alternatives are unacceptable to one or all involved?
- How are alternatives weighed, ranked, and prioritized?

Act on the Choice
- Be empowered to make a difficult decision.
- Give yourself permission to set aside less acceptable alternatives.
- Be attentive to the emotions involved in the process.

Evaluate Outcomes of Action
- Has the ethical dilemma been resolved?
- Have other dilemmas emerged related to the action?
- How has the process affected those involved?
- Are further actions required?

Figure 14-2 A Guide for Decision Making. Burkhardt, M. A. & Nathaniel, A. K. (2002) Ethics and Issues in Contemporary Nursing. Second Edition. Clifton Park, NY: Delmar Learning.

STOP AND THINK

A nurse administered the wrong medication to a patient. The patient then had to be transferred to the intensive care unit and required a longer stay in the hospital. The nurse freely admitted the mistake to her nurse manager. The manager recommended that the two of them go talk with the patient and explain what happened. Then the administration heard about the incident and advised the manager against telling the patient immediately about the error. The situation was also referred to the hospital ethics committee. How can the nurse make the right decision? Who is the nurse an advocate for? Where does loyalty belong when the patient, the staff nurse, the organization, and self are all involved? Use the guide for decision making and the ethics test discussed earlier in this chapter to decide.

CASE STUDY 14-1

To better relate the study of ethics to yourself, take the self quiz below. Do you agree or disagree with the following statements?

1. I would report a nursing coworker's drug abuse.
2. I see no harm in taking home a few nursing supplies.
3. I would tell the truth to a patient who asked if he was dying.
4. I would tell a patient who asked what narcotic pain medicine he was receiving.
5. It is unacceptable to call in sick to take a day off, even if only done once or twice a year.
6. I would accept a permanent, full-time job even if I knew I wanted the job for only 6 months.
7. If I received $100 for doing some odd jobs, I would report it on my income tax returns.
8. When applying for a nursing position, I would cover up the fact that I had been fired from a recent job.
9. I would report the family of a child when the child has findings not consistent with the reported story.
10. I see no harm in giving ordered drugs on a temporary basis to a drug-addicted patient who presents to the emergency department out of narcotics.

(C. S. Faircloth, RN, Personal Communications, March 13, 2003).

REAL WORLD INTERVIEW

One of my most difficult cases involved a man in his early 40s who was in a coma, ventilator dependent, and declared brain dead. The patient was from a different culture, and when the family arrived 6 weeks later from the country abroad, they refused to allow him to be removed from the ventilator. His parents said they were told by the gods that their son would be well several months in the future. After 2 months in the hospital, the administration began to put pressure on the family to transfer the patient.

—Emily Davison, RN

Case Manager

ethically principled and that supports upholding the standards of conduct set by the health care professions. Characteristics of ethical leadership identified by Cassidy (1998) are integrity and courage. These are essential attributes for health care leaders if they are to create an ethical model in the organization.

Organizational Benefits

Ethical behavior and socially responsible acts are not always free. Investing in work/life programs, granting social leaves of absence, and telling patients the absolute truth about potential problems may not have an immediate return (DuBrin, 2000). Nevertheless, recent evidence suggests that high ethics and social responsibility are related to good financial performance (Positive Leadership, 1998). Another perspective on the relationship between profits and social responsibility is that it works two ways. More profitable firms can better afford to invest in social responsibility initiatives, and these initiatives, in turn, lead to more profits (Waddock & Graves, 1997). Being ethical also helps avoid the costs of paying huge fines for being unethical, and a big payoff from socially responsible acts is that they often attract and retain socially responsible employees and customers (DuBrin, 2000).

Creating an Ethical Workplace

Establishing an ethical and socially responsible workplace is not simply a matter of luck and common sense. Nurse managers can develop strategies and programs to enhance ethical and socially responsible attitudes. These may include:

1. Formal mechanisms for monitoring ethics, such as an ethics program or ethics hotline.

2. Written organizational codes of conduct.

3. Widespread communication in the hospital to reinforce ethically and socially responsible behavior.

4. Leadership by example: if people throughout the firm believe that behaving ethically is "in" and behaving unethically is "out," ethical behavior will prevail.

5. Encouraging confrontation about ethical deviations. Unethical behavior may be minimized if every employee confronts anyone seen behaving unethically.

6. Training programs in ethics and social responsibility, including messages about ethics from executives, classes on ethics at colleges, and exercises in ethics (DuBrin, 2000).

7. Instituting an ethics committee made up of interdisciplinary representatives from nurs-

ing, medicine, administration, clergy, consumers, psychiatry, social work, nutritional services, pharmacy, as well as an ethicist. Additional persons may be invited on an as-needed basis. See Figure 14-3. Ethical dilemmas may be referred to the ethics committee by anyone.

These committees provide guidance to patients and their families as well as the health care team. Additional organizational elements needed to support an ethical workplace are seen in Table 14-3.

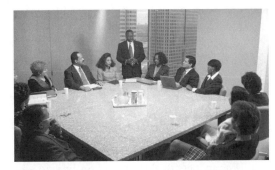

Figure 14-3 Ethics Committee at Work (Photo courtesy of Photodisc)

TABLE 14-3
ORGANIZATIONAL ELEMENTS NEEDED TO SUPPORT AN ETHICAL WORKPLACE

- Have clear job descriptions; hiring, licensing, and credentialing policies; and education and training requirements for RNs, MDs, LPN/LVNs, UAP, RRTs, PTs, social workers, case managers, and other health care staff. The organization must ensure that all staff are safe, competent practitioners before assigning them to patient care. Orient all staff to each other's roles.
- Provide continuous education for all staff to maintain competency.
- Provide standards for ongoing supervision and periodic licensure/ credentialing/competency verification and evaluation of all staff.
- Have clear policies and procedures for delegation and chain of command reporting lines for all staff from RN to charge nurse to nurse manager to nurse executive and, as appropriate to risk management, the hospital ethics committee, the hospital administrator, physicians, the chief of the medical staff, the board of directors, the State Licensing Board for Nursing and Medicine, and the Joint Commission on Accreditation of Health Care Organizations.
- Clarify MD accountability, e.g., if the MD delegates a nursing task to a nonlicensed person, the MD is responsible for monitoring that care delivery. This must be spelled out in hospital policy. If the RN notes that the UAP is doing something incorrectly, the RN has a duty to intervene and to notify the ordering practitioner of the incident. The RN always has a responsibility to protect patient safety.
- Provide standards for regular RN evaluation of UAP and LPNs/LVNs and reinforce the need for UAP and LPN/LVN accountability to the RN. RNs must delegate and supervise. They cannot abdicate this professional responsibility.
- Develop physical, mental, and verbal "No Abuse" policy to be applied to all patients and staff.
- Consider applying for Magnet Status for your hospital. This status is awarded by the American Nurses Credentialing Center to agencies that have worked to improve nursing care (http://www.nursingworld.org).
- Consider a shared governance model of nursing practice to empower nursing decision making.
- Maintain ongoing monitoring of incident reports, sentinel events, and other elements of risk management and performance improvement of the process and outcome of patient care.
- Develop an organizational structure and multidisciplinary committees that foster the development of good communication and evidence-based patient care practices.

ETHICAL CODES

One mark of a profession is the determination of ethical behavior for its members. Several nursing organizations have developed codes for ethical behavior. The International Council of Nurses Code for Nurses appears in Table 14-4.

The American Nurses Association has also developed a Code for Nurses. See the "Exploring the Web" section at the end of this chapter for a site to view this document on-line.

THE FUTURE

Ethical issues in the future that will challenge nursing practice include the allocation of resources, advanced technologies, an aging population, and an increase in behavior-related health problems. These issues all magnify the importance of professional nurses providing leadership that emphasizes ethical behavior in all practice settings.

LITERATURE APPLICATION

Citation: No abuse zone. (2002, March). *Hospitals and Health Networks*, 26, 28.

Discussion: An astounding number of health care workers, 62% to 96%, say that they experienced or witnessed abusive behavior in the past year from a supervisor, a doctor, or even a patient. For example, a nurse working the night shift gets a medication order she can't read and calls the physician at 2 A.M. for clarification. He yells at her and hangs up without answering the question. The nurse is afraid to call back and gives a fatal dose of the wrong drug.

This article discusses guidelines for a five-stage process to rid health care workplaces of abusive behavior. Deborah Anderson, president of Respond 2 Inc., St. Paul, Minnesota, is developing the guidelines in conjunction with the Hennepin Medical Society, Minneapolis, Minnesota. The Respond 2, Inc. five-stage process includes: building a team that meets monthly, surveying employees with an assessment tool about their experiences with workplace abuse, devising a plan to deal with workplace abuse, evaluating outcomes with a resurvey, and infusing the workplace with an atmosphere of collegiality by changing policies and procedures that affect culture, hiring, employee orientation, training, reporting processes, performance evaluation, and appropriate patient safety and quality-related initiatives. In developing this five-stage process, it is imperative that strong support be in place from the leaders of the organization.

Implications for Practice: This five-stage process can be very useful in developing a no-abuse workplace.

TABLE 14-4
INTERNATIONAL COUNCIL OF NURSES CODE FOR NURSES

The fundamental responsibility of the nurse is fourfold: to promote health, to prevent illness, to restore health, and to alleviate suffering.

The need for nursing is universal. Inherent in nursing is respect for life, dignity, and rights of man. It is unrestricted by considerations of nationality, race, creed, color, age, sex, politics, or social status.

Nurses render health services to the individual, the family, and the community and coordinate their services with those of related groups.

Nurses and People

The nurse's primary responsibility is to those people who require nursing care.

The nurse, in providing care, promotes an environment in which the values, customs, and spiritual beliefs of the individual are respected.

The nurse holds in confidence personal information and uses judgment in sharing this information.

Nurses and Practice

The nurse carries personal responsibility for nursing practice and for maintaining competence by continual learning. The nurse maintains the highest standards of nursing care possible within the reality of a specific situation.

The nurse uses judgment in relation to individual competence when accepting and delegating responsibilities.

The nurse, when acting in a professional capacity, should at all times maintain standards of personal conduct that reflect credit upon the profession.

Nurses and Society

The nurse shares with other citizens the responsibility for initiating and supporting action to meet the health and social needs of the public.

Nurses and Coworkers

The nurse sustains cooperative relationships with coworkers in nursing and other fields. The nurse takes appropriate action to safeguard the individual when his care is endangered by a coworker or any other person.

(continues)

Table 14-4 *(continued)*

Nurses and the Profession

The nurse plays the major role in determining and implementing desirable standards of nursing practice and nursing education.

The nurse is active in developing a core of professional knowledge.

The nurse, acting through the professional organization, participates in establishing and maintaining equitable social and economic working conditions in nursing.

From *ICN Code for Nurses: Ethical Concepts Applied to Nursing,* International Council of Nurses, 1973, Geneva: Imprimeries Populaires. Reprinted with permission of International Council of Nurses.

LITERATURE APPLICATION

Citation: Raines, M. L. (2000). Ethical decision making in nurses: Relationships among moral reasoning, coping style, and ethics stress. *JONA's Healthcare Law, Ethics, and Regulation, 2*(1), 29-40.

Discussion: The increasing complexities of health care have led to many ethical dilemmas for nurses. Results from a survey of oncology nurses showed that the nurses experienced an average of 32 different types of ethical dilemmas within the past year. These dilemmas resulted in the nurses experiencing increased stress. The types of ethical issues experienced most frequently were related to pain management, cost containment, decisions in the best interest of the patient, and quality-of-life decisions. The survey also looked at coping strategies that nurses use to deal with stress. Findings indicated nurses used a wide range of positive coping strategies and support resources to help them work through stress. The nurses' primary support consisted of other nurses, but their support resources also included social workers and spouses.

Implications for Practice: Nurses need to develop strategies and have a dependable support system to assist them in coping effectively with the stressful situations encountered in practice.

KEY CONCEPTS

- Society created the profession of nursing for the purpose of meeting specific health needs.

- A personal philosophy stems from an individual's beliefs and values. This personal philosophy will influence an individual's philosophy of nursing.
- Ethics committees provide guidance for decision making about ethical dilemmas

that arise in health care settings.

- The Burkhardt and Nathaniel guide for decision making is a helpful tool.
- Nurse leaders who are dedicated to ethical principles can influence organizational ethics.
- Ethics is the branch of philosophy that concerns the distinction of right from wrong on the basis of a body of knowledge, not just on the basis of opinions.
- Ethical theories offer guidance on ethical living.
- Ethical principles include autonomy and confidentiality, beneficence, nonmaleficence, fidelity, autonomy, respect for others, veracity, and advocacy.
- Ethical values and virtues influence patient care.
- Values clarification is an important step in helping one understand what is truly important.
- The Patient's Bill of Rights encourages more effective patient care.
- The International Council of Nurses' Code for Nurses influences patient care.
- Organizations have a responsibility to society to practice ethically.

KEY TERMS

autonomy	justice
beneficence	morality
bioethics	nonmaleficence
compassion	philosophy
discernment	respect for others
ethical dilemma	values
ethics	veracity
fidelity	

REVIEW QUESTIONS

1. The nurse manager has an ethical responsibility to
   A. the patient.
   B. the organization.
   C. the profession.
   D. the patient, the organization, the profession, and society.

2. The primary role of an ethics committee is to
   A. decide what should be done when ethical dilemmas arise.
   B. prevent the physician from making the wrong decision.
   C. provide guidance for the health care team and family of the patient.
   D. prevent ethical dilemmas from occurring.

3. Ethical dilemmas may be referred to the ethics committee by
   A. physicians only.
   B. nurses, physicians, lawyers, all health care team members, and families of patients.
   C. lawyers only.
   D. hospital administration only.

4. Mrs. Jones rides the elevator to the fifth floor where her husband is a patient. While on the elevator, Mrs. Jones hears two nurses talking about Mr. Jones. They are discussing the potential prognosis and whether he should be told. The nurses are violating which of the following ethical principles?
   A. Autonomy
   B. Confidentiality
   C. Beneficence
   D. Nonmaleficence

REVIEW ACTIVITIES

1. You have a patient who has been labeled as a malingerer who asks what pain medication he is receiving. The nurse knows it is a placebo. Should the nurse tell the patient what the medication is?

   Divide your class into two groups. One group proposes telling the truth and presents the ethical principles that support this position. The other group takes the opposite view and presents the arguments that support this position.

2. An elderly woman, age 88, is admitted to the Emergency Department in acute respiratory distress. She does not have a living will, but her daughter has power of attorney (POA) for health care and is a health care professional. The patient has end-stage renal disease, end-stage Alzheimer's disease, and congestive heart failure. Her condition is grave. The doctors want to intubate her and place her on a ventilator. The sons agree. The daughter states that their mother would not want to be on a machine just to prolong her life.

Divide into groups and discuss the ethical theories and principles that can be applied to this situation. Use the Burkhardt and Nathaniel guide to decision making to help you.

3. As a hospice nurse, you are involved with pain control on a regular basis. Many of the medications prescribed for the management of pain also depress respirations.

Divide into groups and determine a protocol for the use of these medications, keeping in mind that the purpose of hospice is to promote comfort. Support your decisions with ethical theories and principles.

 EXPLORING THE WEB

- See what this Web site says about nursing competencies and ethics. *http://www.ana.org*. Search "ethics" and "competency."
- Use the International Council of Nurses Web site to find the ICN Code for Nurses: *http://www.icn.ch*. Click on the ICN code of ethics.

- Visit *www.aha.org* to view the American Health Association's Bill of Rights.

 REFERENCES

American Hospital Association. (1992). *A patient's bill of rights.* Chicago: Author.

Bowditch, J. L., & Buono, A. F. (1997). *A primer on organizational behavior* (4th ed.). New York: Wiley.

Burkhardt, M. A., & Nathaniel, A. K. (2002). *Ethics & issues in contemporary nursing* (2d ed.). Clifton Park, NY: Delmar Learning.

Cassidy, V. R. (1998). Ethical leadership in managed care. *Nursing Leadership Forum, 3*(2), 52–57.

Chinn, P. L. (1995). *Peace and power: Building communities for the future* (4th ed.). New York: National League of Nursing Press.

Corley, M. (1998). Ethical dimensions of nurse physician relations in critical care. *Nursing Clinics of North America, 33,* 325–337.

DeLaune, S. C., & Ladner, P. K. (2002). *Fundamentals of nursing.* Clifton Park, NY: Delmar Learning.

DuBrin, A. J. (2000). *The active manager.* Mason, OH: Southwestern College Publishing.

International Council of Nurses. (1973). *Code for nurses.* Geneva: Author.

Positive Leadership. (1998, October 5). Research reported in sample issue.

Raines, M. L. (2000). Ethical decision making in nurses: Relationships among moral reasoning, coping style, and ethics stress. *JONA's Healthcare Law, Ethics, and Regulation, 2*(1), 29–40.

Raths, L., Harmin, M., & Simon, S. (1978). *Values and teaching* (2d ed.). Columbus, OH: Merrill.

Sullivan, E., & Decker, P. (2001). *Effective leadership and management in nursing* (5th ed.). Upper Saddle River, NJ: Prentice-Hall.

Waddock, S. A. & Graves, S. B. (1997). The corporate social performance-financial performance link. *Strategic Management Journal*, 303–319.

 SUGGESTED READINGS

American Nurses Association. (2002). *Code of ethics for nurses with interpretive statements.* Washington, DC: American Nurses Publishing.

Austin, W. (2001). Nursing ethics in an era of globalization. *Advanced Nursing Science, 2*, 1–18.

Bishop, A., & Scudder, J. (2001). *Nursing ethics: Holistic caring practice.* Sudbury, MA: Jones & Bartlett.

Bosek, M. (1999). Ethics in practice. *JONA's Healthcare Law, Ethics, and Regulation, 1*(3), 16–19.

Fry, S. T., Johnston, J., Greenfield, S., & Johnston, M. J. (2002). *Ethics in nursing practice: A guide to ethical decision making* (2d ed.). Malden, MA: Blackwell.

Fry, S. T., & Veatch, R. M. (2000). *Case studies in nursing ethics* (2d ed.). Sudbury, MA: Jones & Bartlett.

Kendrick, K. D. & Robinson, S. (2002). Tender loving care as a relational ethic in nursing practice. *Nursing Ethics, 3*, 291–300.

McDaniel, C. (1998). Enhancing nurses' ethical practice: Development of a clinical ethics program. *Nursing Clinics of North America, 33*(2), 299–312.

Meany, M. (2001). From a culture of blame to a culture of safety—the role of institutional ethics committees. *Bioethics Forum, 2*, 32–42.

Peter, E., & Morgan, K. P. (2001). Explorations of a trust approach for nursing ethics. *Nursing Inquiry, 8*, 3–10.

Seifert, P. C. (2002). Ethics in perioperative practice—duty to self. *AORN Journal, 2*, 306–310, 312–313.

Tuckett, A. G. (2000). Virtuous principles as an ethic for nursing. *Contemporary Nurse, 2*, 106–114.

Woods, M. (1999). A nursing ethic: The moral voice of experienced nurses. *Nursing Ethics, 5*, 423–433.

CHAPTER 15

They always say
time changes
things, but you actu-
ally have to change
them yourself.
(Andy Warhol)

Cultural Diversity and Spirituality

OBJECTIVES

Upon completion of this chapter, the reader should be able to:

1. Define culture.
2. Discuss the composition of the U.S. population.
3. Identify key cultural nursing theories.
4. Review strategies for working with a multicultural team.
5. Discuss organizational culture.
6. Integrate understanding and respect for spiritual and religious beliefs of different peoples into patient care.

Mr. Wu is brought into the Emergency Department with diaphoresis, nausea, and vomiting, and he is clutching his left chest. He is speaking with his wife in Chinese and says he understands only a little English. His wife understands none. Fortunately, Charles Lin, a nurse practitioner, is working this shift and is able to communicate in Chinese with the Wu family. Living in Chinatown, Mr. Wu often sees a Chinese doctor who prescribes various herbs for his heart problems. While in the Emergency Department, Mr. Wu refuses to take Western medicine and wishes to see an acupuncturist for his pain.

What are your thoughts on how best to provide care for Mr. Wu?

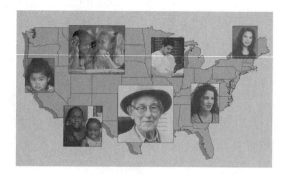

What can you do as a member of the health care team to help Mr. Wu understand what is happening?

Why would Mr. Wu refuse the medication if he entered the hospital?

The United States is a country consisting of many cultures, races, religions, and belief sets. The United States is becoming increasingly diverse and global, with many minority cultures and races developing into majority cultures and races. Newer religions take their place alongside traditional faiths. Both cultural and spiritual differences in people are potential causes for misunderstanding, confusion, and conflict, arising from intolerance and ignorance of these differences. It is imperative that health care providers have an awareness, knowledge, and appreciation for others whose beliefs, values, and practices are different. Culture, religion, and spirituality are often closely intertwined and interdependent, especially in the delivery of health care to an ill patient and the patient's family or community. This chapter discusses key points to keep in mind when working and providing care in a culturally diverse environment. Several nursing theorists are discussed, and trends in diversity are outlined. A section on spirituality will aid in providing the holistic care of a client. Finally, selected beliefs of major world religions are presented.

DEFINING CULTURE, ETHNICITY, ETHNOCENTRISM, VALUES, AND ACCULTURATION

Before one defines a specific culture, one must take into account a person's total environment and his or her relationship to the community. Culture is not defined by the individual; instead, **culture** is defined by the behaviors, norms, belief sets, values, and folkways of a specific group. We grow up with our culture's influences, yet cultural patterns may be altered as we age, or as we move to other communities. As people are exposed to practices within their culture, certain factors are incorporated, shaping one's viewpoints and attitudes (Erlen, 1998). Cultural patterns may be explicit, such as wearing certain clothing, or implicit, such as following religious expectations on certain holidays. Figure 15-1 shows ways in which people differ.

Leininger (1997) states that certain cultural behaviors guide decisions in an expected patterned response, suggesting that practices are

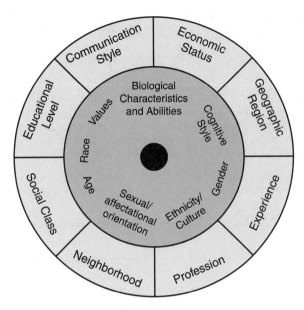

Figure 15-1 Ways in Which People Differ

learned through direct and indirect observations of others. She believes one's cultural background affects the reactions that are generated by any given situation. A patient's cultural background influences that patient's perceptions of health, wellness, and illness (Spector, 2000; Purnell & Paulanka, 1998). See Table 15-1 for selected characteristics of culture.

Ethnicity is a cultural group's perception of itself (group identity). This self-perception influences how the group's members are perceived by others. Ethnicity involves a sense of belonging and a common social heritage that is passed from one generation to the next. Members of an ethnic group demonstrate their shared sense of identity through common customs and

TABLE 15-1
SELECTED CHARACTERISTICS OF CULTURE

- *Culture is learned and taught.* Cultural knowledge is transmitted from one generation to another. A person is not born with cultural concepts but instead learns them through socialization.
- *Culture is shared.* The sharing of common practices provides a group with part of its cultural identity.
- *Culture is social in nature.* Culture develops in and is communicated by groups of people.
- *Culture is dynamic, adaptive, and ever-changing.* Adaptation allows cultural groups to adjust to meet environmental changes. Cultural change occurs slowly and in response to the needs of the group. It is this dynamic and adaptable nature that allows a culture to survive.

STOP AND THINK

You are the team leader when Mr. Wu arrives on your unit from the Emergency Department. He is diagnosed with a myocardial infarction (MI) and is admitted for telemetry monitoring as well as intravenous medications. As you enter the room to do an initial assessment, the certified nursing assistant (CNA) comes out frustrated and tells you, "I do not know what we are going to do with Mr. Wu. He will not let anyone near him."

What is your response to the CNA? What is your first priority regarding care for Mr. Wu? How would you proceed with your assessment? What do you identify as your challenges in caring for Mr. Wu?

traits. **Ethnocentrism** is the belief that one's own culture or ethnic group is better than all other groups, without considering the merits of the other group.

Race refers to a grouping of people based on biological similarities. Members of a racial group have similar physical characteristics such as blood group, facial features, and color of skin, hair, and eyes. There is often overlap between racial and ethnic groups because the cultural and biological commonalities support one another (Giger & Davidhizar, 1999). The similarities of people in racial and ethnic groups reinforce a sense of commonality and cohesiveness.

Values are those standards with which a society is maintained. Generally, values are what our families, community, and society teach as right versus wrong, moral or immoral, ethical or unethical (Yukl, 1994). Cultural values have meaning for a particular group and are the desirable behaviors that are reinforced by the culture. Sometimes, a value may be understood and accepted only by the members of a specific culture, with outside cultures questioning the rationale behind the value. For example, in the American culture, it is generally accepted that the female in a household may hold a job outside the home for a variety of reasons; in other cultures, women are strongly discouraged from working outside the home at all.

The United States once prided itself on its perceived identification as a melting pot, a soci-ety in which all cultures would live and take on American cultural values and characteristics. However, in recent years, the emphasis has shifted to maintaining one's cultural identity and acknowledging the differences (Spector, 2000). Members of a minority culture will usually be identified as members of that minority culture; however, they may take on the positive or negative characteristics of the dominant culture. **Acculturation** is the process by which individuals adjust and adapt either to their host culture or a subculture by altering their own cultural behaviors. Acculturation may be seen in America's Chinatowns: the parents who immigrated may maintain their own native language and customs, such as seeing a Chinese doctor for a physical ailment. The children of the immigrants may speak English as their primary language, with a Chinese dialect as a secondary language, and may seek medical attention from a Western-trained physician for care.

U.S. DIVERSITY

The United States has always welcomed, even encouraged, peoples of diverse cultures, races, and ethnicities. According to 1998 census data, 14% of the United States population, or 31.8 million people, speak a primary language in their home other than English. Thiederman (1996) believes, however, that almost 97% of all people living in the United States can speak some English. The states with the highest percentage of those who speak another primary language are: 36% in New Mexico; 31% in California; and 20% in Arizona, Hawaii, New Jersey, New York, and Texas (Stapleton, 1998).

The U.S. ethnic profile is changing quickly. What was once the majority population may no longer be the dominant race, culture, or ethnic group. It is noted by the U.S. Bureau of the Census that immigrant populations are increasing and may be the majority population in some cities and states. Federally defined racial/ethnic groups for census purposes are white, black, Asian/Pacific Islander, Hispanic, and American Indian/Eskimo. An Asian/Pacific Islander is someone from one of 28 Asian countries or the 25 identified Pacific Islander cultures. In the United States, the Chinese, Filipino, and Japanese are the three largest Asian/Pacific Islander groups. The term *Hispanic* identifies anyone with Spanish as a native language or a linkage to Spain, Latin America, or Mexico. Those members comprising the American Indian/Eskimo population are from one of more than 500 tribes and villages within the United States; almost half live outside a reservation (*Federal Register*, 1996).

According to the 1990 United States Census, by the year 2080 the U.S. cultural mix will be at least 50% minority ethnic groups: Hispanics, 23.4%; African Americans, 14.7%; Asians and others, 12%. Minority groups are becoming the majority group in many areas of the United States, such as in the urban areas of Miami, San Antonio, Washington, D.C., and Los Angeles.

Racial and Ethnic Diversity of Health Care Providers

Unfortunately, the face of American health care providers does not mirror the population that they care for on a daily basis. Studies have illustrated that the health care industry does not reflect the national trend of racial and ethnic diversity, especially in the physician, nursing,

and administrator ranks (Association of American Medical Colleges, 1998). A National Sample Survey completed in 1996 reflects the current demographics of RNs. In 1996, 90% of the total registered nurse workforce was white, non-Hispanic; 4%, black, non-Hispanic; 3%, Asian/Pacific Islander; 2%, Hispanic; and 1%, American Indian/Eskimo (Figure 15-2). Moore (1997) identified that 12% of students entering medical school in 1995 were either black, Indian, Mexican-American, or Puerto Rican. The Association of American Medical Colleges in 1998 identified that only 10% of this minority population became medical students (American Academy of Pediatrics, 2000).

CULTURAL THEORIES

Cultural nursing theories and conceptual models provide a framework for addressing the needs of individual patients and their families while maintaining awareness of cultural differences. **Cultural competence** is defined by the American Academy of Nursing (1992) as care that is sensitive to issues related to culture, race, gender, and sexual orientation. This care is provided by nurses who use cultural nursing theory, models, and research principles in identifying health care needs. The American Medical Association advocates culturally effective health care, taking into consideration the relationship between the provider and patient. Additionally, the Joint Commission on Accreditation on Healthcare Organizations (JCAHO) has commented in its standards on Patient Rights and Organization Ethics that patients have a right to care that is considerate and respectful of their personal values and beliefs (Joint Commission on Accreditation of Healthcare Organizations, 2000).

Transcultural Nursing

Nursing has developed several models of care delivery to help explain relationships between the nurse and culturally diverse patients and their families. Perhaps the best-known model and theory come from Madeleine Leininger,

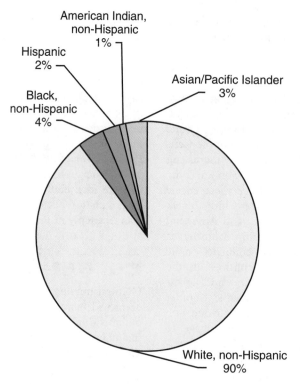

American Indian,
non-Hispanic
1%

Hispanic
2%

Black,
non-Hispanic
4%

Asian/Pacific Islander
3%

White, non-Hispanic
90%

Figure 15-2 Racial and Ethnic Mix of Registered Nurse Population in the United States, 1996

identified as the founder of transcultural nursing theory, who began her research of transcultural nursing in the 1960s. According to Leininger (1978), **transcultural nursing** is the comparative study and analysis of different cultures and subcultures in the world with respect to their caring behavior, nursing care and health-illness values, beliefs, and patterns of behavior with the goal of developing a scientific and humanistic body of knowledge to provide culture-specific and culture-universal nursing care practices. Leininger (1997) states that several precepts are inherent in the practice of transcultural nursing. Caring is the first concept: all cultures have expressions of caring and caring behaviors. However, what is defined as caring in one culture may be perceived very differently in another culture. The second concept is that each culture identifies what it considers adequate and necessary care. Most important, application of tran-

scultural nursing to direct patient care requires an acute awareness of each culture's lifestyle patterns; values; beliefs and norms; symbols and rituals; verbal and nonverbal communications; caring behaviors; shared meanings; and rituals of health, wellness, and illness (Leininger, 1997).

Giger and Davidhizar Model

Giger and Davidhizar's Transcultural Assessment Model (1999) offers a method of completing a cultural assessment and evaluating the meanings of cultural variations. Giger and Davidhizar identify five central concepts in their assessment model: transcultural nursing and provision of culturally diverse nursing care; culturally competent care; cultural uniqueness of individuals; culturally sensitive environments;

and culturally specific illness and wellness behaviors. The authors state that transcultural nursing is patient centered and research focused.

Giger and Davidhizar (1999) describe six concepts that are apparent in every cultural group and that need to be reviewed by nurses when they perform a complete cultural assessment. These six concepts are communication, space, social organization, time, environmental control, and biological variations. The communication concept includes an assessment of both spoken and unspoken language; the space concept includes an assessment of how close people stand to one another, including touch. For example, if we come from a cultural background that encourages touch and closeness, we need to be aware that the members of numerous other cultures require considerably more space and less touch to feel comfortable, especially around strangers. Assessment of social organization reviews cultural identifications such as race, ethnicity, and family patterns.

Every culture has specific ideas about the concept of time and its application in social and personal situations. What may be interpreted as being on time for one culture may be perceived as either extremely early or even late for another culture. Cultural differences are also noted in time orientations of what is future, present, or past time. The concept of environmental control assesses the perceived influence individuals have on their surroundings and their ability to maintain certain cultural health practices. One critical feature of the Giger and Davidhizar model is its inclusion of assessment of biological variations among cultures. Many ethnic and cultural groups are predisposed to certain diseases, have identifying physical characteristics, and have genetic distinctions.

Cultural Competence

Campinha-Bacote (1994) defines cultural competence as a process in which the nurse and patient, family, or community continuously work together to provide optimal care in a culturally diverse environment. Campinha-Bacote identi-

fies four elements necessary to provide culturally competent care. The first element—cultural awareness—builds a sensitivity to another's culture by encouraging self-analysis of one's own prejudices and biases. The goal is for the nurse to move beyond any ethnocentric values to be able to fully appreciate another's culture.

The second element in Campinha-Bacote's model is obtaining cultural knowledge. In this element, nurses increase their familiarity with various cultures, especially values, practices, and lifestyles. Cultural skill is the third element, which involves a cultural assessment of the patient, including his or her perceptions of health and illness, and identifying possible teaching opportunities. The final element illustrated in this model is the cultural encounter, when the nurse has occasion to experience a culture to refine or modify existing knowledge about a specific cultural group (Campinha-Bacote, Yahle, & Langenkamp, 1996).

Spector's Model

Spector (2000) has expanded on several models to describe the degree to which people's lifestyles reflect their traditional culture, whether European, Asian, African, Hispanic, or others. In Spector's view, it is assumed that ethnic groups keep their traditional values, beliefs, and norms; this is known as having consistent heritage. The heritage becomes inconsistent when acculturation occurs.

Spector identifies three categories in her model, the Cultural Heritage Model: culture, religion, and ethnicity. The other six categories in Spector's model are similar to Giger and Davidhizar's model: space, time, communication, biological variations, social organization, and environmental control.

In completing a cultural assessment of a patient using this model, the nurse would perform an assessment in each of the nine categories in Table 15-2. The nurse would begin with the six categories from the Giger and Davidhizar model, then assess the remaining three categories in the Spector model. The cultural

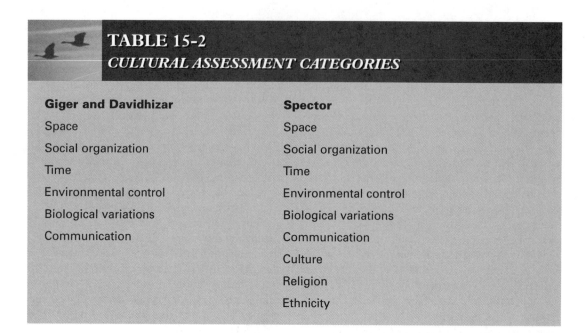

TABLE 15-2
CULTURAL ASSESSMENT CATEGORIES

Giger and Davidhizar	Spector
Space	Space
Social organization	Social organization
Time	Time
Environmental control	Environmental control
Biological variations	Biological variations
Communication	Communication
	Culture
	Religion
	Ethnicity

category calls for assessment of the language spoken in the culture, any unique folkways, traditions, and practices. The religion category calls for assessment of the historical religious beliefs held by the patient and others in the group, as well as formal religious participation. The final category, ethnicity, involves assessment of the symbolic meanings, values, and traditions of a group and includes migratory status, race, kinship ties, food preferences, and internal and external perceptions of group distinctiveness (Spector, 2000). See Table 15-3 for a nursing checklist for providing culturally sensitive care. See Table 15-4 for a cultural resource guide for patient care.

MANAGING A CULTURALLY DIVERSE TEAM

Being different in race, culture, gender, age, sexual affections, or abilities may not always be seen as positive by some people in an organization. Some may think that being different is a deficit, showing obvious or sometimes not-so-

obvious discomfort and displaying prejudices. Others might negate any differences among people, treating everyone the same, regardless of their abilities, values, beliefs, cultural backgrounds, or potential contributions. There is no one best way to manage a multicultural team. It is critical to remember that each culture has developed its own patterned responses to conflict management, stress, joy, fear, work habits, and communication. The following are a few suggestions for working effectively with a multicultural team:

- When problem solving, be sure to include people who are from different cultural backgrounds, experiences, and abilities. By including a variety of team members, you will obtain a variety of ways to look at an issue, with a variety of ways to solve it.
- Not everyone responds to conflict in the same manner. Some may avoid conflict, whereas some may want to confront it. Understand how your team works and what the team members' expectations are for the final result. Model respectful behavior.
- Strive to understand what diversity can bring to the group. Focus on the cultural

TABLE 15-3
NURSING CHECKLIST FOR CULTURALLY SENSITIVE CARE

1. Assess and incorporate family history of health care:
   - Fluency in English
   - Extent of family support or disintegration of family
   - Community resources
   - Level of education
   - Change of social status as a result of coming to this country
   - Intimate relationships with people of different backgrounds
   - Level of stress
   - Spector and Giger and Davidhizar categories from Table 15-2

2. Affirm patient strengths and potential for growth.

3. Recognize informal caregivers (family members and significant others) as an integral part of treatment.

4. Demonstrate caring behaviors rather than just tolerating cultural variations in patient's behavior.

TABLE 15-4
CULTURAL RESOURCE GUIDE

Culture Group and Language	Belief Practices	Nutritional Preferences	Communication Awareness	Patient Care/ Handling of Death
American. English.	Family-oriented.	Beef, chicken, potatoes, vegetables; fast foods, ethnic foods.	Talkative, shake hands, not much touching during conversation. Prefer to gather information for decision-making. Some hugging and kissing, mainly between women.	Family members and friends visit in small groups. Expect high-quality care.

(continues)

Table 15-4 *(continued)*

Culture Group and Language	Belief Practices	Nutritional Preferences	Communication Awareness	Patient Care/ Handling of Death
Mexican. Spanish. May speak one of 50 dialects.	Pray, say rosary, have priest in time of crisis. Limited belief in "brujeria" as a magical, supernatural, or emotional illness precipitated by evil forces.	Corn, beans, chiles, yellow rice.	Tend to describe emotions by using dramatic body language. Very dramatic with grief, but otherwise diplomatic and tactful. Direct confrontation is rude.	May believe that outcome of circumstance is controlled by external force; this can influence patient's compliance with health care. Women do not expose their bodies to men or other women.
Cuban. Spanish.	Catholic with Protestant minority. Santeria, which can include animal sacrifice.	Bread, café con leche, coffee; roast pork, black beans, and rice; plantains, chicken, and rice.	Some may have a tendency to be loud when having a discussion. Use their hands for emphasis and credibility.	Culture requires visiting the sick; the extended family supports the immediate family. It is an insult to the patient if there is not a large family/friend presence.
African-American. English.	Belong to Baptist and other Protestant sects: Muslim	Pork not eaten by Islamics.	Use eye contact to establish trust and demonstrate respect. Silence may indicate lack of trust toward caregiver.	Jehovah Witness will refuse blood transfusion. Are reluctant to donate blood or organs.
Filipino. English, Spanish, and Tagalog (80 dialects).	Seek both faith healer and Western physician when ill. Belief that many diseases are the will of God.	Theory of hot and cold food. Certain foods in the Philippines are traditionally eaten hot or cold, e.g., milk is only taken HOT. Fish, rice, vegetables, and fruit. Meals have to be HOT.	Value and respect elders. Loving and family-oriented. Set aside time just for family.	Family decision important. Ignore health-related issues; often non-compliant. In spite of Western medicine, they often leave things in the hands of God, with occasional folk medicine. Home remedies; herbal tea, massage, and sleep.

(continues)

Table 15-4 *(continued)*

Culture Group and Language	Belief Practices	Nutritional Preferences	Communication Awareness	Patient Care/ Handling of Death
				May subscribe to supernatural cause of disease.
Chinese. Many dialects spoken; one written language.	Harmonious relationship with nature and others; loyalty to family, friends, and government. Public debate of conflicting views is unacceptable. Accommodating, not confrontational. Modesty, self-control, self-reliance, and self-restraint. Hierarchical structure for interpersonal and family interaction.	Often lactose intolerant. Soy sauce, MSG, and preserved foods. Diet consisting of vegetables and rice. Tofu (bean curd) can be prepared in various ways.	Quiet, polite, and unassertive. Suppress feelings of anxiety, fear, depression, and pain. Eye contact and touching are sometimes seen as offensive or impolite. Self-expression and individualism are discouraged.	Women uncomfortable with exams by male physicians. May not adhere to fixed schedule. May fear medical institutions. Use a combination of herbal and Western medicine at the same time. Traditional: acupuncture, herbal medicine, massage, skin scraping, and cupping. Alcohol may cause flushing.
Korean. Hangul.	Family-oriented. Believe in reincarnation. Believe in balance of two forces: hot and cold.	High fiber, spicy seasoning. Speak little during meal. Often lactose and alcohol intolerant.	Reserved with strangers. Use eye contact with familiar individuals. First names used only for family members. Proud and independent. Children should not be used as translators due to reversal of parent/child relationship.	Family needs to be included in plan of care. Prefer non-contact. Respond to sincerity.

(continues)

Table 15-4 *(continued)*

Culture Group and Language	Belief Practices	Nutritional Preferences	Communication Awareness	Patient Care/ Handling of Death
Vietnamese. Vietnamese language has several dialects.	Family loyalty is very important. General respect and harmony. Supernatural is sometimes used as an explanation for disease.	Rice often with green leafy vegetables, fish sauce added for flavor. Meat used sparingly. Tea is main beverage. Often lactose and alcohol intolerant.	Communication— formal, polite manner; limit use of touch. Respect conveyed by nonverbal communication. Person's name used with title, i.e., "Mr. Bill," "Director James."	Negative emotions conveyed by silence and reluctant smile; will smile even if angry. Head is sacred—avoid touching. Back rub— uneasy experience. Common folk practices—skin rubbing, pinching, herbs in hot water, balms, string tying. Misunderstanding about illness—drawing blood seen as loss of body tissue; organ donation causes suffering in next life. Hospitalization is last resort. Flowers only for the dead.

Courtesy of Bonnie Clipper Salzberg, St. David's Medical Center, Austin, TX.

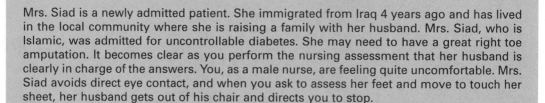

CASE STUDY 15-1

Mrs. Siad is a newly admitted patient. She immigrated from Iraq 4 years ago and has lived in the local community where she is raising a family with her husband. Mrs. Siad, who is Islamic, was admitted for uncontrollable diabetes. She may need to have a great right toe amputation. It becomes clear as you perform the nursing assessment that her husband is clearly in charge of the answers. You, as a male nurse, are feeling quite uncomfortable. Mrs. Siad avoids direct eye contact, and when you ask to assess her feet and move to touch her sheet, her husband gets out of his chair and directs you to stop.

What is your first reaction? How would you handle the situation? What should you consider in your plan of care for Mrs. Siad and her family?

REAL WORLD INTERVIEW

One of the positive things that has happened in my life is that I have been in the military. While in the military, I have worked with many multicultural and multiethnic people. Respect ties everything together. Respect the people you work for and who you work with. Take care of your patients as you would want yourself or your family taken care of. If you work with respect for others, you will conquer prejudices and differences between people.

—Janice Couch, RN Clinical Manager

LITERATURE APPLICATION

Citation: Gooden, M. B., Porter, C. P., Gonzalez, R. I., & Mims, B. L. (2001). Rethinking the relationship between nursing and diversity. *American Journal of Nursing, 101*(1), 63–65.

Discussion: The authors believe that—to safeguard human dignity, to circumvent uncertainty and discomfort, and to respect individuality—nursing has embraced the ethic of caring as the sine qua non of the profession, along with concepts of "diversity" and "multiculturalism," as perspectives for interpersonal relations with patients of all races and ethnicities. But regrettably, disabilities, sexual orientation, gender, social class, physical appearance (such as obesity), and ideologies (such as differing political or religious views) have yet to be incorporated into nursing's concept of diversity.

Nurses might begin to initiate discussion among themselves about diversity by defining racial and ethnic minorities as a subset of the population that has a disproportionately high risk of exposure to factors that compromise health (such as environmental toxins, poverty, lack of health care access, and poor housing).

The American Nurses Association (ANA) has written a series of position statements (for example, *Discrimination and Racism in Health Care, Discrimination against Gays and Lesbians in the Military, Decade of Disabled Persons, Cultural Diversity in Nursing Care*); it has created councils and task forces to address issues of diversity in health care; and it has worked diligently for legislation to improve the health of members of racial and ethnic minorities (the Agenda for Health Care Reform and the Nurse Education Act are two examples). Moreover, the ANA's commitment to the incorporation of the concept of diversity into its activities is evidenced by its participation as the only nursing organization on the Steering Committee to Eliminate Racial and Ethnic Disparities in Health, cosponsored by the Department of Health and Human Services and the American Public Health Association.

Implications for Practice: If the nursing profession is to close the health-disparity gap and improve the welfare of the citizens in the United States, it is imperative that nurses rethink the relationship between nursing and diversity.

differences and build an appreciation for what everyone can contribute.

- Do not assume that all members of a certain ethnic group, gender, age, or culture act and respond in the same manner. Do not label one culture as preferred over another.
- Value everyone's differences and recognize their similarities. Seek out experiences with those whose cultural background is different from your own.
- Pay close attention to both verbal and non-verbal communication for cultural cues. Confront, acknowledge, and work with prejudices so that effective communication can occur.
- Ask for clarification. Do not assume.
- Alter your assumptions about others based on their membership in certain groups. For example, do not conclude that all males from a particular culture act a certain way toward females just because they are a member of a certain ethnic group.
- Assist those who are not of the majority cultural group to be successful. As a starting point, include them in informal networking within the organization's culture.

ORGANIZATIONAL CULTURE

Organizational culture is the system of shared values and beliefs that actively influence the behavior of organization members. The term *shared* is important because it implies that many people are guided by the same values and that they interpret them in the same way. Values develop over time and reflect an organization's history and traditions. Culture consists of the culture of an organization, such as being helpful and supportive toward new members (DuBrin, 2000).

Five dimensions of organizational culture are of major significance in influencing organizational culture (Ott, 1989).

1. Values. Values are the foundation of any organizational culture. The organization's philosophy is expressed through values, and values guide behavior on a day-to-day basis.

2. Relative diversity. The existence of an organizational culture assumes some degree of similarity. Nevertheless, organizations differ in how much deviation can be tolerated.

3. Resource allocation and reward. The allocation of money and other resources has a critical influence on culture. The investment of resources sends a message to people about what is valued in the organization.

4. Degree of change. A fast-paced, dynamic organization has a culture different from that of a slow-paced stable one. Top-level managers, by the energy or lethargy of their stance, send messages about how much they welcome innovation.

5. Strength of the culture. The strength of a culture or how much influence it exerts is partially a by-product of the other dimensions. A strong organizational culture guides employees in many everyday actions. It determines, for example, whether an employee will inconvenience himself or herself to satisfy patients. If the organizational culture is not so strong, employees are more likely to follow their own whims—they may decide to please a patient only when convenient.

SPIRITUALITY

Religion and spirituality play a large role in many peoples' lives—they influence what people wear, who they can marry, when they seek medical advice, and when they can peacefully die. It is often when people are sick that they seek comfort from religious or spiritual beliefs, seeking strength in their faith or beliefs.

Defining Spirituality and Religion

Spirituality and *religion* are two distinct terms, yet they are closely interrelated. Stoll (1989) defines spirituality "as my being: my inner person. It is who I am—unique and alive. My spirituality motivates me to choose meaningful relationships and pursuits. Through my spirituality I give and receive love; I respond to and appreciate God, other people, a sunset, a symphony and spring." Stoll identifies two key dimensions of spirituality in her discussion: the dimension of her relationship with a higher being and the dimension of her relationships with herself and other people, identifying her place in nature. The term **spiritual** refers to a belief in a higher power, an awareness of life and its meaning, and the centering of a person with his or her purpose in life. Spiritual does not necessarily mean following an organized religion, but it may mean valuing oneself, one's environment, and those who are part of that surrounding environment. One can be spiritual yet not be a member of a recognized religious group.

Religion is an organized and public belief system of worship and practices that generally has a focus of a god or supernatural power. Religion generally offers an arrangement of symbols and rituals that are meaningful and understood by those who follow and participate in the beliefs and values of the religion. Often, there are religious rituals that mark significant events and passages in a person's life: birth, adulthood, marriage, and death. However, being a member of a religious group does not make someone spiritual (Long, 1997).

Spiritual Distress

One area of cultural assessment that may produce discomfort for the nurse is the area of spiritual/religious assessment. Many times religion and religious upbringing are topics that are not freely discussed because they are thought to be private information, not to be readily shared. This may be one reason some health care providers may not feel comfortable in assessing their patient's religious beliefs. The North American Nursing Diagnosis Association (NANDA) has identified three nursing diagnoses that address the spiritual care of the patient: spiritual distress (distress of the human spirit), risk for spiritual distress, and readiness for enhanced

spiritual well-being (North American Nursing Diagnosis Association, 2001).

Spiritual distress includes questioning the purpose of life and its meaning, refusing to participate in one's usual religious practices, and seeking unusual assistance rather than the usual spiritual or religious support (Tucker, Canobbio, Paquette, & Wells, 1996). Spiritual distress may occur when there is a conflict between what an individual wants or desires to occur and the beliefs of the individual's religion, such as when a Catholic patient uses birth control. Other examples include when an unexpected negative patient outcome occurs, and the patient gets angry at her God, believing that she was being punished or that she was unworthy of getting better.

To provide spiritual care, the nurse does not need focused religious education, just an awareness that a spiritual assessment, much like a cultural assessment, is useful for complete patient care and optimal outcomes. If the nurse becomes aware that the patient is suffering from spiritual distress, then the nurse can decide whether to address it directly with the patient or the patient's family, or whether to bring someone to the patient who may be more helpful, such as the patient's own religious representative.

Spiritual Assessment

Nurses need to ensure that they ask the questions that may lead to better patient outcomes. In a Duke University study of older adults, it was discovered that those patients who participated in religious activities were 40% less likely to have high blood pressure (Gale Group, 2000). There is more and more interest in the effect that spirituality and religion play on a person's physical health and well-being (Levin, Larson, & Puchalski, 1997). An integral part of a patient's initial assessment should include data about a patient's spiritual and religious beliefs. This is more than identifying which church a person attends and who his or her next of kin is. Several spiritual assessment tools are found in the literature (Reed, 1991; Dossey, Keegan, & Guzzetta, 2000; Leininger, 1997; O'Brien, 1999). These tools assist the nurse in assessing patient spirituality.

REAL WORLD INTERVIEW

It is sometimes hard for nurses to address completing a spiritual patient assessment if they don't want to look like they are imposing their own beliefs on their patients. Maybe they feel uncomfortable even talking about the topic with patients if they are not even acknowledging their own spirituality. Their comfort level with their own spirituality is going to affect their patient assessments.

—Janice Wyatt, RN, Clinical Manager

Religious Beliefs Related to Health Care

The following section offers a brief description of the major religions of the world. A nurse should be attentive to the spiritual needs and customs of patients and their families in order to provide holistic nursing care. Note that members of each religion vary in their adherence to their religion's beliefs.

Buddhism

Buddhism follows the teaching of Buddha. Buddhist rituals include chanting of last rites at bedside immediately following death. Buddhism discourages drug and alcohol use, and some sects are vegetarian. Illness is seen as a result of negative karma. Cleanliness is viewed as very important. Buddhists are often hesitant to receive treatment such as surgery on holy days.

Christianity

Members of the Christian church profess a belief in Jesus Christ. There are many denominations within the Christian religion, such as Roman Catholic, Baptist, and Episcopalian. These denominations may even have opposite ideas and rituals. A Roman Catholic patient may have beliefs and values that are very different from those of a member of an Episcopalian church, yet both are professed Christians.

Health care practices vary widely, as do religious activities and even social expectations and traditions. Many Christians use the Bible to guide them in everyday life. A patient may turn to the Bible as a source of encouragement, especially during difficult times. Other Christians do not. Because of the wide variety of Christian religions, it is imperative that nurses make sure they have an understanding of a patient's belief set when they perform a spiritual assessment. For example, Jehovah's Witnesses will not submit to any blood transfusions, yet other Christian religions have no qualms about accepting this procedure. Seventh-day Adventists have dietary restrictions that include caffeine and alcohol. Roman Catholics don't believe in abortion.

Hinduism

Hinduism is believed to be one of the oldest religions in the world. Fasting occurs on specific days of the week, according to which god the Hindu person worships. Most Hindus accept modern medical practices; however, many believe that a person's illness is a result of sins committed in a previous life. Many Hindus are vegetarians. Last rites are carefully prescribed, and family members are often particular about who touches a body after death. A Hindu will most likely be cremated.

Judaism

Judaism is a religion based on the word and laws of God, as written in the book of the Old Testament. There are several different Jewish ideologies. Central to Jewish beliefs is that there is one God. Anyone born of a Jewish mother is considered to be Jewish, as is anyone who formally converts to Judaism. Holy days are many, with the Sabbath beginning on Friday evening at sundown and lasting through sundown on Saturday.

Depending on the ideology followed, some Jewish people have dietary restrictions, known as kosher dietary laws. These laws prohibit the eating of certain meats and eating milk and meat products together during a meal. Upon death, the body is ritually cleansed and buried as soon as possible after death. Autopsy is prohibited in the Jewish faith.

Islam

The religion of Islam comprises many sects of the Islamic faith. Followers perform ritual washing after prayer, which occurs five times a day. Followers of Islam do not eat any pork products, nor do they drink alcoholic beverages. One important ritual is the fasting period in the ninth month of the Muhammadan year, called *Ramadan*; during this period, one fasts during the daytime. Family must be with a dying person. The dying person must confess his sins and ask forgiveness. The family washes the body and only family and friends may touch the body. They usually oppose autopsy. Islamic patients may hold a fatalistic view that interferes with or hinders compliance with the treatment plan.

Agnosticism and Atheism

Two other terms may arise when a nurse cares for a patient and completes a spiritual assessment. If patients state they are **agnostic,** they are not committed to belief in the existence or nonexistence of a god or a supreme being, or perhaps they believe that no one has effectively proven that a god exists. If patients state they are

atheists, they do not believe in the existence of a god or a supreme being.

KEY CONCEPTS

- As a result of changing demographics in the United States, a majority race or ethnicity today may soon become a minority.
- Health care providers need to more closely mirror the diversity of their patients. Concerted efforts are being made to recruit diverse students to both the medical and nursing professions.
- Culture has a significant influence on the delivery of care for patients, including their interpretations of health and illness and when and how they seek medical attention.
- Diversity characteristics include such things as age, race, ethnicity/culture, sexual/affectional orientation, gender, physical abilities, and so on.
- Transcultural nursing provides a framework for understanding such things as caring behavior, health-illness values, and so on.
- Working on a multicultural team requires an understanding of culture.
- Some nursing theorists on culture include Leininger, Giger and Davidhizar, Campinha-Bacote, and Spector.
- Understanding a patient's beliefs about health care and illness affects the outcomes of care and leads to culturally competent care.
- Spirituality and religion are different entities yet are important for the holistic care of a patient.
- Patients often consider spiritual and religious beliefs to be personal information, which may interfere with gathering a spiritual assessment.
- Nurses need to be aware of their own spirituality and beliefs to feel comfortable in discussing spirituality or religious beliefs with a patient.
- Patients practice many religious beliefs.

KEY TERMS

acculturation

agnostic

atheist

cultural competence

culture

ethnicity

ethnocentrism

race

religion

spiritual

spiritual distress

transcultural nursing

values

REVIEW QUESTIONS

1. Which are important issues to consider when working with a multicultural team?
   A. Everyone should be focused on the same goals and objectives.
   B. All nurses should be from the same professional background.
   C. Everyone should have the same values about health care.
   D. Everyone in the United States should have the same beliefs because they all are living in the United States.

REVIEW ACTIVITIES

1. You are a nurse in an HIV clinic that sees a variety of patients from all cultures and ethnicities.

   What type of information is necessary for you to take care of your patients? What do you see as some of the challenges in working with your patient population?

2. The hospital where you work is in a predominantly white, non-Hispanic area. Lately, there has been an influx of migrant farmworkers from Mexico because local farms cannot find local workers.

   What do you perceive as some of the health needs of the migrant farmworkers? What do you see as potential barriers to care for these workers? How would you facilitate the provision of care for these workers and their families?

3. On the unit where you work as a nurse, one particular nurse is adamant about sharing her Christian religious beliefs with patients and their families, regardless of their background, religion, or culture. A Jewish family is upset because the nurse was teaching Protestant beliefs to their ill father.

   What will you discuss with the family? Are there any potentially positive outcomes of this situation? What will you say to your nurse coworker? Should anything else be done?

EXPLORING THE WEB

- This Web site breaks down the population of the United States: *http://www.census.gov*
- Language and cultural effects on health care delivery are the focus of this site: *http://www.diversityrx.org*
- Looking for a listing of transcultural nursing references? Try these two sites: *http://www.sunyit.edu*. Click on "library and resources" and type in "transcultural nursing." *http://www.iun.edu*
- The following site has a variety of culture and ethnicity links: *http://www.cultural-diversity.org*

REFERENCES

American Academy of Nursing. (1992). AAN expert panel report. *Nursing Outlook, 40*(6), 277–283.

American Academy of Pediatrics. (2000). Enhancing the racial and ethnic diversity of the pediatric workforce. *Pediatrics, 105*(1), 129–131.

Association of American Medical Colleges. (1998). *Minority medical students in medical education: Facts and figures IX*. Washington, DC: Author.

Campinha-Bacote, J. (1994). Cultural competence in psychiatric nursing: A conceptual model. *Nursing Clinics of North America, 29*, 1–8.

Campinha-Bacote, J., Yahle, T., & Langenkamp, M. (1996). The challenge of cultural diversity for nurse educators. *The Journal of Continuing Education in Nursing, 27*(2), 59–64.

Dossey, B. M., Keegan, L., & Guzzetta, C. E. (2000). *Holistic nursing: A handbook for practice* (3rd ed.). Gaithersburg, MD: Aspen.

DuBrin, A. J. (2000). *The active manager*. Clifton Park, NY: Delmar Learning.

Erlen, J. A. (1998). Culture, ethics and respect: The bottom line is understanding. *Orthopaedic Nursing, 17*(6), 79–82.

Federal Register. (1996, November 13). Notice. 61 *Federal Register* 58211–58216.

Gale Group. (2000). Cleveland Medical School programs incorporate spirituality as a prescription for healing. *Jet, 97*(17), 16.

Giger, J. N., & Davidhizar, R. E. (1999). *Transcultural nursing*. Baltimore: Mosby.

Gooden, M. B., Porter, C. P., Gonzales, R. J., & Mims, B. L. (2001). Rethinking the relationship between nursing and diversity. *American Journal of Nursing, 101*(1), 63–65.

Joint Commission on Accreditation of Healthcare Organizations. (2000). *Comprehensive manual for hospitals: The official handbook*. Oakbrook Terrace, IL: Author.

Leininger, M. (1978). *Transcultural nursing: Concepts, theories and practices*. New York: Wiley.

Leininger, M. (1997). Transcultural nursing research to transform nursing education and practice: 40 years. *Image: Journal of Nursing Scholarship, 29*, 341–347.

Levin, J. S., Larson, D. B., & Puchalski, C. M. (1997). Religion and spirituality in medicine: Research and education. *Journal of the American Medical Association, 278*(9), 792–793.

Long, A. (1997). Nursing: A spiritual perspective. *Nursing Ethics, 4*, 496–510.

Moore, J. D. (1997, December 15). The unchanging of healthcare. *Modern Healthcare*, 30–34.

North American Nursing Diagnosis Association. (2001). *NANDA's nursing diagnosis: Definitions and classifications 2001–2002*. Philadelphia: Author.

O'Brien, M. E. (1999). *Spirituality in nursing*. Sudbury, MA: Jones and Bartlett.

Ott, J. (1989). *The organizational culture perspective*. Chicago: Dorsey Press.

Purnell, L. D. & Paulanka, B. J. (1998). *Transcultural health care*. Philadelphia: F. A. Davis.

Reed, P. G. (1991). Preferences for spirituality related nursing interventions among terminally ill and nonterminally ill hospitalized adults and well adults. *Applied Nursing Research, 4*(3), 122–128.

Spector, R. (2000). *Cultural diversity in health and illness*. Norwalk, CT: Appleton & Lange.

Stapleton, S. (1998). Emphasis on cultural competence. *American Medical News, 41*(9), 3.

Stoll, R. (1989). The essence of spirituality. In V. Carson (Ed.), *Spiritual dimensions of nursing practice* (pp. 4–23). Philadelphia: Saunders.

Thiederman, S. (1996). Improving communications in a diverse healthcare environment. *Healthcare Financial Management, 50*(11), 72–75.

Tucker, S., Canobbio, M., Paquette, E., & Wells, M. (1996). *Patient care standards: Collaborative planning guides*. St. Louis, MO: Mosby.

Yukl, G. (1994). *Leadership in organizations* (3rd ed.). Englewood Cliffs, NJ: Prentice Hall.

Warhol, A. (1975). *The philosophy of Andy Warhol: From A to B and back again*. New York: Harcourt, Brace, Jovanovich.

 # SUGGESTED READINGS

American Association of Colleges of Nursing. (1997). *Statement on diversity and equality of opportunity*. Washington, DC: Author.

American Association of Colleges of Nursing. (1998). *Essentials of baccalaureate education for professional nursing practice*. Washington, DC: Author.

Barnes, D. M., Craig, K. K., & Chambers, K. B. (2000). A review of the concept of culture in holistic nursing literature. *Journal of Holistic Nursing, 3,* 107–221; discussion 221–226.

Brown, G. (2001). Culture and diversity in the nursing classroom: An impact on communication and learning. *Journal of Cultural Diversity, 1,* 16–20.

Carpenito, L. J. (1999). *Handbook of nursing diagnosis* (8th ed.). Philadelphia: Lippincott.

Coile, R. C., Jr. (2001). Magnet hospitals use culture, not wages, to solve nursing shortage. *Journal of Healthcare Management, 4,* 224–227.

Davidhizar, R., & Giger, J. N. (2001). Teaching culture within the nursing curriculum using the Giger-Davidhizar Model of Transcultural Nursing Assessment. *Journal of Nursing Education, 6,* 282–284.

Lauver, D. R. (2000). Commonalities in women's spirituality and women's health. *Advances in Nursing Science, 22*(3), 76–88.

Leininger, M. (2002). Culture care theory: A major contribution to advance transcultural nursing knowledge and practices. *Journal of Transcultural Nursing, 3,* 189–192.

Mendyka, M. (2000). Exploring culture in nursing: A theory-driven practice. *Holistic Nursing Practice, 1,* 32–41.

Neuhauser, P. C. (2000). Culture.com: Leading the way to e-nursing. *Journal of Nursing Administration, 12,* 580–582.

Pew Health Professions Commission. (1995). *Critical challenges: Revitalizing the health professions for the twenty-first century.* San Francisco: UCSF Center for the Health Professions.

Polifko-Harris, K. (1995). *The influence of national culture on work-related values and job satisfaction between American and Filipino registered nurses.* Unpublished doctoral dissertation, Old Dominion University, Norfolk, VA.

Polifko-Harris, K. (2000). Managing a culturally diverse workforce. In L. M. Simms, S. A. Price, & N. E. Ervin (Eds.), *Professional practice of nursing administration* (pp. 567–581). Clifton Park, NY: Delmar Learning.

Rayman, K. M., Ellison, G. C., & Holmes, G. (1999). Toward a caring culture in professional nursing. *Seminar in Nurse Management, 4,* 188–192.

Rooda, L. (1993). Knowledge and attitudes toward culturally different patients: Implications for nursing education. *Journal of Nursing Education, 32*(5), 209–213.

Stevens, S. (2002). Nursing workforce retention: Challenging a bullying culture. *Health Affairs, 5,* 189–193.

CHAPTER 16

The future belongs to those who believe in the beauty of their dreams. (Eleanor Roosevelt)

NCLEX-RN Preparation and Your First Job

OBJECTIVES

Upon completion of this chapter, the reader should be able to:

1. Discuss preparation for the NCLEX.
2. Detail the process of beginning a successful nursing job search.
3. Develop a resume and cover letter.
4. Identify appropriate preparation for a successful job interview.
5. Discuss potential interview questions and identify acceptable answers.
6. Describe typical components of health care orientation.
7. Discuss elements of performance feedback.

Juliette will be graduating from her nursing education program in 1 month. She is one of the few students in her class who has not even begun looking for a job. She is beginning to wonder whether she should start now rather than wait until she passes her NCLEX-RN. Everyone else around her excitedly speaks about the job market being wide open, but she is just not motivated to start her job search.

Should Juliette begin her job search now? Should she wait until she takes the NCLEX-RN?

What are some of the positive aspects of waiting to begin her job search until she becomes a registered nurse (RN)? What are some of the negative aspects of waiting?

Where are the opportunities for new graduate nurses?

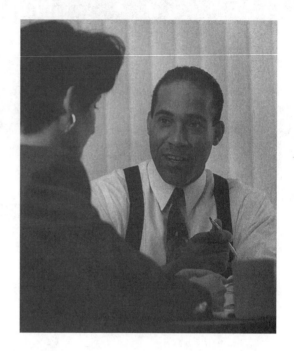

Starting a new career is exciting, but it also may cause a little anxiety, even if you are well prepared. New graduates are no longer under the watchful eyes of their instructors and now must make independent nursing decisions. The focus of this chapter is to give new nursing graduates the tools to pass NCLEX and to seek and obtain a nursing position. Included in this chapter are tips on NCLEX preparation, resume writing, sample interview questions and answers, and hints on how and where to search for a job.

PERSPECTIVES

Data from the National League for Nursing (NLN, 2001) illustrates the following:
- Average age of nurses: 43.4 years
- Average associate professor's age: 52.0 years
- Steady decline in enrollment in nursing education programs from 1995 to 1999 and a 13.6% decline in graduates
- 32% of nursing graduates were BS prepared and 10% were MS prepared in 1999

- Steady decline in the number of NCLEX-RN exams taken from 1994 to 1999

These facts have led to many opportunities for nurses.

PREPARATION FOR NCLEX-RN

NCLEX-RN is the national nursing licensure examination prepared under the supervision of the National Council of State Boards of Nursing. NCLEX is taken after graduation from an accredited nursing program and prior to practice as a registered nurse. The examination follows a test plan formulated on four categories of client needs that registered nurses commonly encounter. The concepts of the nursing process, caring, communication, cultural awareness, documentation, self-care, and teaching/learning are integrated throughout the four major categories of client needs. The percentage of NCLEX questions in each category is identified in Table 16-1.

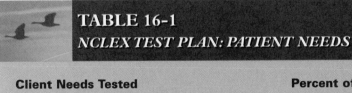

TABLE 16-1
NCLEX TEST PLAN: PATIENT NEEDS

Client Needs Tested	Percent of Test Questions
Safe, effective care environment:	
Management of care	7–13%
Safety and infection control	5–11%
Physiologic integrity:	
Basic care and comfort	7–13%
Pharmacological and parenteral therapies	5–11%
Reduction of risk potential	12–18%
Physiological adaptation	12–18%
Psychosocial integrity:	
Coping and adaptation	5–11%
Psychosocial adaptation	5–11%
Health promotion and maintenance:	
Growth and development through the life span	7–13%
Prevention and early detection of disease	5–11%

NCLEX Questions

Graduates may receive anywhere from 75 to 265 questions on the NCLEX examination during their testing session. Fifteen of the questions are questions that are being piloted to determine their validity for use in future NCLEX examinations. Students cannot determine whether they passed or failed the NCLEX examination from the number of questions they receive during their session.

Factors Affecting NCLEX-RN Performance

Several factors have been identified as being associated with performance on the NCLEX examination. Some of these factors are identified in Table 16-2.

Review Books and Courses

In preparing to take the NCLEX, the new graduate may find it useful to review several of the many NCLEX review books on the market. It is useful to review content and questions developed by different authors of these review books. Review content in the review books in any of your weak content areas. Review books often include a review of nursing content, or sample test questions, or both. They frequently include computer software disks with test questions for review. The test questions may be arranged in the review book by clinical content area, or they

TABLE 16-2
FACTORS ASSOCIATED WITH NCLEX-RN PERFORMANCE

- HESI Exit Exam
- Assesstest
- NLN Comprehensive Achievement Test
- NLN achievement tests taken at end of each nursing course
- Verbal SAT score
- ACT score
- High school rank and GPA
- Undergraduate nursing program GPA
- GPA in science and nursing theory courses
- Competency in American English language
- Reasonable family responsibilities or demands
- Absence of emotional distress
- Critical thinking competency

may be presented in one or more comprehensive examinations covering all areas of the NCLEX. Be sure to actually practice taking the examinations in the review books. Do not just jump ahead to look at the section on correct answers and rationales before answering the questions if you want to improve your examination performance.

Once you have completed a comprehensive examination in the review books, review the answers and rationales for any weak content areas and take another comprehensive exam. Repeat this process until you are doing well in all clinical content areas and in all areas of the NCLEX examination plan. Listings of the NCLEX review books are available at *http://www.amazon.com*. It is helpful to use several of these books and computer software when reviewing for the NCLEX.

NCLEX review courses are also available. Brochures advertising these programs are often sent to schools and are available in many sites nationwide. The quality of these programs can vary, and students may want to ask faculty and former nursing graduates for recommendations. Practice visualization and relaxation techniques as needed. These strategies will assist you in conquering the three areas necessary for successful test taking—anxiety control, content review, and test question practice.

Nursing Exit Exams

Many nursing programs administer an examination to students at the completion of their nursing program. Some of these exams are the NLN Achievement test and the HESI Exit Exam. New graduates who examine their feedback from one of these examinations have important information regarding their strengths and weaknesses that can help them focus their review for the NCLEX. A strategy for examining this feedback and organizing this review is outlined in Table 16-3.

REAL WORLD INTERVIEW

My best advice to anyone preparing for the NCLEX is to take lots of practice tests. I answered close to 1,500 questions in preparation and I feel it did me a world of good. I kept my nursing textbooks handy and when I ran into something I didn't know, I looked it up.

—*Amanda Meadows, RN, BSN*

TABLE 16-3
PREPARATION FOR THE NCLEX-RN TEST

Name: _____

Strengths: _____

Weak content areas identified on NLN examination, HESI Exit Exam, Assesstest or comprehensive exam from NCLEX review book:

_____

_____

_____

Weak content areas identified by yourself or others during formal nursing education program (include content areas in which you scored below a grade of B in class or any factors from Table 16-2):

_____

_____

_____

Weak content areas identified in any area of the NCLEX test plan, including the following:

Safe, effective care environment

Physiological integrity

Psychosocial integrity

Health promotion and maintenance

Weak content areas identified in any of the top 10 patient conditions in each of the following categories:

Adult health

Women's health

Mental health nursing

Children's health

(Consider the 10 top diagnoses, medications, diagnostic tools and tests, nursing interventions, treatments, and procedures used for each of the patient categories.)

Weak content areas identified in the following areas:

Therapeutic communication tools   Delegation

Defense mechanisms   Setting priorities

Growth and development   Other

Management

(continues)

Table 16-3 *(continued)*

Organize Your Study

Your study schedule could look like the following:

Day 1: Practice adult health test questions. Score the test, analyze your performance, and review test question rationales and content weaknesses.

Day 2: Practice women's health test questions. Repeat above process.

Day 3: Practice children's health test questions. Repeat above process.

Day 4: Practice mental health test questions. Repeat above process.

Day 5: Continue with content review and question practice in all weak content areas. Continue this process until you are doing well in all areas of the test.

REAL WORLD INTERVIEW

A dean that I know talks about the fact that she failed what was called in those days "the boards." She tells her students that it was the most traumatic event of her life (or at least *one* of the most traumatic events). When you have given it "your all" to complete a nursing curriculum, you want to be a successful NCLEX candidate. The HESI Exit Exam can help you achieve that goal. Look at your score printout and review any subject area that has a HESI score of less than 85. Remember, HESI scores are NOT percentage scores, but research data indicate that those who have HESI scores of 85 or above have a 94% probability of passing the NCLEX-RN (Nibert, Young, & Adamson, 2002).

— *Susan Morrison, PhD, RN*

— *President Health Education Systems, Inc. (HESI)*

Tips for NCLEX

Some final tips for NCLEX are shared in Table 16-4.

BEGINNING A JOB SEARCH

The critical first step in your job search is preparation. Know what clinical area you are interested in and what skills you have that may fit that area.

Consider what type of hospital you want to work in; that is, a large university teaching hospital, a small private community hospital, and so forth.

Magnet Hospitals

In 1993, the American Nurses Credentialing Center (ANCC) established the Magnet Services Recognition Program. The ANCC Magnet Program has certified 50 hospitals in the United States and is now expanding internationally. It

TABLE 16-4
SELECTED NCLEX TIPS

- Remember Maslow's Hierarchy of Needs.
  - Meet physical needs first: airway, breathing, circulation, safety.
- Don't choose a psychological answer as the correct answer if your patient has a higher priority physical need.
- Remember the nursing process—assess your patient first, then plan, implement, and evaluate.
  - Do in this order: assess, plan, implement, evaluate.
- In answering questions, assume you have the doctor's order for any possible choices. NCLEX is usually looking for the correct nursing action.
- Assume you have perfect staffing, plenty of time, and all the necessary equipment for any possible answer choices on the test.
- Assume you are able to give perfect care, "by the book"—don't let your personal experience direct you to choose an answer that is less than high-quality care.
- Remember to care for the patient first and then check the equipment.
- Know 10 most common diseases with medicines, labs, diagnostic tools, procedures, treatments used in each of the 10 most common diagnoses for adult medical, surgical, women, children, and psychiatric disorders.
- Know common lab norms, e.g., K, BS, CBC, hematocrit, pro time, PTT, ABG, SG of urine, digoxin level, lithium level, BUN, and creatinine.
- Know communication techniques—look for answers that offer patients your support and keep them talking.
- Know the defense mechanisms.
- Know growth and development, e.g., developmental tasks for each age, toys for each childhood stage, etc.
- Know management rules:
  - Don't delegate assessment, teaching, or evaluation.
  - It is okay to delegate care for a stable patient with expected outcomes.
  - It is okay to delegate tasks that involve standard, unchanging procedures.
- Prepare mentally with:
  - Anxiety control
  - Relaxation techniques
  - Regular exercise
  - Avoiding negative people
  - Thinking positively
- Remember—you graduated from and met the criteria of a nationally and/or state accredited nursing program. You can pass one more test!

has had proven success in raising the standards of nursing practice. The characteristics of ANCC Magnet hospitals include high nurse-to-patient ratios, substantial nurse autonomy and control over the practice setting, positive nurse and physician relationships, nurse participation in organizational policy decisions, and strong nursing leadership.

Not only are nurses in Magnet hospitals more likely to rate their care environment as

STOP AND THINK

You are taking your NCLEX-RN in 6 weeks. Using Table 16-3, identify your plan of study. How will you identify your strengths and weaknesses? How can you work to improve any weaknesses?

excellent, but there is also some evidence that patient outcomes are better in Magnet hospitals. In one study, patients with AIDS in Magnet hospitals had a significantly lower mortality rate than those on dedicated AIDS units or in scattered bed arrangements in non-Magnet hospitals. The Magnet hospitals' better outcomes in this instance were attributed to their higher nurse-to-patient ratios (Aiken, 2002).

Nursing Residency Programs

Consider looking for a 1-year nursing residency program like the one currently being implemented through a partnership between the American Association of Colleges of Nursing (AACN) and the University HealthSystem Consortium (UHC). In addition to developing clinical judgment and leadership skills for new nurses at the point of care, the goal of the residency program is to strengthen the new nurse's commitment to practice in the inpatient setting by making the first critical year a positive working and learning experience (JCAHO, 2001).

Multistate Licensure Compact

The multistate licensure compact allows a nurse to have one license (in his or her state of residency) and to practice in other states (both physically and electronically), subject to each state's practice law and regulation. Under mutual recognition, a nurse may practice across state lines unless otherwise restricted. View guidelines of the multistate licensure compact at *http://*

www.ncsbn.org. Find the nurse licensure compact map and click on it.

Where to Look

The first place many nurses think to begin a job search is the local newspaper. Other places include employment bulletin boards, telephone lines, and job fairs. Many health care employers have an employment bulletin board, telephone line, or Web site that identifies job openings on a weekly basis. It is often helpful to begin a job tracking file. See Figure 16-1.

Electronic Media and the Internet

There are several sources of on-line employment. These sources include search engines; job boards; and agency and company sites such as those for a specific hospital, health care agency, or health care company. Electronic media sites can also include health care journals. Following are some examples of search engines:

- Dogpile (allows you to search multiple search engines at one time; this site is known as a metasearch engine):
  http://www.dogpile.com
- Excite: *http://www.excite.com*
- WebCrawler: *http://www.webcrawler.com*
- Infoseek: *http://www.infoseek.com*
- Google: *http://www.google.com*

Some examples of job boards specific to health care include the following:

- *http://www.healthcareerweb.com*
- *http://www.medjobs.com*
- *http://www.monster.com*

Agency and Referral Source	Telephone Number	Contact Name	Resume Sent/Date	Thank-You Letter	Follow-Up

Figure 16-1 Tracker for Job Leads

- *http://www.aone.org* (This site requires membership to use.)

A few examples of other sites with job openings include the following:

- *http://www.rn.com*
- *http://www.careercity.com*

DEVELOPING A RESUME

Resumes are generally the first opportunity a prospective employer has to see who you are and what your qualifications are for a given position.

A **resume** is a brief summary of your background, training, and experience as well as your qualifications for a position (see Figure 16-2). It should be viewed as a marketing tool to sell yourself to a prospective employer. Generally, a resume should be no longer than one to two pages on good quality white or ivory paper. It needs to contain concise information that clearly identifies your specific skills, strengths, and experiences. A resume should be honest, neat, easy to read, and have no errors. In companies that are highly desirable to work at, the resume is also often used as a screening tool so that a recruiter's time can best be spent wisely with potential employees who are seen as welcome team members.

There is no one perfect resume style. It is agreed that an effective resume (1) gets the employer's interest; (2) identifies critical areas such as education, work experience, and special qualifications; (3) should be tailored to the employer's needs; (4) creates a favorable first impression about you and your abilities; (5) communicates that you are someone who is a good fit for the position; and (6) is visually appealing. A good resume takes time to prepare. Avoid abbreviations. You should ensure that what is presented on paper is truthful and presents you as a capable person who is able to make immediate and sustained contributions to an organization.

The statement "References available upon request" can be placed on the last line of a resume. You can either provide a listing of references on the application, or bring a separate reference list to a job interview. Include at least three professional references, with names, titles, addresses, and phone numbers—but only after receiving permission from these persons to use them as references. Do not use family, friends, or neighbors as references. Notify your references when you interview to let them know they may be contacted.

Table 16-5 is a summary of action verbs for resume preparation.

Writing a Cover Letter

A resume should always have a letter of introduction, known as the cover letter. It is a one-page letter designed to entice the prospective employer to become interested enough to read the resume. It does not reiterate the entire resume but presents highlights and a summary of the essential points found on the resume. Figure 16-3 is an example of a cover letter.

Developing an Electronic Resume

There are several ways to create an electronic resume, including writing the resume using standard word processing software such as Microsoft Word or WordPerfect. Type the resume using the word processing software and then save it in one of three formats: ASCII plain text (.txt), rich-text (.rtf), or as hypertext (.html). ASCII text files are the most common types of data files found on the Internet. This type allows for simplicity in reading the text but does not allow any type of text formatting such as boldface characters, bullets, underlining, or italics. The recipient receives plain, clear text without any identifying marks, tabs, or visually appealing formatting. If you want to highlight a specific area, then use a character like an asterisk (*).

Table 16-6 identifies the steps to follow in creating an electronic resume.

A SUCCESSFUL INTERVIEW

A registered nurse is considered a professional, with professional dress expected for the interview. A good rule of thumb is to wear what you would consider business attire (Figure 16-4). For women, a suit with skirt, a tailored pantsuit, or a neat dress is appropriate. For men, a neatly tailored shirt with tie, pants, and perhaps a sport

Caitlin O'Malley
2424 Sailing Avenue
Cherry Hill, NJ 08080
(609) 444-2212 (home)
cat24@excite.net

OBJECTIVE: An entry-level position as a pediatric registered nurse

EDUCATION: Associate of Science in Nursing, May 2004
Freedom Community College, Philadelphia, PA

Highlights: * Maintained 3.66 GPA, Dean's list
* Class president
* Preceptorship on the Oncology Unit at the Children's Hospital of Philadelphia

EXPERIENCE: Patient Care Assistant, Labor and Delivery
St. Mary's Medical Center, Philadelphia, PA
(August 2002–present)

Duties: * Assist in the preparation of the operating room
* Provide basic patient care monitoring, including vital signs, phlebotomy, glucose screening
* Prepare and stock patient rooms

Life Guard and Camp Counselor
Camp Perry, Point Pleasant, NJ
(Summers 1999–2002)

Duties: * Supervise waterfront for 150 campers along with three additional lifeguards
* Perform basic camp counselor duties, including direct supervision of campers ages 9 to 14

CERTIFICATION: Certified as a Basic Life Support Provider, 1999–present

PROFESSIONAL
ORGANIZATIONS: National Student Nurses Association
American Red Cross, Blood Drive Volunteer
Philadelphia Free Clinic, Registration Volunteer
Hospice Volunteer

Figure 16-2 Resume

TABLE 16-5
LIST OF ACTION VERBS FOR RESUME

accomplished	delivered	identified	operated	reorganized
achieved	demonstrated	increased	organized	revamped
administered	designed	initiated	oversaw	revised
analyzed	developed	innovated	performed	simplified
approved	directed	instituted	planned	solved
built	earned	launched	proposed	streamlined
communi-cated	eliminated	listed	provided	supervised
	established	maintained	purchased	taught
completed	evaluated	managed	redesigned	terminated
conceived	expanded	mastered	reduced	trained
conducted	explored	motivated	reengineered	transformed
coordinated	generated	negotiated	reinforced	utilized
created				

coat would be appropriate to wear to an interview for a staff nurse position. It is best to dress conservatively rather than in a trendy manner. Makeup, perfume, and jewelry should be minimal. Be sure to turn off all cell phones and pagers so that all your attention can be directed at the interviewer. Use good eye contact with your interviewer. Practice potential interview questions ahead of time. Use the interview time to highlight your strengths and abilities. See Table 16-7.

Questions to Ask During an Interview

You will also be offered the opportunity to ask questions of the interviewer, so be prepared with several that clearly illustrate your interest in the organization and your willingness to become a valued team member. It is best to have your questions written down so that if you are under a little stress, you do not forget to ask specific

questions. See Table 16-8 for some sample questions that you might want to investigate.

Writing a Thank-You Letter

After your interview, you should send a thank-you letter to the interviewer. Many people do not take the time to write a personal note, and this will set you apart from other potential employees as someone who is professional and sincerely interested in joining the organization. Figure 16-5 illustrates a thank-you letter as a follow-up to an interview.

ORIENTATION TO YOUR NEW JOB

Many health care organizations divide nursing orientation into general and unit-specific sections. According to a report in the *Chicago Tribune,* half

Caitlin O'Malley
2424 Sailing Avenue
Cherry Hill, NJ 08080
(609) 444-2212

April 10, 2004

Ms. Vanetha Raj, BSN, RN
Nurse Recruiter
Shore Memorial Hospital
100 Seashore Drive
Point Pleasant, NJ 07726

Dear Ms. Raj:

This letter is in response to your advertisement in the April 10, 2004 issue of the Philadelphia Inquirer for a registered nurse in the pediatrics ward. I completed my pediatric clinical rotation at Children's Hospital of Philadelphia and since that time I have had a strong interest in developing a career in pediatric nursing.

I am currently enrolled in the Associate of Science in Nursing program at Freedom Comunity College and plan to graduate in May 2004. My GPA in nursing is currently a 3.66, and I am active in professional activities such as the Nursing Student Association, Omicron Delta, and as a mentor to undergraduate nursing majors. I am highly motivated and enjoy working with children and their families. I look forward to learning as much as I can about the nursing profession in my new position.

Thank you for your time and consideration of my resume. I look forward to speaking with you in the near future to discuss the potential of employment as a registered nurse at Shore Memorial Hospital. I will be calling within the next week to check on the status of my application. I may be reached at home at (609) 444-2212.

Sincerely,

Caitlin O'Malley

Figure 16-3 Cover Letter

TABLE 16-6
CREATING AN ELECTRONIC RESUME

Step 1: In the word processing program, set margins so that 6.5 inches of text are displayed. This is seen easily by the majority of e-mail programs.

Step 2: Write the resume using a font in 12-point type, such as Courier 12 or Times New Roman 12.

Step 3: Save the resume as a text-only file with line breaks. Do not use the Tab key. Use the space bar instead. Use the left justification format.

Step 4: Open this new file in a text editor such as Microsoft Notepad.

Step 5: Review the resume. This is how the recipient will see the resume once it is transmitted via e-mail. Pay careful attention to unsupported formats or those formats that your word processing program may not be able to read. You may have to add ASCII-supported characters such as asterisks to make the resume easier to view. Proofread!

Step 6: Copy and paste the resume in the body of a test e-mail message. Maybe send it back to yourself or a friend who uses a different e-mail program to see how the recipient views your resume.

Step 7: When sending a resume electronically, a cover letter should also accompany the resume. Rather than sending both the cover letter and the resume in the text area, or as separate attachments, the preferred approach is to send the cover letter in the text portion of the e-mail, and attach the resume.

Adapted from *Electronic resumes and online networking* (p. 72), by R. Smith, 1999, Franklin Lakes, NJ: Career Press.

of all hospitals have reduced orientation programs for newly graduated nurses. Once hired, new nurses receive an average of 30 days training, in contrast with 3 months of hands-on training provided 5 years ago (Berens, 2000). General orientation includes information and skills measurement, which all nurses new to the facility need, regardless of their eventual unit assignment. Figure 16-6 is a sample schedule for the first week of general orientation at one medical center.

General orientations are outcome based, requiring the orientee to demonstrate competency, perhaps by written medication or knowledge tests or skills measurement (Burke, 2000).

Unit-based orientation, whether it follows the general orientation or is interspersed throughout, focuses on the specific competencies a new nurse needs to care for the diagnoses and ages of patients typical to the assigned unit. Many organizations have developed unit-specific competency tools that list those skills orientees need to demonstrate. These lists provide a useful road map with which to plan a learner-specific orientation. Figure 16-7 is an excerpt from an Emergency Department's unit-based orientation tool. It is also useful to identify your own learning needs and to study them on your own. See Table 16-9.

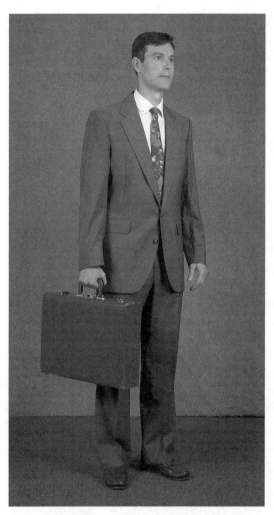

Figure 16-4 Interview attire should be neat and professional.

Preceptors

Preceptors can play a key role in introducing the new nurse to coworkers and other members of the health team. The orientee needs to be introduced to the specific functions and roles of those people who interact daily with the nurses on the unit (Marrelli, 1997). This helps the new nurse identify relationships within the unit and between the unit and the larger health care organization.

A good preceptor is clinically experienced, enjoys teaching, and is committed to the role. Good preceptors need to be familiar with the organization's policies and procedures and willing to share knowledge with their orientees (Meinecke, 2000). The best preceptors are active and purposeful with their charges (Marquis & Huston, 2000). They model behaviors and think out loud in the hearing range of their orientees (Fey & Miltner, 2000).

Reality Shock

In 1974, Kramer described "reality shock" and discussed the difficulties some new graduates have in adjusting to the work environment. Kramer identified a conflict between new graduates' expectations and the reality of their first nursing position. A skilled preceptor can assist new nurses through this transition by offering them opportunities to validate their impressions. The support of other new nurses in a similar situation, such as those participating in the same core orientation, is particularly helpful (Marquis & Huston, 2000).

Mentors

Developing a mentoring relationship with a more experienced, successful nurse is another strategy for professional growth and help in setting long-term goals. A mentor coaches a novice nurse and helps the novice develop skills and career direction (Shaffer, Tallarica, & Walsh, 2000). A mentor may introduce the new nurse to professional networking opportunities and may assist the new nurse in workplace problems.

To find a mentor, a new nurse needs to communicate a willingness to learn and grow. A newer nurse usually needs to seek out a prospective mentor rather than wait to be approached by one. An ideal mentor is an experienced nurse who is willing to support and counsel other nurses when asked (Shaffer et al., 2000). This may lead to a formal structured relationship or a more informal role-modeling association.

TABLE 16-7
INTERVIEW QUESTIONS

Question	Potential Response
Tell me about yourself.	Do not go into a long list, but have two to three traits that are solid (e.g., "I am a positive person and look for new learning experiences").
Why do you want to work here?	Describe several attributes of the work environment, the staff, or the patients (e.g., "I enjoyed my rotation on 5 West—the staff worked as a team and I am looking for that type of support in my first position" or "I am interested in your excellent orientation program for new graduates" or "I want to work at a Magnet hospital").
What do you want to be doing in 5 years?	Identify a long-term goal and figure out how to achieve it with progressive responsibilities and achievements.
What are your qualifications?	Discuss education and experiences that you have had that qualify you for the new position.
What are your strengths?	This is a favorite question. Look at the job description. What qualities do you have that are required? Are you able to work under stress, are you organized, are you eager to learn new skills, do you enjoy new challenges? Do you work well with others? Do you have good communication skills? Are you a hard worker?
What would your references say?	You may want to ask your references this question. Would they say you are focused? A team player? A problem solver? Good at project completion?
Are you interested in more schooling?	Many who have just graduated may want to say no, but an employer wants someone who is interested in life-long learning, especially in the nursing profession.
What has been your biggest success?	Think of a success ahead of time that may fit with the organization. It does not have to be in nursing.
What has been your greatest failure?	Again, think ahead, but this time, make sure you can state what you learned from the negative experience. After all, to fail is to learn, so state what you would do differently next time and why.
If applicable, why do you want to leave your current job?	You can say that you are seeking new responsibilities, experiences, and challenges. Give an example of a new experience you are looking for.

TABLE 16-8
SAMPLE QUESTIONS TO ASK DURING AN INTERVIEW

1. How can I prepare myself to work on this unit and do a good job?

2. May I have a copy of the job description and performance appraisal form? When will I be evaluated?

3. Is there a clinical ladder program?

4. Who is my preceptor?

5. What shift will I be scheduled to work? Will I rotate shifts? Are special requests for time off honored?

6. What holidays and weekends am I scheduled to work?

7. What type of benefits are offered with this position? (Health, dental, retirement, holiday time, sick time, continuing education opportunities, educational reimbursement)

8. What type of orientation or internship will I receive? How long is it? Does it address how to work well with other practitioners?

9. What is the salary? When do raises occur? Is there a shift differential? Is there a differential for advanced nursing degrees?

10. Is this a Magnet hospital? Do you monitor nurse sensitive outcomes?

PERFORMANCE FEEDBACK

Everyone needs feedback about their performance, particularly when they are in a new position. Some preceptors and managers recognize new employees for their progress, but in many cases, the new nurse needs to solicit their feedback. A concrete mechanism to measure one's own performance is through the objective learning materials, job descriptions, and competency-based orientation tools provided by nurse educators. New nurses must successfully pass the written and technical parts of orientation. While in orientation, and at least annually thereafter, new graduates should meet at regular intervals with their preceptor and manager to review progress (Fey & Miltner, 2000).

At each of these sessions, it is important for the new nurse to solicit feedback. Ask, "How do you think I'm doing? Am I at the level you would expect? What should I focus on next?"

Answers to questions such as these allow the orientee to measure progress and set goals for the future.

A sample performance goals outline might look like the following:

By the next scheduled performance assessment, nurse Joanne Johnson will do the following:

- Successfully complete the advanced pediatric assessment course
- Assume the primary nurse role for patients with an anticipated length of stay of greater than 3 days
- Become an active participant on a unit-based or hospitalwide committee
- Attend a pediatric nursing conference

360-Degree Feedback

Some health care organizations have moved to an evaluation program known as **360-degree feedback**. In the 360-degree feedback system,

Caitlin O Malley
2424 Sailing Avenue
Cherry Hill, NJ 08080
(609) 444-2212

April 26, 2004

Ms. Vanetha Raj, BSN, RN
Nurse Recruiter
Shore Memorial Hospital
100 Seashore Drive
Point Pleasant, NJ 07726

Dear Ms. Raj:

Thank you for the time you spent with me as I interviewed for a position as a registered nurse at Shore Memorial Hospital. I enjoyed meeting the pediatric nurse manager and several of the staff nurses yesterday and was especially impressed with the sense of professionalism among the staff.

I have requested that my transcripts be sent directly to your office and I will have three of my instructors complete the reference forms you gave me. I look forward to hearing from you soon about my second interview and will contact you in two weeks as directed.

Sincerely,

Caitlin O Malley

Figure 16-5 Follow-Up to Interview Letter

an individual is assessed by a variety of people in order to provide a broader perspective (Marriner-Tomey, 2000). For example, a nurse may complete a self-assessment and submit a packet detailing the year's progress. This may include documentation of in-services completed in the assessment period, samples of charting, and details related to committee work. The appraisal process also includes peer reviews, evaluation by the nurse's immediate supervisor, and patient interviews (Edwards & Ewen, 1996).

Corrective Action Programs

Sometimes, performance evaluation indicates the need for significant improvement. Most

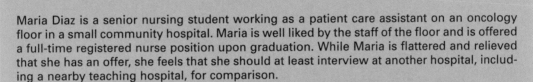

CASE STUDY 16-1

Maria Diaz is a senior nursing student working as a patient care assistant on an oncology floor in a small community hospital. Maria is well liked by the staff of the floor and is offered a full-time registered nurse position upon graduation. While Maria is flattered and relieved that she has an offer, she feels that she should at least interview at another hospital, including a nearby teaching hospital, for comparison.

How would Maria begin her job search at other hospitals? What are the key elements to securing an interview at other hospitals? Once Maria has an interview, what type of questions should she be prepared to answer from the interviewer? What type of questions should Maria be prepared to ask?

health care organizations have a prescribed corrective action program. One of the first steps in helping employees improve their performance is identifying whether the poor performance is developmental or related to a failure to follow policies or procedures. For example, a nurse may be having difficulty completing assignments in an appropriate time frame. The manager needs to coach the nurse, assisting the nurse with whatever support will help the nurse improve (Grensing-Pophal, 2000). Another category of corrective action is disciplinary corrective action. Most organizations have a series of progressive steps for corrective action in cases in

LITERATURE APPLICATION

Citation: McNeese-Smith, D. K. (2000). Job stages of entry, mastery, and disengagement among nurses. *Journal of Nursing Administration, 30*(3), 140–147.

Discussion: Career stages have been conceptualized by a number of researchers. McNeese-Smith surveyed practicing nurses to identify characteristics common to nurses in each stage. The author found that nurses in the entry stage seek to identify with the expectations of their new job. If they receive support from their supervisor and develop realistic goals, they move into the mastery stage. In the mastery level, the focus is on accomplishment and professional growth. At some point while in this stage, nurses begin to perceive themselves as experts.

The third stage, disengagement, begins only if nurses believe their current position no longer offers challenges or growth. The high esteem of the nurse in the mastery phase is replaced by boredom and declining performance. At this point, the nurse usually leaves the position.

Implications for Practice: Nurses move through stages in their professional development. Those who remain actively involved and seek professional growth avoid disengagement.

RN Orientation Template
Week One

Monday Perdiems/Weekend Staff attend May 21	Tuesday Perdiems/Weekend attend May 22 0745 meet in main lobby	Wednesday Perdiems/Weekend attend May 23	Thursday Perdiems/Weekend attend May 24	Friday May 25
Human Resource/ Safety Education	8:00-11:30 Intro/Tour Nursing at AMC Education Opportunities	08:00-11:00 Documentation Standards of Care, protocols, I/O, graphic, Clinical Pathways Unit Day Prep *(ED exempt: modules)*	08:00-09:30 Modules	07:30-10:30 SMS Computer/P Building-If needed
Remember to sign in on your unit if you want to get paid for the days you attend orientation.	11:30-12:00 Tina Raggio-Project Learn		09:30-11:00 Epidemiology *Carolyn Scott*	10:30-12:00 **Independent Activities on Unit of Hire or Modules**
	12:00-1:00 Lunch	11:00-11:30 Restraints	11:00-11:30 Lunch	12:00-1:00 Meet with Director **Main 4 Office Lunch Provided**
	1:00-2:00 Delegation/Assigning *Donna Harat*	11:30-12:00 Back Video Nurse Scheduling	11:30-2:30 SMS Computer Class	1:00-2:00 Pastoral Care **Room U477**
	2:00-4:30 Modules	12:00-1:00 Lunch	3:00-4:00 Math Calculation Class (**optional-check with Educator**)	2:00-4:00 Modules
	some orientees may need to attend the SMS Computer class in the P building from 11:30-2:30-check with Educator	1:00-4:30 Skills Lab Afternoon Emergency Care and Mock Code (ACLS or PALS exempt and does not apply to NICU), IV/Phlebotomy Skills, Accucheck, PCA Pump	4:00-4:30 Planning for next week/core orientation/orientee assessment forms	

Required Modules:

Age Specific ☐	IV Therapy ☐	Blood and Blood Products ☐	RN Medication ☐ ☐	Patient Rights ☐
Peds or Adult Emergency Care☐		Latex Allergy☐	Patient Classification ☐	
Order Transcription (not for ED, PACU)☐		Pain Management☐	Documentation ☐	CPR: (see handout)

Dept of Education #262-3705

Figure 16-6 Registered Professional Nurse General Orientation Schedule Template—Week One (Courtesy of Albany Medical Center, Albany, NY)

Name	Preceptor	Unit/Dept. Emergency Dept Date:

At the completion of orientation the RN will perform technical nursing skills specific to the age and characteristics of the patients served consistent with the Standards of Nursing Practice.

Self Evaluation Scale 1 2 3	RN Technical Skill Checklist	Method of Validation/ Code	Date Met/ Initials

	1. Cardiovascular
	  A. Initiate IV therapy
	    1. Adult, non-trauma
	    2. Trauma patient
	    3. Pediatric
	    4. Newborn
	    5. Phlebotomy percutaneous approach
	
	  B. Blood sampling:
	    1. arterial line
	    2. blood sampling: port-a-cath
	    3. Triple lumen/ trauma cath/ central line
	
	  C. Central venous line management: securing/ dressing/caps/ tubing
	    1. Trauma catheter/ triple lumen
	    2. Implanted device external access (i.e., Hickman)
	    3. PICC line
	    4. Port-a-cath
	
	  D. Infusion pumps
	    1. IV pumps
	    2. Syringe pumps
	    3. Programmable pediatric pump
	    4. Patient Controlled Analgesia
	
	  E. Spacelab bedside and Central monitors
	    1. Cardiac rhythm interpretation
	
	  F. Defibrillator operation
	    1. Zoll
	    2. Physiocontrol 10 and 9
	
	  G. External transcutaneous pacer–Zoll
	
	  H. Transvenous pacer pack: Emergent
	
	  I. Transvenous pacer pack: Urgent
	    1. Pulse generator
	    2. Ushkow's lead
	
	  J. Blood Products administration
	
	  K. Level I blood warmer and rapid infuser
	
	  L. Spun Hct
	
	  M. Utilization of doppler for vascular assessment		

	2. Gastro-intestinal
	
	  A. Tubes & Drains
	    1. Salem sump/ Nasogastric tube (age appropriate size)
	      a. Measuring
	      b. cetacaine administration
	      c. securing
	    2. Gastric decontamination/ lavage (Code Blue)		

Figure 16-7 Emergency Department Competency-Based Orientation Tool Sample Page, Excerpt (Courtesy of Albany Medical Center, Albany, NY)

TABLE 16-9
*PERSONAL IDENTIFICATION OF ORIENTATION NEEDS
ON A SPECIFIC UNIT*

Review the following on your unit:

10 most common medical diagnoses

10 most common nursing diagnoses

10 most common medications and IV solutions

10 most common diagnostic tests

10 most common laboratory tests

10 most common nursing and medical interventions and treatments

LITERATURE APPLICATION

Citation: McNeese-Smith, D. K. (2000). Job stages of entry, mastery, and disengagement among nurses. *Journal of Nursing Administration*, 30(3), 140–147.

Discussion: Career stages have been conceptualized by a number of researchers. McNeese-Smith surveyed practicing nurses to identify characteristics common to nurses in each stage. The author found that nurses in the entry stage seek to identify with the expectations of their new job. If they receive support from their supervisor and develop realistic goals, they move into the mastery stage. In the mastery level, the focus is on accomplishment and professional growth. At some point while in this stage, nurses begin to perceive themselves as experts.

The third stage, disengagement, begins only if nurses believe their current position no longer offers challenges or growth. The high esteem of the nurse in the mastery phase is replaced by boredom and declining performance. At this point, the nurse usually leaves the position.

Implications for Practice: Nurses move through stages in their professional development. Those who remain actively involved and seek professional growth avoid disengagement.

LITERATURE APPLICATION

Citation: Snodgrass, S. G. (2001, June 10). Wish you were a star? Become one! *Chicago Tribune*, D1.

Discussion: The most logical way to predict your future is to create it, so if you want to be a star, start by becoming a top performer now. Companies are drawn to those who use up-to-date skills and leadership to produce measurable results. Organizations seek such people out. Surprisingly, few people understand this. You can begin to position yourself now with exceptional performance.

Start by delivering more than you promise and consistently outperform yourself. Exceed expectations on a regular basis, seek more responsibility, value teamwork and diversity, provide leadership, and always go beyond the call of duty. Communicate effectively and know how to network with others. Be resourceful, comfortable with ambiguity, and open to saying, "I don't know, but I'll find out." In addition, take initiative and persevere until you reach quantifiable results. Finally, assume some personal risk by thinking outside the box and exploring bold, new solutions to challenges. Provide yourself with a margin of confidence through lifelong learning. Be open, flexible, and adapt to new ideas. Spend time with those who challenge your thinking.

You should also be creative, seek innovative solutions, and supplement your past experience with a fresh perspective. Learn how to put your ideas into action and be persistent because achieving results takes time. In addition, do your homework. Understand the business agenda and close any gaps between what you are and what you could be. In other words, define your goals, then create and implement a personal development plan. Finally, demonstrate respect for others, and apply the golden rule. Achieving great results with great behavior enables your star to rise. You can begin the process right now with these specific steps:

- See the big picture. Know why your job was created, how it relates to your organization, and what opportunities it contains. You can positively influence outcomes through performance and achievement.
- Invest in your organization; make decisions as if you owned the company. Determine which actions promise the most significant impact, and then pursue them with zeal.
- Push your comfort zone by seeking challenges, finding the positive in negative situations, taking action, and learning from the past.
- Make time for people; understand the culture, values, and beliefs of the organization; keep things in perspective; and have fun.
- Inspire those around you to exceed expectations; also, convey a sense of urgency, and consistently drive issues to closure.

After you do all this, how do you ensure that you will be noticed? Ask how your company identifies and rewards top performers. Inquire as to whether there is a high-potential category. You should pursue an environment in which the best are recognized and valued. It should be an organization that provides career growth, lifelong learning, and development opportunities.

continues

Literature Application *(continued)*

You also want meaningful work, an opportunity to contribute, and an environment that prizes new ideas and fresh perspectives. In addition, you deserve honest feedback and the opportunity to provide the same in return. Finally, seek an organization that energizes and empowers you, encourages your good health, respects your point of view, and honors your performance. Many such organizations abound.

Implications for Practice: Though a business professional wrote this article, the advice rings true for nurses as well.

REAL WORLD INTERVIEW

I remember my first job in nursing about 40 years ago. It was as a staff nurse on a general medical-surgical unit. I had a wonderful preceptor, Ed Fuss, RN. He worked with me and helped me until gradually I could assume my full role as a staff nurse on the unit. It took a while. It was very stressful to care for the 42 patients on that unit. After my orientation period, I would sometimes be the only RN, though I would have several licensed practical nurses and nurse aides working with me. I had to quickly learn appropriate delegation techniques.

Nursing has been a great career for me. I have worked as a nurse in Indiana, Illinois, Pennsylvania, New York, Oklahoma, Wisconsin, and Texas. I have had many nursing positions and now work part time in the emergency department as a staff nurse. I find I can move quickly into the culture of a new unit by being friendly, helping others on the unit, and keeping my nursing skills up to date. I notice that people in other professions often complain about being concerned that they will lose their job. In nursing, I have not had to worry about job layoffs. I always have been able to get an interesting nursing job doing something I like.

I have had nurse friends who have worked as nurse practitioners, nurse chaplains, traveling nurses, nurse educators, nurse administrators, flight nurses, missionary nurses, nurse lawyers, informatics nurses, nurses in a homeless shelter, nurses on a cruise boat, etc. There are all kinds of nursing opportunities. I also like stopping at the scene of an accident and knowing I can help. It has been my privilege to be a nurse. How many other professions can say they save lives for a living!

—*Patricia Kelly-Heidenthal*, RN, MSN

which employee performance does not improve. For example, a manager may begin by providing a verbal warning to an employee whose attendance is minimally acceptable. If the nurse's attendance problem continues, the nurse may receive a written warning. Without improve- ment, this could proceed to a suspension, final warning, and eventually termination. In a union environment, the employee may have the right to union representation after a verbal reprimand.

Nurses who receive a verbal warning from their manager should immediately demonstrate a commitment and plan for improvement in order to avoid any progression toward corrective action. It is useful, although not always easy, to avoid taking the corrective action personally and look on the feedback as an opportunity for improvement.

KEY CONCEPTS

- Organizational orientation is both general and unit based. Orientation is a time for developing strong relationships with preceptors and members of other disciplines, as well as for mastering competencies needed for safe patient care.
- Nurses receive performance feedback both informally and as part of periodic evaluations. This input is valuable in developing personal goals.
- Corrective action programs can be used to coach an employee who is having performance problems and to foster change in an employee who is failing to follow agency policies.
- A Magnet hospital may offer wonderful opportunities for nurses.
- Newspapers, electronic media and the Internet, job fairs, and employment hot lines are all possible avenues for job opportunities.
- An effective resume will (1) get the employer's interest; (2) identify critical areas such as education, work experience, and special qualifications; (3) be tailored to the employer's needs; (4) create a favorable first impression about you and your abilities; (5) communicate that you are someone who is a good fit for the position; and (6) be visually appealing.
- The purpose of a cover letter is to entice the prospective employer to become interested enough to read the resume.
- In dressing for an interview, it is best to dress professionally and conservatively rather than in a trendy or casual manner.
- When preparing for an interview, practice answering potential interview questions with a colleague, friend, or family member before the actual interview so that you have practiced answers to difficult questions.

- In addition to asking questions about shifts and rotation schedules, it is important to ask questions about other aspects of your prospective job, such as the salary, benefit package, educational opportunities, orientation and preceptorship, and evaluation practices.

KEY TERMS

resume   360-degree
                            feedback

REVIEW QUESTIONS

1. Which of the following is the best response to the interview question "What are your strengths?"
   A. "I have many. Where do you want me to begin?"
   B. "I have strong communication skills, both written and verbal, and I am someone who values completing a task."
   C. "I think I am well liked and get along with everyone."
   D. "Well, I am just a new nurse without many strengths right now, but I will be learning with this new job."

2. What is the primary function of a cover letter?
   A. To entice the prospective employer to become interested enough to read the resume
   B. To have a letter to include with your resume
   C. To include references that are not listed on a resume
   D. To reiterate all that is on your resume

3. General orientation includes which of the following?
   A. Information all nurses new to a facility need
   B. Mastery of unit-specific processes

C. Patient care for a specific diagnostic group of patients

D. Patient care for a specific age group of patients

4. Preceptors who work with new nursing graduates should have all of the following characteristics EXCEPT

A. be clinically experienced.

B. enjoy teaching.

C. committment to the preceptor role.

D. ability to float to specialty units.

REVIEW ACTIVITIES

1. You are graduating in 2 months from an ADN program. Develop a resume using the format in this chapter.

2. You are interested in the concept of 360-degree feedback. Who could you ask to give you feedback on your clinical performance to achieve 360-degree feedback?

3. Review a recent nurse salary survey—for example, see Charles, Piper, Mailey, Davis, and Baigis (2000) in the References section. How do nursing salaries in your area compare?

4. While looking on a Web site for a hospital out of state, you notice that you can submit a resume electronically for a job position that you are interested in applying for. What are the differences between an electronic resume and a traditional paper resume? Develop an electronic resume using the suggestions found in this chapter.

5. You are a new nurse who has been asked to interview for a position on the orthopedic floor. Develop a cover letter expressing interest in the position. Develop a listing of possible interview questions.

6. Review the *AJN Career Guide, January 2001,* How to Interview on Your Terms, pp. 16–18 (Russo, 2001). How can this guide help prepare you for interviewing for a nursing position?

EXPLORING THE WEB

- There are many Web sites specific to nursing employment opportunities. Try some of these:
  http://www.americanmobile.com
  http://www.rnwanted.com
  http://www.healthopps.com
  http://www.healthcareers-online.com
  http://www.healthcaretraveler.com

- Look up several of these nursing sites:
  Association of Pediatric Oncology Nurses:
  http://www.apon.org
  Association of Rehabilitation Nurses:
  http://www.rehabnurse.org
  Association of Women's Health, Obstetric and Neonatal Nurses:
  http://www.awhonn.org
  Trauma Nursing:
  http://www.emergency.com

- Review these generalized Web sites for nursing issues:
  http://www.nursingworld.org
  http://www.nursingcenter.com
  http://nursing.net
  http://www.nurseweek.com
  http://www.medzilla.com
  http://www.medsearch.com

- Review these good examples of letters of application in a variety of situations:
  http://www.career.vt.edu

- Check this site for job opportunities:
  http://healthcare.monster.com

- Check these Web sites:
  Library references by e-mail:
  http://www.ci.austin.tx.us and type in library reference.
  Online journal articles:
  http://www.medscape.com

- Nursing articles are available online at:
  http://www.nursingcenter.com. Click on library of nursing journals.
  http://www.nursingmanagment.com

- Check these sites:
  National Student Nurses' Association:
  http://www.nsna.org

Magnet listing of hospitals: *http://www.nursingworld.org.* Type in the word magnet.

- Check this guide to education and careers in nursing, which includes the most comprehensive directory of nursing schools with full school profiles, and detailed nursing Q&As: *http://www.allnursingschools.com*

REFERENCES

Aiken, L. (2002). Superior outcomes for magnet hospitals: The evidence base. In M. L. McClure & A. S. Hinshaw (Eds.), *Magnet hospitals revisited: Attraction and retention of professional nurses* (pp. 61–81). Washington, DC: American Nurses Publishing.

Albany Medical Center. (2001). Emergency department competency-based orientation tool sample pages excerpt. Albany, NY: Author.

Albany Medical Center. (2001). Registered professional nurse general orientation schedule template—week one. Albany, NY: Author.

Berens, M. J. (2000). Training often takes a back seat. *Chicago Tribune.*

Burke, A. (2000). Organization-wide competency and education. *Nursing Management 31*(2), 20–25.

Charles, J. P., Piper, S., Mailey, S. K., David, P., & Baigis, J. (2000). Nurse salaries in Washington, D.C. and nationally. *Nursing Economic$, 18*(5), 243–249.

Edwards, M. R., & Ewen, A. J. (1996). *360 feedback.* New York: American Management Association.

Fey, M. K., & Miltner, R. S. (2000). A competency-based orientation program for new graduate nurses. *Journal of Nursing Administration, 30,* 126–132.

Grensing-Pophal, L. (2000). Give-and-take feedback. *Nursing Management, 31*(2), 27–28.

Joint Commission on Accreditation of Healthcare Organization (JCAHA). (2001). *Health care at the crossroads.* Oakbrook Terrace, IL: Author.

Kramer, M. (1974). *Reality shock: Why nurses leave nursing.* St. Louis, MO: Mosby.

Marquis, B. L., & Huston, C. J. (2000). *Leadership roles and management functions in nursing* (3rd ed.). Philadelphia: Lippincott.

Marrelli, T. M. (1997). *The nurse manager's survival guide* (2nd ed.). St. Louis, MO: Mosby.

Marriner-Tomey, A. (2000). *Guide to nursing management and leadership* (6th ed.). St. Louis, MO: Mosby.

McNeese-Smith, D. K. (2000). Job stages of entry, mastery, and disengagement among nurses. *Journal of Nursing Administration, 30*(3), 140–147.

Meinecke, J. (2000). Orientation: Six ways to avoid throwing new nurses to the wolves. *Nursing Management, 31*(2), 30.

National League for Nursing (NLN). (2001). Press release. Retrieved January 31, 2001, from *http://www.nln.org.*

Nibert, A., Young, A., & Adamson, C. (2002). A fourth validity study of the HESI Exit Exam. *Computer Information for Nursing, 20(6),* 261–267.

Russo, E. (2001). How to interview on your own terms. In *AJN career guide,* 2001 (pp. 16–18). Philadelphia: Lippincott.

Shaffer, B., Tallarica, B., & Walsh, J. (2000). Win-win mentoring. *Nursing Management, 31(1),* 32–34.

Smith, R. (1999). *Electronic resumes and online networking.* Franklin Lakes, NJ: Career Press.

Snodgrass, S. G., (2001, June 10). Wish you were a star? Become one! *Chicago Tribune,* D1.

SUGGESTED READINGS

Alspach, J. (1984). Designing a competency-based orientation for critical care nurses. *Heart and Lung, 13*, 655–662.

Beeman, P. B., & Waterhouse, J. D. (2001). NCLEX-RN performance: Predicting success on the computerized examination. *Journal of Professional Nursing, 4*, 158–165.

Bozell, J. (1999). *Anatomy of a job search—a nurse's guide to finding and landing the job you want.* Philadelphia: Springhouse.

Briscoe, V. J., & Anema, M. G. (1999). The relationship of academic variables as predictors of success on the National Council Licensure Examination for Registered Nurses (NCLEX-RN) in a selected associate degree program. *Association of Black Nursing Faculty Journal, 4*, 80–83.

Connelly, L. M., Yoder, L. H., & Miner-Williams, D. (2000). Hidden charges: Top competencies to develop in a charge nurse. *Nursing Management, 31*(5), 27–29.

Diehl-Oplinger, L., & Kaminski, M. F. (2000). Need critical care nurses? Inquire within. *Nursing Management, 31*(3), 44–46.

Dimitrov, D. M., & Shelestak, D. (2001). Learning outcomes related to success on NCLEX-RN. *Nurse Education, 3*, 108.

Eddy, L. L., & Epeneter, B. J. (2002). The NCLEX-RN experience: Qualitative interviews with graduates of a baccalaureate nursing program. *Journal of Nursing Education, 6*, 273–278.

Johnson, C. (2000). We made a mistake. *Nursing Management, 31*(4), 22–24.

Kennedy, J. L. (1999). *Resumes for dummies.* Foster City, CA: IDG Books Worldwide.

Lauchner, K. A., Newman, M., & Britt, R. B. (1999). Predicting licensure success with a computerized comprehensive nursing exam: The HESI Exit Exam. *Computers in Nursing, 17*(3), 120–125.

Lee, L. A. (2000). Buzzwords with a basis: Motivation, mentoring, empowerment. *Nursing Management, 31*(10), 24–27.

Morrison, S., Free, K. W., & Newman, M. (2002). Do progression and remediation policies improve NCLEX-RN pass rates? *Nurse Education, 2*, 94–96.

National Council of State Boards of Nursing, Inc.; 676 North St. Clair Street, Suite 550; Chicago, Illinois 60611-2921; *http://www.ncsbn.org;* (312) 787-6555 or (800) 325-9601.

Nibert, A. T., & Young, A. (2001). A third study on predicting NCLEX success with the HESI Exit Exam. *Computer Nursing, 4*, 172–178.

Poorman, S. G., & Webb, C. A. (2000). Preparing to retake the NCLEX-RN: The experience of graduates who fail. *Nurse Education, 4*, 175–180.

Ringerman, E. S., & Ventura, S. (2000). An outcomes approach to skill mix change in critical care. *Nursing Management, 31*(10), 42–46.

Ross, C. A. (2000). Benefits of cooperative learning groups when preparing for the NCLEX-RN examination. *Nurse Education, 3*, 124.

Seven tips to improve nurse performance. (2000). *Management Briefings for Nurse Leaders, 1*(5), 7.

Siktberg, L. L., & Dillard, N. L. (2001). Assisting at-risk students in preparing for NCLEX-RN. *Nurse Education, 3*, 150–152.

Smith, J. E., & Crawford, L. H. (2002). The link between entry-level RN practice and the NCLEX-RN® examination. *Nurse Education, 3*, 109–112.

Spann, K. (2000). How do you rate your team's teamwork? *Nursing Management, 31*(1), 45.

Stark, M. A., Feikema, B., & Wyngarden, K. (2002). Empowering students for NCLEX(R) success: Self-assessment and planning. *Nurse Education, 3*, 103–105.

Urden, L. D., & Rogers, S. (2000). Out in front. *Nursing Management, 31*(7), 27–30.

Wendt, A. (2001). End-of-life competencies and the NCLEX-RN examination. *Nursing Outlook, 3*, 138–141.

CHAPTER 17

Career Planning and Achieving Balance

TO NURSE

To Care

To Solace

To Touch

To Feel

To Hurt

To Need

To Heal others,

As well as ourselves

(Carol Battaglia,

1996)

OBJECTIVES

Upon completion of this chapter, the reader should be able to:

1. Identify strategies for professional growth.
2. Discuss certification and clinical ladders.
3. Define health.
4. Identify the six concepts of health, i.e., physical, intellectual, emotional, professional, social, and spiritual health.
5. Describe selected strategies to maintain physical, intellectual, emotional, professional, social, and spiritual health.

You have just started in your new nursing position. You are excited and want to do a good job as well as plan for the future. You want to continue to grow professionally and yet have a life outside nursing also. There are many questions you are thinking about. Where do you see yourself 1, 5, or 10 years from now? What opportunities exist for certification and additional education? How can you ensure some balance and less stress in your life both inside and outside nursing?

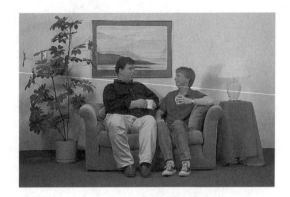

The 20th century was a unique time in nursing's history; the profession struggled to assume its rightful role in the health care arena with its members performing traditional as well as new nursing roles, and it significantly upgraded its educational, clinical, research, and managerial focus. This chapter examines emerging opportunities for new graduates. It also discusses planning for future nursing opportunities and strategies for healthy living.

STRATEGIES FOR PROFESSIONAL GROWTH

New nurses are more likely to stay in their positions if they are challenged and have opportunities for professional growth ("Getting X-ers to Stay," 2000).

Professional growth and practice require competent staff. **Competency** is defined as possession of a required skill, knowledge, qualification, or capacity (*Webster's Universal Encyclopedic Dictionary*, 2001) and is best determined in practice by a group of one's peers. Alspach (1984) defines competency as a determination of an individual's capability to perform to defined expectations (p. 656). Competency of professional staff can be ensured through credentialing processes developed either at an agency or through certification by a national nursing organization. See Table 17-1.

Certification

Certification is the process by which a nongovernmental agency or association certifies that an individual licensed to practice a profession has met certain predetermined standards specified by that profession for practice. The process of certification allows nurses to demonstrate a specific educational or clinical expertise for their patient population. Many certifications last up to 5 years and the nurse may recertify by either retesting or completing the needed number of continuing education contact hours. Many different organizations issue certification credentials for nursing. See the *American Journal of Nursing Career Guide 2001* for a listing of more than 80 certifications available to nurses ("Your Guide to Certification," 2001).

Clinical Ladder

A clinical or career ladder may be in place in an agency. Although the criteria may vary, most programs have three or four distinct levels. **Clinical ladders** offer the nurse the opportunity to seek promotion in a specific track, within a clinical, educational, research, or managerial focus. For example, to be promoted from a new Graduate Level I to a Level II RN, the nurse may be required to complete a specialty course such as Advanced Cardiac Life Support (ACLS) or EKG interpretation, join a unit- or hospital-based committee, and finish the preceptor course. Besides offering opportu-

TABLE 17-1
SELECTED NURSING CERTIFICATIONS AND ORGANIZATIONS

Certification examples	ACLS	advanced cardiac life support
	BLS	basic life support
	CEN	certified emergency nurse
	CCRN	critical care registered nurse
	CRNA	certified registered nurse anesthetist
	NRP	neonatal resuscitation program
Selected certifying organizations	PALS	pediatric advanced life support
	ANCC	American Nurses Credentialing Center
	AANA	American Association of Nurse Anesthetists
	ACCN	Association of Critical Care Nurses
	ANA	American Nurses Association
	AWHONN	Association of Women's Health, Obstetric, and Neonatal Nurses
	NANN	National Association of Neonatal Nurses
	NAPNAP	National Association of Pediatric Nurse Associates and Practitioners
	WOCN	Wound, Ostomy, and Continence Nurses Society

nity for promotion, these programs offer an objective way to measure a nurse's achievements. Clinical ladders can be time-consuming to complete yet they provide valuable information. See Figure 17-1.

Nontraditional and Advance Practice Nursing Roles

Although many new graduates will be interested in traditional nursing positions, other new roles have emerged for nurses. See Table 17-2.

Some of these roles can be self-developed using the base of a basic nursing program. Other roles require additional education and/or certification. See a listing of various nursing education programs at *http://www.allnursingschools.com*.

HEALTHY LIVING— ACHIEVING BALANCE

Nursing is a caring profession. Nurses spend their days helping others, many times at the expense of themselves. But, if there is nothing left for nurses, they will not be able to maintain the strength to care for their patients.

Definition of Health

Health as a concept has been in the literature since the inception of modern nursing. Florence Nightingale described health as "being well and using every power the individual possesses to the fullest extent" (Nightingale, 1969 [1860], p. 334). The World Health Organization (1998)

Colorado Differentiated Practice Model

The Colorado Differentiated Practice Model for Nursing has a separate clinical ladder for the six preparatory backgrounds depicted on the conceptual model (Diagram 1). A nurse selects the education clinical ladder according to the nursing credential s/he has attained.

The framework for each educational ladder has four distinct stages. These stages allow nurses to self-pace their advancement. A nurse is placed in a stage according to his or her own competency and experience.

Each nursing ladder has four weighted components as follows:
- Competency Statements 60%   • Institutional Goals 15%
- Skills 10%   • Professional Activities 15%

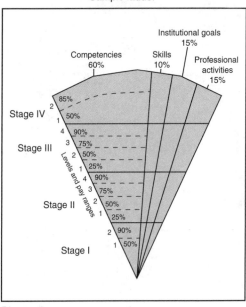

Conceptual model

Sample ladder

Diagram 1

Diagram 2

Figure 17-1 Colorado Differentiated Practice Model (Courtesy Marie E. Miller, Colorado Nursing Task Force, 2001)

describes **health** as a "state of complete physical, social, and mental well-being, and not merely the absence of disease or infirmity. Health is a resource for everyday life, not the object of living."

Goals for Healthy People 2010

In January 2000, more than 1,500 individuals, health professionals, and organizations convened in Washington, D.C. to discuss goals for health promotion and disease prevention for the United States population (U.S. Department of Health and Human Services, 2001). Healthy People 2010 has developed two overall goals for the nation: (1) to encourage those of all ages to increase their life expectancy as well as improve their overall quality of life and (2) to eliminate disparities among various pockets of the population. Ten leading health indicators will be used to measure the overall goals for the nation Table 17-3).

REAL WORLD INTERVIEW

There are five levels of our clinical ladder, which is similar to Benner's novice to expert model. The RN1s or novices are the new graduates and people in orientation. The experts are the clinical specialists. A lot of them have also become nurse practitioners so that the organization can receive some reimbursement for their patient care services. This is a good thing because otherwise I'm afraid we wouldn't have these expert nurses anymore. They are the true mentors for nursing staff, especially when you are working with a very complex or difficult patient situation.

Staff nurses also mentor each other. During orientation, your preceptor guides you along the path from RN I to RN II. When you decide you'd like to advance to RN III, you can choose another mentor. RN IIIs provide much more clinical leadership for staff and for the overall unit. I decided I was ready to be promoted to that level when other staff consistently were coming to me for clinical guidance and with patient care questions. Now, as an RN III, I am the chairperson of our unit-credentialing committee, which is part of the quality council of our shared governance model.

Our clinical ladder uses a portfolio as the main tool to evaluate the nurse's readiness to advance. When you are an RN I in orientation, you are first introduced to the idea of a portfolio and how to put it together. It is difficult at first, as people do not know what is expected. However, after that first time when you are promoted from an RN I to an RN II, it becomes easier. You just build on what is already in the portfolio.

A portfolio should include the following:

Licenses

Your resume

Letters of reference

Evaluations

Clinical documentation of patient care

Validations for competencies related to technical skills (medication administration, IV therapy)

Examples of participation in development of the team plan of care

Exemplars

CEU certificates

Presentations

Publications

The portfolio tells the story of your practice. When a group of people are ready for promotion, the members of the credentialing committee meet. We review the portfolios and make recommendations related to advancement. The nurse manager is a member of this committee. She always reviews the portfolio and gives us her feedback even if she is unable to attend the credentialing meeting. I enjoy reading the exemplars the best. Exemplars are mini-stories that paint the pictures of each nurse's practice, and they are all so different.

Stacey Conley, RN, BS, Staff Nurse

STOP AND THINK

Many nurses are certified in their area of specialty. You are planning to take a certification examination in the future, but are not sure you really want to spend the time required to prepare for it. Some reflections on what certification might do for you are useful:

What is the reason you want to take this examination? Will becoming certified make a difference in your job? Will becoming certified allow you to further progress in your position? Is certification required for licensure?

TABLE 17-2
SELECTED NONTRADITIONAL ROLES AND ADVANCE PRACTICE NURSING ROLES

Nurse practitioner	Nurse entrepreneur
Clinical nurse specialist	Parish nurse
Certified nurse-midwife	Travel nurse
Nurse educator	Case manager
Informatics nurse	Flight nurse

AREAS OF HEALTH

Health is a complex and dynamic state of being. A healthy person must balance various aspects in life to achieve and maintain good health. When one area of life is affected, other areas of health are also affected. There is overlap among each area, but for purposes of discussion in this chapter, health has been divided into the following six elements: physical health, intellectual health, emotional health, professional health, social health, and spiritual health (Figure 17-2). The tool in Table 17-4 will assist you in identifying your health trends in each of the six areas of health.

Physical Health

Physical health, the first element of health, encompasses nutrition as well as exercise coupled with a balanced amount of sleep. Physical health also includes health promotion and disease prevention behaviors such as avoiding smoking, maintaining a healthy body mass index with healthy nutrition and exercise, and having annual Pap smears and other screening procedures that detect health problems early.

Body Mass Index Calculation

You can assess your body weight in relation to your height by calculating your body mass index (BMI). You can calculate this at *http://www. nhlbi.nih.gov*. The National Institute of Health (n.d.) has established the following guidelines for interpretation of the BMI:

REAL WORLD INTERVIEW

Becoming a flight nurse after being a pediatric intensive care nurse for $7^1/_2$ years was a huge role change, especially because of the autonomy I now have. I am responsible for performing an assessment on a patient, and then delivering care based on my findings. The care a flight nurse delivers is based on diagnosis-specific standards of care. Many times the patient diagnosis is known, such as when a patient is being transferred from a hospital, but it is the flight nurse's responsibility to ensure that the previous care initiated is still appropriate for this patient. The physical environment is also very different from my previous role. Many of the patients I encounter are located in a very small community hospital with limited resources. When I have a flight mission at an accident scene, the patient may be in an ambulance, trapped in a vehicle, on the ground, or in their house. Once the patient is initially assessed and stabilized, they are moved to the confined and noisy environment of the helicopter. I think that the biggest change from being a staff nurse to a flight nurse is the limited resources available while on a call. Although physician consult is only a radio or phone call away, I am expected to make autonomous clinical decisions in order to save the patient valuable time in receiving lifesaving therapies. At times, I must rely solely on my own experience and that of my partner.

Allison Goodell, BSN, RN, NREMT-P, Flight Nurse

CASE STUDY 17-1

It is March of your last year at college. You have been offered a position as a staff nurse at a hospital where you really wanted to work. For the past several weeks during your last clinical rotation, however, you have had the opportunity to work with an advance practice nurse. You start to think that perhaps this is what you would like to do in the future. How can you begin to plan for this?

Consider the following:
- What additional education and experience do you need before moving into this role?
- Have the clinical rotations you had as a student prepared you to work toward an advance practice role?
- What resources are available to you that would provide information in guiding your decision?
- Will spending more time working as a staff nurse better prepare you to be an advance practice nurse?

- 30 and above is obese
- 25 to 29.9 is overweight
- 18.5 to 24.9 is optimal health
- Below 18.5 is considered underweight

Nutrition and Exercise

Following nutritional guidelines is not enough to maintain physical health. Exercise is another essential ingredient for healthy living. Exercise

REAL WORLD INTERVIEW

As NPs face the new millennium, it is advisable to listen to the wisdom of the famous author on China, Pearl Buck, who said, "To understand today, you have to search yesterday." Further, to envision the future, think "outside the box" creatively, constructively, and globally. Unfortunately, most people hate change; so do professionals. By their very nature, professionals can become myopic, territorial, and conservative. Some that are so resistant to change become arrogant, self-important, and greedy. Nursing must face the future differently. Tomorrow's practitioners will face globalization, not only of economics but of every field of human endeavor. Demographics, technological advances, transportation, and communication will expand beyond imagination and at lightning speed. Health information will no longer belong exclusively to the health professions. The Internet will see to that. The challenge for NPs is to be proactive rather than reactive in creating a social, cultural, political, and physical environment in which to successfully live, work, and thrive as a responsible member of the new society and as an advocate for our patients and their families. So, thoroughly examine the past, keep the enduring human values of caring, compassion, and courage in nursing, listen to your best teachers—the patients—and create your own future accordingly.

Loretta Ford, EdD, RN, FAAN

Founder, Nurse Practitioner Program

TABLE 17-3
HEALTHY PEOPLE 2010 INDICATORS

Physical activity	Responsible sexual behavior	Environmental quality
Overweight and obesity	Mental health	Immunization
Tobacco use	Injury and violence	Access to health care
Substance abuse		

provides many benefits. It can improve cardiovascular function by lowering cholesterol and blood pressure and strengthening heart muscle. Exercise can boost the immune response to disease. Weight-bearing exercises are especially helpful for calcium uptake in bones. Exercise also improves flexibility and endurance and decreases fat deposition. Exercise can also make you feel better mentally. With exercise usually come fewer depressive thoughts, less anxiety, an increase in self-confidence, and increased mental acuity (Maraldo, 1999). Try to exercise a minimum of three times a week for 30 minutes at a time.

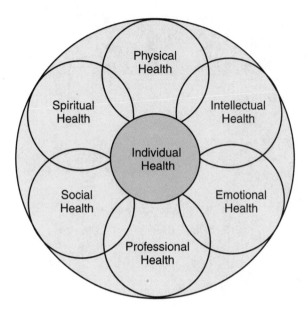

Figure 17-2 Elements of Health

Sleep

Sleep is another component of physical health. It is not uncommon for nurses to sleep less than 8 hours per night. Nurses who work nights may find it especially difficult to sleep for an uninterrupted block of time. Nurses who are constantly changing shifts are more susceptible to sleep deprivation. It is estimated that it can take from 4 to 6 weeks to change sleeping patterns. In spite of this, nurses may work various shifts within a week. If it is necessary to swing to a different shift, it is best to rotate from days to evenings to nights. People generally adapt better if shift rotation is done clockwise (Rogers, 1997).

Sleep-deprived individuals become petulant and find it difficult to remember or concentrate on the simplest tasks. If sleep deprivation occurs for a very long period of time, paranoia and hallucinations can occur. Other effects include overeating, hypersexuality, and increased susceptibility to viral infections (Davidhizar, Poole, & Giger, 1996; Turek & Zee, 1999). A period of 24 hours of wakefulness is equivalent to a blood alcohol level of 0.10% (Dawson & Reid, 1997) in terms of impaired cognitive and psychomotor skills. Even more frightening are the potential negative effects for patients. Taffinder, McManus, Russell, and Darzi (1998) found that surgeons who were sleep deprived committed 20% more errors and took approximately 14% longer to perform simulated surgery than when well rested.

Intellectual Health

Intellectual health is the second element of health and encompasses those activities that maintain intellectual curiosity. Intellectually healthy people are able to think critically and make sound decisions. They read, have hobbies, learn from experience, and are flexible and remain open to new ideas. For purposes of this chapter, the term *intellectual health* also includes doing personal financial planning.

TABLE 17-4
HEALTH ASSESSMENT TOOL

	Yes	No
Physical Health		
1. I exercise at least 30 minutes 3 times a week.		
2. I eat three balanced meals a day.		
3. I sleep 8 hours a night.		
4. My immunizations are up-to-date.		
5. I avoid risky behaviors, e.g., smoking, drugs, tanning booths, unprotected sex.		
6. I have regular health screenings and do Pap tests or monthly testicular self-examinations.		
Intellectual Health		
7. I plan to purchase real estate soon.		
8. I read at least one book a month and try to practice critical thinking.		
9. I have a 401K or 403b savings plan for retirement.		
10. I know how much money I have invested in Social Security.		
11. I have invested in diversified mutual stock and bond funds.		
12. I save 10% of my income for the future.		
13. I have a hobby I enjoy.		
Emotional Health		
14. I have developed strategies to deal with my own anger.		
15. I have developed strategies to deal with the anger of others.		
16. I work well with others.		
17. I practice stress management techniques.		
18. I try to be empathetic and sense what others are feeling.		
19. I try to find a reason to laugh daily.		
20. I use my preferences to make decisions and set goals.		

continues

Table 17-4 (continued)

	Yes	No

Professional Health

21. I have professional goals including certification and additional nursing education.

22. I have a mentor.

23. I have attended at least three workshops in the past year.

24. I subscribe to three nursing journals.

25. I belong to at least one professional organization.

26. I use appropriate personal protective equipment.

27. I never recap a needle.

28. I use good body mechanics when transferring patients.

29. I follow standards of care when handling gaseous waste, disinfectants, and chemotherapy.

30. I follow standards of care in dealing with radiation equipment and environmental hazards.

Social Health

31. I go out with my friends at least once a week.

32. I see my family regularly.

33. I have at least one friend I can confide in.

34. I have a wide diversity of professional, family, neighborhood, and church friends.

35. Not all my friends are nurses.

36. I do volunteer work.

Spiritual Health

37. I pray or meditate every day.

38. I believe in a higher power.

39. I attend meetings at a place of worship regularly.

40 I read spiritual books or spend time in quiet meditation daily.

41. I maintain a daily journal.

42. I seek help from professional counselors as needed.

STOP AND THINK

Consider the Healthy People 2010 Indicators. How is your personal behavior related to each of the indicators? How can you do better? How can you help your family, friends, and community do better? Keep a diary for 1 week on how you are doing on five or more of the indicators. See Figure 17-3 for a sample diary. At the end of the week, assess to see how well you have taken care of yourself. Is this a typical week? Do you need to make any changes? Were there any surprises? You can also record for several weeks and compare the outcomes.

	Physical Activity	Overweight and Obesity	Tobacco Use	Responsible Sexual Behavior	Mental Health	Other
Monday						
Tuesday						
Wednesday						
Thursday						
Friday						
Saturday						
Sunday						

Figure 17-3 Healthy People 2010 Diary

Personal Financial Planning

The first step in personal financial planning is to identify your annual salary. Mee and Carey (2000) surveyed 2,784 nurses throughout the country and found that the average salary for nurses with 5 or fewer years of experience was $33,054.00, and the mean starting wage was $15.41 per hour.

Next, begin to think about the percentage of your salary you want to save; most experts recommend 10% to 15% yearly. There is no better time than now to invest in your future. See Table 17-5. Now is the time to begin saving for such things as a home, your children's education, and even retirement no matter what your age.

Savings for retirement are three-pronged: (1) Social Security funds, (2) employee retirement funds, and (3) additional personal savings. You should annually check the accuracy of your Social Security account by reviewing the information sent to you by the Social Security Administration, available at *http://www.ssa.gov.*

Employee Retirement Funds. The most common retirement funds are the 401K or 403b plans. The only difference between the two is that the 403b is a plan offered by a nonprofit organization and the 401K is offered by a for-

TABLE 17-5
TIME VALUE OF MONEY

A nurse who invests $2,000 yearly at an 8% annual rate of return, beginning at age 20 will earn over $850,000 by age 65 versus a nurse who makes the same yearly investment but begins at age 30. The latter nurse will earn only about $350,000 by age 65.

profit organization. Otherwise, the two plans are exactly alike. For purposes of this discussion, the term *401K* will be used.

Both the employee and employer contribute retirement money to a **401K**. This is a great way to save because many health care institutions will match the funds that you contribute. Once your money is put into the fund, it is tax sheltered, meaning you do not pay any taxes on the amount contributed until it is withdrawn. For example, if you earn $35,000 per year and contribute $3,500 to the 401K, you will be taxed on only $31,500 of income. If the money is withdrawn before you reach the age of $59\frac{1}{2}$, you will pay a 10% federal penalty. This is an incentive to keep the money in the account until retirement; the 401K plan should be considered a long-term investment.

Once the money is in the fund, you must decide how the company administering the plan will invest it for you. You have two basic choices: bond mutual funds and stock mutual funds. Each of these investment opportunities has risks and benefits (Orman, 1997). Many advisors recommend diversifying and including a mix of these funds in your planning depending on your age. Several reliable information sources rank mutual funds for quality. These include the annual ratings by *Consumer Reports* and the Morningstar ratings available through the Internet. (See "Exploring the Web" at the end of this chapter.)

Individual Retirement Account (IRA). Another type of retirement fund is the individual retirement account (IRA). This account is an option for anyone with sufficient employment income. Contributions could not exceed $3,000 per year (for 2002). This fund may or may not be tax deductible, depending on what other retirement accounts you held and which type of IRA you opened (Tyson, 2000). There are two kinds of IRAs: the traditional IRA and the Roth. The **Roth IRA** was first introduced in 1998. A Roth IRA is taxed prior to the investment but grows tax-free and there is no penalty for early withdrawal (Orman, 1999). Orman highly recommends the Roth IRA and the 401K for investments.

Personal Savings and Real Estate.
After investing in retirement funds, you also have a few more options for investment. You can open a **money market account**, checking account, and/or a savings account.

You also have the option to invest in stock or bond mutual funds or individual stocks or bonds outside of your retirement account. You can start your research by reviewing Valueline at your local library (see "Exploring the Web" at the end of this chapter). The key to successful investment is to diversify, meaning to spread your money around in many different types of investment options, stocks, bonds, mutual funds, and so on.

Finally, talk to a real estate agent about a low-money-down home loan and you will be on your way to financial security.

How to Educate Yourself

There are many ways to learn more about investments. Brokerage firms offer classes periodically. Try taking a course on personal finance at a local college. You can also go to the Internet (see "Exploring the Web" at the end of this chapter).

Another option is to hire a financial planner, but that can become expensive (Barker, 2000). The last suggestion is to read. Many of the books on the best-sellers list discuss personal finance. Suze Orman (1997) is an author who many find easy to understand and very relevant. Subscriptions to *Money, Barron's,* and *Kiplinger Magazine* can be educational.

Emotional Health

Emotional health is the third element of health. Our emotions express how we are feeling about an event. Emotions can be intense and evoke a strong response. Our challenge as human beings is to acknowledge the emotion and then respond appropriately. Truly, emotions are one of our greatest gifts and add spice to our lives (Dossey & Keegan, 2000).

Emotional Intelligence

Emotional intelligence refers to the capacity for recognizing our own feelings and those of others, for motivating ourselves, and for managing emotions well in ourselves and in our relationships. It describes abilities distinct from, but complementary to, academic intelligence. Many people who are book smart but lack emotional intelligence end up working for people who have lower IQs but excel in emotional intelligence skills (Goleman, 1998).

Emotional intelligence includes these five basic emotional and social competencies:

- Self-awareness: Knowing what we are feeling in the moment, and using those preferences to guide our decision making; having a realistic assessment of our own abilities and a well-grounded sense of self-confidence
- Self-regulation: Handling our emotions so that they facilitate rather than interfere with the task at hand, being conscientious and delaying gratification to pursue goals, and recovering well from emotional distress

- Motivation: Using our deepest preferences to move and guide us toward our goals, to help us take initiative and strive to improve, and to persevere in the face of setbacks and frustrations
- Empathy: Sensing what people are feeling, being able to take their perspective, and cultivating rapport and attunement with a broad diversity of people
- Social skills: Handling emotions in relationships well and accurately reading social situations and networks; interacting smoothly; using these skills to persuade and lead, negotiate and settle disputes, for cooperation and teamwork (Goleman, 1998)

Anger

Anger is a universal, strong feeling of displeasure that is often precipitated by a situation that frustrates or prevents a person from attaining a goal or getting what is wanted from life. Anger is influenced by one's beliefs. Ellis (1997) describes anger as an irrational response that arises from one of four irrational ideas: (1) that the treatment one received was awful (awfulizing), (2) feeling that one can't stand having been treated so irresponsibly and unfairly (can't stand-it-itis), (3) believing that one should not, must not behave as he did (shoulding and musting), and (4) because one acted in a terrible manner, he is a terrible person (undeservingness and damnation). He maintains that beliefs remain rational as long as the evaluation of the action does not involve an evaluation of the person. Rational and appropriate responses are feelings of disappointment. Anger, on the other hand, can be unmanageable and self-defeating. Ellis believes that we all have the ability to choose our response to anger.

Anger can be dealt with in one of several ways. Three methods that may work from time to time but that may have serious and potentially destructive drawbacks are denying and repressing anger, which may lead to resentment; expressing anger, which may lead to defensiveness on the part of the respondent; and turning the other cheek, which may lead to continued mistreatment and lack of trust. Because anger stems from carrying things further and viewing the situation as awful, terrible, or horrible, Ellis (1997) advocates disputing irrational beliefs.

Ways to Cope with Anger. When confronted with an angry person, it is wise to think the problem through rationally and then respond in a calm manner. Grensing-Pophal (1998) recommends three steps in resolving conflict. First, listen attentively to the other person. Choose a quiet, private room where you will not be interrupted. Listen without bias and without mentally preparing your next response. Second, think about what the speaker has said as if you were a third party. Try to be objective and work out a solution that is agreeable to both parties. Third, respond without anger and work toward a resolution.

Humor and Stress Management

Laughter is the best medicine. Laughter has many benefits: it's free; it's a natural tranquilizer that is nonfattening and sodium free; and, best of all, it's contagious (Grensing-Pophal, 1998) (Figure 17-4). Humor can also affect you physiologically. It can enhance the immune system and boost the cardiovascular and respiratory systems (Lannon, 2000). Try to laugh daily. Laughter is a critical stress reliever. See Table 17-6 for other stress management techniques.

Avoiding Thought Distortions

Research on thinking processes has shown that people sometimes make mistakes in the way they perceive information and think about the world around them. When people are depressed, their automatic thoughts are loaded with distorted thinking. If one can recognize this distorted thinking (Table 17-7), one can begin to turn life in a more positive direction.

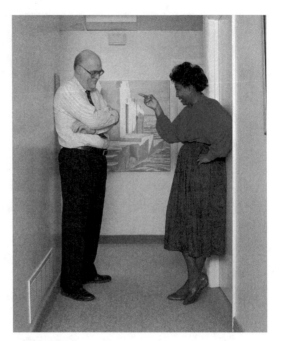

Figure 17-4 Laughter is an effective stress reliever.

Professional Health

Professional health is the fourth element of health. A person is professionally healthy when he is satisfied with his career choice and thinks that there is continual opportunity for growth. The professionally healthy individual is goal directed and seeks every opportunity to obtain knowledge and new learning experiences. This may include going back to school for more education, becoming certified in your clinical practice area, and avoiding occupational hazards.

Occupational Hazards Common among Nurses

An important aspect of professional health is avoidance of occupational hazards. The U.S. Bureau of Labor Statistics (1999) states that the incidence of nonfatal occupational injuries and illnesses for 1999 was 7.5 per 100 full-time workers for those employed in health care

TABLE 17-6
STRESS MANAGEMENT TECHNIQUES

Meditate.	Do relaxation exercises.	Be polite to all.
Think peaceful thoughts.	Do something different for lunch.	Take a walk.
See things as others might.	Give yourself a pat on the back.	Read.
Forgive your mistakes.	Join a support group.	Join a club.
Do not procrastinate.	Talk about your worries.	Sing a song.
Set realistic goals.	Be affectionate.	Forgive and forget.
Do a good deed.	View problems as a challenge.	Listen to music.
Vary your routine.	Get/give a massage.	Take a hot bath.
Appreciate what you have.	Say a prayer.	Call an old friend.
Focus on the positive.	Expect to be successful.	Let go of the need to be perfect.

LITERATURE APPLICATION

Citation: Healy, C., & McKay, M. (1999). Identifying sources of stress and job satisfaction in the nursing environment. *Australian Journal of Advanced Nursing, 17*(2), 30–35.

Discussion: One hundred twenty-nine nurses from a large private hospital filled out questionnaires related to job stress and job satisfaction. The findings from the questions indicated that a burdensome workload was the nurses' primary concern followed by unclear treatment protocols, conflict with doctors, and dealing with dying patients. Sixty-six of the 129 who completed questionnaires also submitted written descriptions of stressful work situations. This subgroup of 66 nurses elaborated on situations not covered in the initial questionnaire. Conflict among the nursing staff was identified as the most stressful occurrence. The conflict among the staff was caused by the inexperience of some nurses, criticism from other nurses, concern regarding other nurses' practice, and lack of support. The second most commonly cited stressful circumstance was the enormous workload.

Implications for Practice: Nursing administration needs to be aware of the stress and workload of nurses. Providing nursing leaders with quantifiable data concerning nursing responsibilities is most helpful. Nurses are at risk for job burnout as a result of the intensity and duration of the stressors at work. A high level of stress may also affect the quality of patient care. Nurses need to address the staffing issues and continue to care for themselves.

TABLE 17-7
THOUGHT DISTORTIONS

Thought distortion	Example
All-or-nothing thinking: seeing things only in absolutes	If I leave this job, no one will respect me.
Overgeneralization: interpreting every small setback as a never-ending pattern of defeat	Everyone here is so smart; I'm a real loser.
Dwelling on negatives: ignoring multiple positive experiences	I made a mistake. I'm not good enough to be a nurse.
Jumping to conclusions: assuming that others are reacting negatively without definite evidence	I don't know why I study. Everyone thinks I'm going to fail the NCLEX anyway.
Pessimism: automatically predicting that things will turn out badly	It's only a matter of time before everything falls apart for me.
Reasoning from feeling: thinking that if one feels bad, one must be bad	My head hurts because I'm a bad person.
Obligations: living life around a succession of too many "shoulds," "shouldn'ts," "musts," "oughts," and "have-tos."	I should marry Joe. Everyone likes him.

Compiled from Frisch & Frisch (2002).

facilities. This is the second highest rate of occupational injury among workers employed in the service industry. Nurses are at risk for injury on the job.

There are numerous suggestions for safeguarding against various hazards in the workplace. Occupational hazards can be divided into four major categories: (1) infectious agents, (2) environmental agents, (3) physical agents, and (4) chemical agents. See "Exploring the Web" at the end of this chapter and Table 17-8.

Social Health

Social health is another significant element of health. The essence of social health is interacting with other people. Having the ability to relate to others is essential for life. Few can survive completely alone. We relate to people at various levels—some we know intimately and others are mere acquaintances. These relationships occur within the immediate and extended family; at work; and within the local, national, and international community. These relationships give meaning to our lives. There are times when relationships cause distress and pain and other times when they bring great joy. We strive toward harmony in all relationships. It is human nature to seek out others and grow in relationships (Dossey & Keegan, 2000).

Impact of Social Relationships

Try to interact socially with friends in person as often as possible. Cell phones and e-mail are

TABLE 17-8
SAFEGUARDS FOR OCCUPATIONAL HAZARDS

Infectious Agents
- Do not recap needles.
- Use needle-free intravascular access devices.
- Place needle disposal containers near point of use of needles.
- Use personal protective equipment.
- Report all needle-stick injuries immediately.

Physical Agents
- Follow standards of care for dealing with radiation/laser equipment.
- Assess work area for amount of noise.
- Eliminate excessive noise in the workplace.
- Implement good body mechanics. Get equipment and help to lift heavy patients.

Environmental Agents
- Develop a zero tolerance, no abuse policy to protect nurses and all staff.
- Develop a violence reduction plan to protect nurses.
- Rotate shifts clockwise—day to evening to night (Rogers, 1997).
- Assess for dangerous chemicals, mold, and fungus in your workplace.
- Review Occupational Safety and Health Administration (OSHA) standards at your facility for environmental agents.
- Develop an agency/facility plan to work with victims of terrorism.
- Maintain air quality, avoid fumes from glutaraldehyde, ethylene oxide, and laser plume smoke.

Chemical Agents
- Utilize effective ventilation systems.
- Develop standards of care for handling gaseous waste, chemotherapy, disinfectants, and anesthetics.
- Protect pregnant nurses from handling chemotherapy during the first trimester.
- Use appropriate nonlatex barrier protections.
- Develop policies and procedures to ensure safety from latex allergies.

helpful forms of communication, but nothing is more effective than face-to-face conversation. Be careful, though, to stay away from negative relationships and people who do not treat you well. Sometimes it is difficult to end a friendship, but if the relationship is destructive, it may be in your best interest to end it.

Another way to build relationships is through rituals. For example, celebrate Christmas with friends by seeing *The Nutcracker* or play tennis with a friend once a week. But do not forget about your friends of the past. Phone a friend from the past or contact a family member you have argued with (Hallowell, 2000).

Finally, another way to establish friendships is through volunteerism. For example, join the American Red Cross as a disaster volunteer or pursue another activity that you find rewarding. It is also a good way to be aware of community issues.

Spiritual Health

Spiritual health, the last element of health, is the ability to find strength from within. This strength results from a connection with a higher being or power (Chilton, 1998). It is through our spirituality that we find meaning in life. It is the essence behind how we live our lives. It also is a piece of our lives that needs attention and development.

Religion and Health

Koenig (1999) has extensively researched religion and health. His findings lend some scientific support to the positive effects of prayer and religious involvement. Koenig (1999) found that older adults who are religiously active (based on attendance at religious services) are more physically fit and live longer than those who are less religious. It appears that prayer does have a positive impact on health outcomes. See the "Suggested Readings" for other resources on spirituality.

KEY CONCEPTS

- Clinical ladders can guide nursing development.
- There are numerous types of advance practice nurses (APNs), within both the hospital and community settings. Some examples of these roles include the CNS, NP, and CRNA.
- Some nontraditional role opportunities include the flight nurse, traveling nurse, and parish nurse.
- To provide quality patient care, nurses need to first take care of themselves and maintain a healthy lifestyle.
- Health is not just the absence of disease, it is the state of complete balance of six elements of health, i.e., physical, intellectual, emotional, professional, social, and spiritual health.

- The ability to care for yourself consists of multiple dimensions that overlap and interact constantly. If one dimension is affected, all dimensions are affected.
- Nurses' physical health encompasses good nutrition, proper exercise, and adequate sleep.
- An important piece of intellectual health is adequate financial planning. Now is the time to begin saving.
- Emotional health includes emotional intelligence and laughter.
- Maintaining many different types of relationships helps to keep you healthy.
- Spiritual well-being is another essential element of good health. Spirituality needs to be continually nurtured.
- To stay healthy, you must make a conscious decision to maintain each of the six elements of health.

KEY TERMS

anger
certification
clinical ladders
competency
401K
emotional health
health
intellectual health

money market
  account
physical health
professional health
Roth IRA
social health
spiritual health

REVIEW QUESTIONS

1. You have $1,000 that you would like to deposit into an account. Which of the following would offer the highest interest rate with the greatest flexibility in accessing the money?
   A. Money market account
   B. Passbook savings account

C. Traditional bank checking account
D. Traditional IRA

2. The optimal method for rotating shifts to decrease fatigue is
   A. rotate clockwise.
   B. rotate counterclockwise.
   C. rotate nights to days only.
   D. rotate evenings to days only.

3. The process of certification allows the registered nurse to
   A. demonstrate clinical expertise.
   B. demonstrate educational expertise.
   C. demonstrate clinical and/or educational expertise.
   D. demonstrate advanced nursing degrees.

 REVIEW ACTIVITIES

1. Try doing a short relaxation exercise. Take a deep breath in and let it out. Take slow, deep breaths that originate from the diaphragm. Tighten the muscles in your right arm for 30 seconds and release. Your arm should feel totally limp and relaxed. Do the same with your left arm. Tighten the muscles in your right leg for 30 seconds and release. Repeat with the left leg. Pull in your stomach muscles for 30 seconds and release. Tighten the muscles in your buttocks and release. Continue to breathe in and out deeply. You can practice this brief exercise anytime or anywhere. If you are having a particularly hectic day, take a minute to do a relaxation exercise. You can vary the exercise by flexing any group of muscles you want.

2. Your best friend is getting married next month, and you are the maid of honor. You have already purchased a nonrefundable airline ticket to attend the shower. You work in a very small intensive care unit. You have been working 10- and 12-hour shifts and are near exhaustion. Your head nurse calls you 2 days before you are to leave for the shower and asks you to work the weekend. One of the staff has been involved in a serious car accident, and there is no one else to work. What would you do?

3. You were recently hired on a nursing unit. What equipment and supplies do you need to protect yourself from occupational hazards?

4. Finally, you have graduated and moved to the city of your choice and are working at the health care facility of your choice. You are starting to apply all the knowledge and skills that you gained at school. You are around all types of nursing mentors and role models and are witnessing firsthand the activities of new and experienced staff nurses, as well as those of advance practice nurses. Develop some goals regarding where you will be 1, 3, 5, or 10 years from now. Identify how you will determine your progress.

5. Review the salary survey in the March 2001 issue of *Nursing 2001*, pp. 44–47. How will the information help you plan your future goals?

6. Review the salary survey in the July 30, 2001, issue of *Modern Healthcare*, p. 27. Notice how various health care executives are compensated. How will this information help you plan your future goals?

7. Review the Guide to Certification in the *American Journal of Nursing Career Guide 2001*, p. 40. How will this information help you plan your future goals?

8. Review the article on international nursing in the *American Journal of Nursing Career Guide 2001*, p. 12. How will this information help you plan your future goals?

 EXPLORING THE WEB

1. Calculate your BMI and determine your life expectancy and health risks at *http://www.nhlbi.nih.gov*.

- Try one of the following sites to retrieve information on dietary supplements, nutrition, and alternative medicine: *http://www.nutritionsite.com http://www.alternativemedicine.com http://www.homeopathic.net*

2. Retirement Information Sites:
- *http://www.mpowercafe.com* for information on a 401K
- *http://www.quicken.com*
- Charles Schwab: *http://www.schwab.com* and click on *Retirement Planning*
- Social Security: *http://www.ssa.gov*
- Fidelity Investments: *http://www.fidelity. com* and click on *Retirement Center;* then follow the different retirement options
- Vanguard: *http://www.vanguard.com* and click on *Personal Investors;* then click on the *Planning & Advice* tab
- Valueline: *http://www.valueline.com* and click on *What's New? Retirement Planners*
- Morningstar: *http://www.morningstar.com* and click on *Retirement*

3. Resources for Violence Prevention:
- The ANA's Workplace Violence: Can You Close the Door? Call (800) 274-4ANA *http://www.nursingworld.org*
- Guidelines for Preventing Workplace Violence for Healthcare and Social Service Workers. U.S. Department of Labor, OSHA 3148-1996, available on-line: *http://www.osha-slc.gov*
- Violence Potential Assessment Tool. Contact Victoria Carroll at (970) 416-6811.

4. Resources for Needle Sticks
- General resource links: *http://www.medamicus.com*
- Safer Needle Devices: Protecting Health Care Workers: *http://www.osha-slc.gov*
- American Nurses Association: *http://www.nursingworld.org*
- Centers for Disease Control and Prevention: *http://www.cdc.gov*

5. Resources for Latex Allergy
- ANA's position paper on Latex Allergy: *http://www.nursingworld.org* or call (800) 274-4ANA
- OSHA *http://www.osha-slc.gov*

6. Resource for Back Strain
- Occupational Safety and Health Administration's ergonomics information *http://www.osha-slc.gov* or call (202) 693-1999.

7. General Interest and Nursing Issues:
- Centers for Disease Control: *http://www. cdc.gov*
- National Institutes of Health: *http://www. nih.gov*
- National League for Nursing: *http://www. nln.org*
- ANA certification listing: *http://www.nursingworld.org*
- Center for Nursing: *http://www.nursingcenter.com*
- National Council of State Boards of Nursing: *http://www.ncsbn.org*
- General nursing interest site: *http://www. allnurses.com*
- Health care information: *http://www.medscape.com, http://www.docguide.com*

8. Specialty Issues:
- American Association of Nurse Anesthetists: *http://www.aana.com*
- Flight nursing: *http://www.flightweb.com*
- Small Business Administration: *http://www. sbaonline.sba.gov*
- Service Corps of Retired Executives: *http://www.score.org*
- Traveling nurses: *http://www.springnet.com http://www.healthcareers-online.com*

 REFERENCES

Alspach, J. (1984). Designing a competency-based orientation for critical care nurses. *Heart & Lung, 13,* 655–662.

Barker, R. (2000, January 24). A small price to pay for retirement. *Business Week, 183*–184.

Chilton, B. (1998). Recognizing spirituality. *Image: Journal of Nursing Scholarship, 30*(4), 400–401.

Davidhizar, R., Poole, V. L., & Giger, J. N. (1996). Power nap rejuvenates body, mind. *Pennsylvania Nurse, 51*(3), 6-7.

Dawson, D., & Reid, K. (1997). Fatigue, alcohol, and performance impairment. *Nature, 338*(6639), 235.

Dossey, B. M., & Keegan, L. (2000). Self-assessments: Facilitating healing in self and others. In B. M. Dossey, L. Keegan, C. E. Guzzetta, & L. G. Kolkmeier (Eds.), *Holistic nursing: A handbook for practice* (pp. 361–374). Gaithersburg, MD: Aspen.

Ellis, A. (1997). *Anger: How to live with it and without it.* New York: Citadel Press, Kensington.

Frisch, N., & Frisch, L. (2002). *Psychiatric Mental Health Nursing.* 2nd ed. Clifton Park: Thomson Delmar Learning.

Getting X-ers to stay (2000). Management briefings for nurse leaders, 1(5)3.

Goleman, D. (1998) *Working with emotional intelligence.* New York: Bantam Books.

Grensing-Pophal, L. (1998). Resolving conflicts: It's as easy as 1-2-3. *Nursing98, 28*(9), 63.

Hallowell, E. (2000). Strong relationships really do help ensure good health. *Bottom Line Health, 14*(2), 3–4.

Healy, C., & McKay, M. (1999). Identifying sources of stress and job satisfaction in the nursing environment. *Australian Journal of Advanced Nursing, 17*(2), 30–35.

Koenig, H. G. (1999).The healing power of faith. *Annals of Long-Term Care, 7*(10), 381–384.

Lannon, P. (2000, April 27). Laughter, fun is key to combating stress. *The Doings Newspapers,* 63.

Maraldo, P. (1999). *Women's health for dummies.* Chicago: IDG Books Worldwide.

Mee, C. L., & Carey, K. (2000). Salary survey. *Nursing2000, 30*(4), 58–61.

National Institute of Health (n.d.). *Body mass index calculator.* Retrieved February 2, 2002, from *http://www.nhlbi.nih.gov*

Nightingale, F. (1969). *Notes on nursing.* New York: Dover. (Original work published 1860)

Orman. S. (1997). *The 9 steps to financial freedom.* New York: Crown.

Orman, S. (1999). *The courage to be rich: Creating a life of material and spiritual abundance.* New York: Riverhead Books.

Random House Webster's unabridged dictionary. (1997). New York: Random House.

Rogers, B. (1997). Health hazards in nursing and health care: An overview. *American Journal of Infection Control, 25*(3), 248–261.

Survival of the fittest. (2001). *Consumer Reports, 66*(3), 32–36.

Taffinder, H. J., McManus, I. C., Russell, R. C. G., & Darzi, A. (1998). Effect of sleep deprivation on surgeons' dexterity on laparoscopy simulator. *The Lancet, 352,* 1191.

Turek, F. W., & Zee, P. C. (1999). *Regulation of sleep and circadian rhythms.* New York: Marcel Dekker.

Tyson, E. (2000). *Personal finance for dummies.* Chicago: IDG Books Worldwide.

U.S. Bureau of Labor Statistics. (1999, December). *Workplace injury and illness summary.* Retrieved April 30, 2002, from *http://www. bls.gov/iif/*

U.S. Department of Health and Human Services. (2001). *Healthy People 2010: Goals.* Retrieved January 2, 2002, from *http://www. health.gov.*

Webster's Encyclopedic Universal Dictionary (2001). New York: Barnes and Noble.

World Health Organization. (1998). *Health education and promotion.* Retrieved January 19, 2002, from *http://www.who.int.*

Your guide to certification. (2001, January). *American Journal of Nursing Career Guide 2001—Part 2,* 40–49.

SUGGESTED READINGS

Benson, H. (2000). *The relaxation response.* New York: Avon Books.

Boston Women's Health Book Collectice. (1998). *Our bodies, ourselves for the new century.* New York: Simon & Schuster.

Breathmach, S. B. (1995). *Simple abundance.* New York: Time Warner.

Carroll, V. (1999). Workplace violence. *American Journal of Nursing, 99*(3), 60.

Chopra, D. (2000). *How to know God.* New York: Harvey Books.

Dickerson, P. S., & Nash, B. A. (1999). Hospital extra. Nurse entrepreneurs as educators. *American Journal of Nursing, 99*(6), 24A, 24D.

Dickerson, S. S., Peters, D., Walkowiak, J. A., & Brewer, C. (1999). Active learning strategies to teach case management. *Nurse Educator, 24*(5), 52–57.

Donner, G. J., & Wheeler, M. M. (2001). Career planning and development for nurses: The time has come. *International Nursing Review, 2*, 79–85.

Dugas, C. (1999, December 3). Retirement calculators figure it out. *USA Today,* 3B.

Ford, L. C. (1997). Advanced practice nursing. A deviant comes of age . . . the NP in acute care. *Heart & Lung: Journal of Acute & Critical Care, 26*(2), 87–91.

Froman, R. D. (2001). Assessing the credibility of a clinical ladder review process: An interrater reliability study. *Nursing Outlook, 49*(1), 27–29.

Geier, W. (1999). Caring side-by-side with acute care nurse practitioners. *Nursing Management, 30*(9), 32–34.

Grensing-Pophal, L. (1999). Multi-tasking made easy. *Nursing99, 29*(2), 55–56.

Holzer, B. (2000). *Set for life: Financial peace for people over 50.* New York: Wiley.

Knaus, V., Felten, S., Burton, S., Fobes, P., & Davis, K. (1997). The use of nurse practitioners in the acute care setting. *Journal of Nursing Administration, 27*(2), 20–27.

Manthey, M. (1999). Financial management for entrepreneurs. *Nursing Administration Quarterly, 23*(4), 81–85.

Manthey, M. (1999). I never saw myself as a change agent. *Reflections, 25*(2), 19–21.

McWilliam, C. L., Spence Laschinger, H. K., & Weston, W. (1999). Health promotion amongst nurses and physicians: What is the human experience? *American Journal of Health Behavior, 23*(2), 95–103.

Mee, C. L., & Carey, K. W. (2001). Nursing 2001 salary survey. *Nursing2001, 31*(3), 44–47.

Miracle, V. A. (2002). A closing word: The importance of certification. *Dimensions of Critical Care Nursing, 21*(3), 120.

Nolan, M. T., Harris, A., Kufta, A., Opfer, N., & Turner, H. (1998). Preparing nurses for the acute care case manager role: Educational needs identified by existing case managers. *Journal of Continuing Education in Nursing, 29*(3), 130–134, 142–143.

Owen, B. D. (1999). Preventing back injuries. *American Journal of Nursing, 99*(5), 76.

Pearson, L. J. (1999). Annual update of how each state stands on legislative issues affecting advanced practice. *The Nurse Practitioner, 24*(1), 16–82.

Penny, J. T. (1997). What a travel nurse company seeks in you . . . Nursing 97 travel nursing guide. *Nursing 1997, 27*(6), 69.

Phillips, B., & D'Orso, M. (1999). *Body-for-life.* New York: HarperCollins.

Presley, D., & Robinson, G. (2002). Violence in the Emergency Department. *Nursing Clinic of North America, 37*(1), 161–169.

Redfield, S. M. (1999). *Creating a life of joy: A meditative guide.* New York: Time Warner Trade Publishing.

Richardson, C. (1999). *Take time for your life.* New York: Broadway Books.

Ruiz, D. M. (1999). *The four agreements.* San Rafael, CA: Amber-Allen.

Rupp, J. (1998). *The cup of our life; a guide to spiritual growth.* Notre Dame, IN: Ave Maria Press.

Schulmeister, L. (1999). Starting a nursing consultation practice. *Clinical Nurse Specialist, 13*(2), 94–100.

Shriver, M. (2000). *Ten things I wish I'd known.* New York: Time Warner.

Simms, L., Price, S., & Ervin, N. (2000). *Professional practice of nursing administration* (3rd ed.). Clifton Park, NY: Delmar Learning.

Simpson, R. L. (1998). Nursing informatics. From nurse to nursing informatics consultant: A lesson in entrepreneurship. *Nursing Administration Quarterly, 22*(2), 87–90.

Stein, M. K. (1998). *The prosperous retirement.* Boulder, CO, Emstco Press.

Steinhauer, R. G. (2001). International nursing. In *AJN Career Guide 2001—Part 2*, pp. 12–15.

Travel nurse spotlight: Travel nurse web sites. (1999). *Nursing99, 29*(6), 80–81.

Travel nursing spotlight: Agency alternative. (1999). *Nursing99, 29*(6), 78–79.

Trossman, S. (2002). What do credentials mean to you?: Nurses talk about the value of ANCC certification. *American Journal of Nursing, 102*(5), 71–73.

Valanis, B., Vollmer, W. M., & Steele, P. (1999). Occupational exposure to antineoplastic agents: Self- reported miscarriages and stillbirths among nurses and pharmacists. *Journal of Occupational and Environmental Medicine, 41*(8), 632–638.

Ventura, M., & Grandinetti, D. (1999). NP progress report: A survey. *RN, 62*(7), 33–35.

VGM Career Books (ed.). (2001). *Resumes for Nursing Careers.* New York: McGraw-Hill Contemporary Books.

Wilburn, S. (1999). Is the air in your hospital making you sick? *American Journal of Nursing, 99*(7), 71.

Worthington, K. (1999). Toward a latex-safe workplace. *American Journal of Nursing, 99*(11), 71.

Wright, J., & Basco, M. (2001). *Getting your life back: The complete guide to recovery from depression.* New York: Free Press.

Zukav, G. (1999). *The seat of the soul.* New York: Simon & Schuster.

360-degree feedback   Performance evaluation system in which an individual is assessed by a variety of people in order to provide a broader perspective about their performance.

401K   Retirement savings account that both employee and for-profit employer contribute to.

403b   Retirement savings account that both employee and not-for-profit employer contribute to.

accommodating   Satisfying the needs of others, sometimes at the expense of self.

accountability   Liability for actions.

accounting   Activity that nurse managers engage in to record and report financial transactions and data.

acculturation   Process by which individuals adjust and adapt either to their host culture or a subculture by altering their own cultural behaviors.

achievement   Accomplishment of goals through effort.

activities of daily living   Activities related to toileting, bathing, grooming, dressing, feeding, and mobility.

activity log   Time management technique to assist in determining how both personal and professional time is used by periodically recording activities.

administrative law   Body of law created by administrative agencies in the form of rules, regulations, orders, and decisions which protect the rights of citizens.

administrative principles   General principles of management that are relevant to any organization.

affiliation   Associations and relationships with others.

agnostic   Person who is not committed to belief in the existence or nonexistence of a god or a supreme being, or perhaps believes that no one has effectively proven that a god exists.

altruism   The unselfish concern for the welfare of others.

American Nurses Association   Full-service professional nursing organization representing the nation's entire registered nurse population.

assault   Offer to or threat of touching another in an offensive manner without that person's permission.

atheist   Does not believe in the existence of a god or a supreme being.

attending   Active listening to gain an understanding of the patient's message.

auditory   Pertaining to hearing.

authority   Power and/or right to make decisions.

autocratic leadership   Centralized decision-making style with the leader making decisions and using power to command and control others.

autonomy   An individual's right to self-determination and individual liberty.

avoiding   Retreating.

battery   Touching of another person without that person's consent.

benchmark   A quantitative or qualitative standard or point of reference used in measuring or judging quality or value.

benchmarking   Management tool for seeking out the best practices in one's industry so as to improve performance.

beneficence   The duty to do good to others and to maintain a balance between benefits and harms.

bioethics Ethics specific to health care; serves as a framework to guide behavior in ethical dilemmas.

break-even point That point at which income and expenses are equal.

budget A plan that provides formal quantitative expression for acquiring and distributing funds over the ensuing time period.

bureaucratic organization Hierarchy with clear superior-subordinate communication and relations, based on positional authority, in which orders from the top are transmitted down through the organization via a clear chain of command.

capital budget Accounts for the purchase of major new or replacement equipment.

capitation Payment of a fixed dollar amount, per person, for the provision of health services to a patient population for a specified period of time (e.g., one month).

care delivery model Method to organize the work of caring for patients.

case management Strategy to improve patient care and reduce hospital costs through coordination of care.

certification Process by which a nongovernmental agency or association asserts that an individual licensed to practice a profession has met certain predetermined standards specified by that profession for practice.

certified registered nurse anesthetist Advanced clinical nursing specialist who manages the patient's anesthesia needs before, during, and after surgery or other procedures.

change Making something different from what it was.

change agent One who is responsible for implementation of a change project.

civil law That body of law that governs how individuals relate to each other in everyday matters.

clarifying Restating, rephrasing, or questioning a message as part of a process to help make meaning clear.

clinical information system (CIS) Collection of software programs and associated hardware that supports the entry, retrieval, update, and analysis of patient care information and associated clinical information related to patient care.

clinical ladder A promotional model that acknowledges that staff members have varying skill sets based on their education and experience. As such, depending on skills and experience, staff members may be rewarded differently and carry differing responsibilities for patient care and the governance and professional practice of the work unit.

clinical nurse specialist Advanced practice registered nurse, with either a master's or doctoral degree in a clinical specialty, who functions as health care provider, educator, consultant, researcher, and leader.

clinical pathway Care management tool that outlines the expected clinical course and outcomes for a specific patient group.

collaborating Resolving conflict so that both parties are satisfied.

collective action Method to deal with problems by acting as a group with a single voice.

collective bargaining Practice of employees, in a collective group, bargaining with management in reference to wages, work practice, and other benefits.

collective bargaining agent Individual who works with employees and employers to formalize collective bargaining though unionization.

committee Work group with a specific task or goal to accomplish.

common law Body of law that develops from precedents set by judicial decisions that, over time, have the force of law, as distinguished from legislative enactments.

competing Engaging in rivalry to meet a goal.

compromising Finding a middle ground solution where neither party meets all their goals.

computer literacy The knowledge and understanding of computers combined with the ability to use them effectively.

computerized patient record (CPR) Electronic record that includes all information about an individual's lifetime health status and health care; replacement for the paper medical record as the primary source of information for health care, meeting all clinical, legal, and administrative requirements.

conflict Disagreement about something of importance to each person involved.

connection power Strength that comes from the extent to which nurses are connected with others having power.

consensus Situation in which all group members agree to live with and support a decision, regardless of whether they totally agree.

constitution A set of basic laws that specifies the powers of the various segments of the government and how these segments relate to each other.

construction budget Budget that is developed when renovation or new structures are planned.

contingency theory Leadership theory that acknowledges that other factors in the environment influence outcomes as much as leadership style and that leader effectiveness is contingent upon or depends upon something in addition to the leader's behavior.

contract law Rules that regulate certain transactions between individuals and/or legal entities such as businesses. Also governs transactions between businesses.

cost center Departmental subsection or unit for tracking of financial data in an agency.

culture Behaviors, norms, belief sets, values, race, traditions, and folkways of a specific group.

dashboard Documentation tool providing a snapshot image of pertinent information and outcomes reflecting a point in time.

data capture Collection and entry of data into a computer system.

decision making Behavior exhibited in making a selection and implementing a course of action from alternatives.

defamation Intentionally false communication, either published or publicly spoken.

delegation Transferring to a competent individual the authority to perform a selected nursing task in a selected situation (NSCBN, 1995).

Delphi technique Process that groups employ to arrive at a decision, though group members never meet face to face; questionnaires are distributed repeatedly for opinions, then summarized and disseminated again with the summaries given to group members. This process continues until consensus is achieved.

democratic leadership Style in which participation is encouraged and authority is delegated to others.

deontology Ethical theory stating that, in determining the ethics of a situation, a person must consider the motives of the actor, not the consequences of the act.

department clinical information system System that meets the operational information needs of a particular department, such as the laboratory, radiology, pharmacy, medical records, or billing department.

diagnostic-related groups Patient groupings established by the federal government for health care reimbursement purposes; these patient groupings are sorted by patient disease or condition.

differentiated nursing practice Care delivery model that sorts the roles, functions, and work of registered nurses according to some identified criteria, commonly education, clinical experience, and competence.

direct care Time spent providing hands-on care to patients.

direct cost Cost directly related to patient care within a nurse manager's unit.

direct expenses Expenses that are directly associated with patient care (e.g., medical and surgical supplies and drugs).

disease management Systematic, population-based approach to identify persons at risk, intervene with specific program of care, and measure clinical and other outcomes (Epstein and Sherwood, 1996).

economics Study of how scarce resources are allocated among possible uses.

egoism The tendency to be self-centered or to consider only oneself and one's own interests.

employee-centered leadership Leadership style with a focus on the human needs of subordinates.

empowerment Process by which we facilitate the participation of self and others in decision making.

enterprise An organization of any size established as a business venture.

episodic care unit Unit that sees patients for defined episodes of care; examples include dialysis or ambulatory care units.

ethical dilemma A conflict between two or more ethical principles for which there is no easy decision.

ethics The doctrine that the general welfare of society is the proper goal of an individual's actions rather than egoism; the branch of philosophy that concerns the distinction between right from wrong on the basis of a body of knowledge, not just on the basis of opinions.

ethnicity Component of cultural identity that includes several factors such as race, geographic identity, physical features, and language.

ethnocentrism Belief that one's own culture or ethnic group is better than all other groups.

evidence-based care Care that is recognized by nursing, medicine, health care institutions, and health policy makers as care based on state-of-the-art science reports. It is a process approach to collecting, reviewing, interpreting, critiquing, and evaluating research and other relevant literature and practice for direct application to patient care.

evidence-based medicine Means to integrate individual clinical medical experience with external clinical evidence using a systematic research approach (Sackett, Rosenberg, Gray, Haynes, & Richardson, 1996).

evidence-based nursing practice Conscientious, explicit, and judicious use of theory-derived, research-based information in making decisions about care delivery to individuals or groups of individuals and in consideration of individual needs and preferences (Ingersoll, 2000, p. 152).

evidence-based practice Conscientious, explicit, and judicious use of current best evidence in making decisions about the care of individual patients (Sackett, et al., 1996, p. 71).

expert power   Power derived from the knowledge and skills nurses possess.

false imprisonment   Imprisonment that occurs when people are incorrectly led to believe they cannot leave a place.

fee for service reimbursement   Health care reimbursement based on services provided.

feedback   A new message generated by the message receiver in response to the original message from the sender.

fidelity   The principle of promise keeping; the duty to keep one's promise or word.

fixed costs   Expenses that are constant and are not related to productivity or volume.

focus groups   Small groups of individuals selected because of a common characteristic (e.g., a specific patient population, patients in day surgery, new diabetics, and so on) who are invited to meet in a group and respond to questions about a topic in which they are expected to have interest or expertise or experience.

formal leadership   When a person is in a position of authority or in a sanctioned role within an organization that connotes influence.

full-time equivalent   Measure of the work-time commitment of a full-time employee.

functional health status   Ability to care for oneself and meet one's own personal human needs.

functional nursing   Care delivery model that divides the nursing work into functional units that are then assigned to one of the team members.

goal   Specific aim or target that the unit wishes to attain within a specified time span of 1 year.

Good Samaritan laws   Laws that have been enacted to protect the health care professional from legal liability for actions rendered in an emergency when the professional is giving service without pay.

grapevine   An informal communication channel where information moves quickly from person to person and is often inaccurate.

group process   Stages that a group progresses through as it matures, consisting of the following: forming, storming, norming, performing, and adjourning.

Hawthorne effect   Phenomenon of being observed or studied, which results in changes in behavior that might not occur if person or event was not being observed.

health   State of complete physical, social, and mental well-being, and not merely the absence of disease or infirmity (World Health Organization, 1998).

health determinants   Biological, psychosocial, environmental (physical and social), and health system factors or etiologies that may cause changes in the health status of individuals, families, groups, populations, and communities.

health-related quality of life   Those aspects of life that are influenced either positively or negatively by one's health status and health risk factors.

health risk factors   Modifiable and non-modifiable variables that increase or decrease the probability of illness or death.

health status   Level of health of an individual, family, group, population, or community; the sum of existing health risk factors, level of wellness, existing diseases, functional health status, and quality of life.

horizontal integration Integration that occurs when a health care system contains several organizations of one type, such as hospitals.

indirect care Time spent on activities that are patient related but are not done directly to the patient.

indirect expenses Expenses that are related to such items as utilities, such as gas, electric, and phones, that are not directly related to patient care.

informal leader Individual who demonstrates leadership outside the scope of a formal leadership role or as a member of a group, rather than the head or leader of the group.

information power Nurses who influence others with the information they provide to the group are using information power.

inpatient unit Hospital unit that is able to provide care to patients 24 hours a day, 7 days a week.

instrumental activities of daily living Activities related to food preparation and shopping; cleaning; laundry; home maintenance; verbal, written, and electronic community communications; financial management; and transportation, as well as activities to meet social and support needs, manage health care needs, access community services and resources, and meet spiritual needs.

integrated delivery system Network of health care organizations that provides a coordinated continuum of service to a defined population and is willing to be held clinically and fiscally accountable for the outcomes and the health status of the population served. Integrated networks include hospitals, nursing homes, schools, public health departments, and social and community health organizations.

interdisciplinary team Group composed of members with a variety of clinical and educational expertise.

interpersonal communication Communication that is between individuals.

intrapersonal communication Self-talk.

job-centered leaders Leadership style that focuses on work schedules, cost, and efficiency with less attention given to developing work groups and high-performance goals.

justice The principle of fairness that is served when an individual is given that which he or she is due, owed, deserves, or can legitimately claim.

knowledge workers Those workers who are involved in serving others through their specialized knowledge.

laissez-faire leadership Passive and permissive leadership style in which the leader defers decision making.

leader-member relations Feelings and attitudes of followers and leaders regarding acceptance, trust, and credibility of each other.

leadership Process of influence whereby the leader influences others toward goal achievement.

legitimate power Power derived from the position a nurse holds in a group; it indicates the nurse's degree of authority.

living will Document voluntarily signed by patients that specifies the type of care they desire if and when they are in a terminal state and cannot sign a consent form or convey this information verbally.

maintenance or hygiene factors (Herzberg) Elements such as salary, job security, working conditions, status, quality of supervision, and relationships with others that prevent job dissatisfaction.

malpractice   Professional's wrongful conduct in discharge of professional duties or failure to meet standards of care for the profession, which results in harm to another individual entrusted to the professional's care.

management process   Process of planning, organizing, coordinating, and controlling resources and staff to achieve organizational goals.

margin   Profit.

MEDLARS (Medical Literature Analysis and Retrieval System)   Computerized system of databases and databanks offered by the National Library of Medicine.

message   Message originating with the sender, consists of verbal and nonverbal stimuli that are taken in by the receiver.

mission   Call to live out something that matters or is meaningful; an organization's mission reflects the purpose and direction of the health care agency or a department within it.

mission statement   A formal expression of the purpose or reason for existence of the organization.

modular nursing   Care delivery model that is a kind of team nursing that divides a geographical space into modules of patients with each module having a team of staff led by an RN to care for them.

money market account   Similar to a bank checking account though it often requires a larger minimum amount of money to open the account and often has a higher interest rate for your money.

morality   Behavior in accordance with custom or tradition; usually reflects personal or religious beliefs.

motivation   Whatever influences our choices and creates direction, intensity, and persistence in our behavior.

motivation factors (Herzberg)   Elements such as achievement, recognition, responsibility, advancement, and the opportunity for development that all contribute to job satisfaction.

negligence   Failure to provide the care a reasonable person would ordinarily provide in a similar situation.

Nonmaleficence   The principle of doing no harm.

nonproductive hours   Paid time not devoted to patient care; includes benefit time such as vacation, sick time, and education time.

nurse practitioner   Advanced practice nurse who has education beyond the bachelor's degree in a clinical specialty area strongly focused on primary care.

nursing hours per patient day   Standard measure that quantifies the nursing time available to each patient by the available nursing staff.

objective   Measurable step that must be taken to reach a goal.

operational budget   Account for the income and expenses associated with day-to-day activity within a department or organization.

organizational change   Planned alteration in an organization to generally improve efficiency.

outcome elements of quality   Outcome elements of quality are the end products of quality care; outcomes review the status of patients that may result from health care. Outcome elements ask the question, "How is the patient better as a result of health care?"

Pareto principle   Principle, developed by Pareto, a 19th century economist, which states that 20% of effort results in 80% of results, or conversely that 80% of unfocused effort results in 20% of results.

patient acuity Measure of nursing workload that is generated for each patient based on their needs.

patient care redesign Initiative in the 1990s to redesign how patient care was delivered.

patient-centered care Care delivery model in which care and services are brought to the patient.

patient classification system (PCS) System for identifying different patients based on their acuity, functional ability, or resource needs.

patient-focused care A model of differentiated nursing practice that emphasizes quality, cost, and value.

patient-focused clinical information system System in which automation supports patient care processes; typical applications include order entry, results reporting, clinical documentation, care planning, and clinical pathways.

payer Third-party reimburser (insurance company or government).

performance improvement Structured system for creating organization-wide participation and partnership in planning and implementing continuous improvement methods to understand and meet or exceed customer needs and expectations.

personal change Alteration made voluntarily for one's own reasons, usually for self-improvement.

philosophy Statement of beliefs based on core values; rational investigations of the truths and principles of knowledge, reality, and human conduct.

philosophy of an organization A value statement of the principles and beliefs that direct the organization's behavior.

physical health Encompasses nutrition and exercise coupled with a balanced amount of rest; health preventive behaviors such as avoiding smoking; and health screening behaviors that detect health problems early such as an annual Pap smear.

politics Process by which people use a variety of methods to achieve their goals.

population-based health care practice Development, provision, and evaluation of multidisciplinary health care services to population groups experiencing increased health risks or disparities, in partnership with health care consumers and the community in order to improve the health of the community and its diverse population groups.

population-based nursing practice Practice of nursing in which the focus of care is to improve the health status of vulnerable or at-risk population groups within the community by employing health promotion and disease prevention interventions across the health continuum.

position power Degree of formal authority and influence associated with the leader's position in an organization.

power Ability to create, get, and use resources to achieve one's goals.

practice guideline Descriptive tool or standardized specifications for care of the typical patient in the typical situation; these guidelines are developed by a formal process that incorporates the best scientific evidence of effectiveness and expert opinion. Synonyms or near synonyms include practice parameter, preferred practice pattern, algorithm, protocol, and clinical standard (JCAHO, 1999, p. 113).

preferred provider organization (PPO) Contracts with health care providers (practitioners and hospitals) and payers (self-insured employers, insurance companies, government, or managed care organizations) to provide health care services to a defined population for predetermined, fixed fees.

primary health care Services that emphasize the promotion of health and the prevention of illness or disability.

primary nursing Care delivery model that clearly delineates the responsibility and accountability of the RN and reinforces the RN as the primary provider of nursing care to patients.

problem solving Active process that starts with a problem and ends with a solution.

process Set of causes and conditions that repeatedly come together in a series of steps to transfer inputs into outcomes.

process elements of quality Elements that identify what nursing and health care interventions must be in place to deliver quality. Process elements are such things as managing the health care process, utilizing clinical practice guidelines and standards for nursing and medical interventions, passing medications, and so on.

productive hours Hours worked and available for patient care.

profit Determined by the relationship of income to expenses.

progressive discipline System in which the manager and employee's mutual goal is to take steps to correct performance in order to bring it back to an acceptable level; it offers a stepwise process with opportunities for continued feedback and clarification of expectations.

protective factors Patient strengths and resources that the patients can use to combat health threats that compromise core human functions.

public law General classification of law, consisting generally of constitutional, adminis-

trative, and criminal law. Public law defines a citizen's relationship with their government.

quality assurance Quality inspection approach to ensure that minimum standards of care exist in health care institutions, primarily hospitals.

quality improvement Systematic process to continuously improve outcomes based on customers' needs.

quality of life Level of satisfaction one has with the actual conditions of one's life, including satisfaction with socioeconomic status, education, occupation, home, family life, recreation, and the ability to enjoy life, freedom, and independence.

reasonable outcomes Objectives that can and should be achieved even though there are less-than-optimal circumstances and limited resources.

receiver One who takes in a message and analyzes it.

reengineering Turning an organization upside down and inside out through fundamental rethinking and radical redesign of work processes to achieve dramatic improvements in critical performance.

referent power Power derived from how much others respect and like any individual, group, or organization.

reflective thinking Examining and observing ourselves as we perform a task or make a decision about a certain situation.

relative value unit (RVU) Index number assigned to various health care services based on the relative amount of resources (labor and capital) used to produce the service.

religion Organized and public belief system of worship and practices that generally has a focus of a god or supernatural power.

resilience The physical and psychosocial capacity of individuals and groups to adapt, succeed, and persevere over time in the face of recurring threats to psychosocial and physiologic integrity.

resources People, money, facilities, technology, and rights to properties, services, and technologies.

respect for others Acknowledgement of the right of people to make their own decisions.

responding Verbally and nonverbally acknowledging a sender's message.

resume Brief summary of your background, training, and experience as well as your qualifications for a position.

revenue Income generated through a variety of means (e.g., billable patient services, investments, and donations to the organization).

reward/coercive power Power to reward or punish others, as well as power to instill fear in others to influence them to change their behavior; withholding rewards or achieving a goal by causing fear in others often results in resentment.

Roth IRA Individual retirement account that is much less restrictive than an IRA; first introduced in 1998.

secondary health care Services that emphasize detection and early intervention in illness to prevent further illness and disability.

self-scheduling Process by which staff on a unit collectively decide and implement the monthly work schedule.

sentinel event Unexpected occurrence involving death or serious physical or psychological injury to a patient.

shared governance Situation where nurses and managers work together to define their roles and expected outcomes, holding everyone accountable for their role and expected outcomes.

situational leadership A leadership framework that maintains that there is no one best leadership style, but rather that effective leadership lies in matching the appropriate leadership style to the individual's or group's level of motivation and task-relevant readiness.

skill mix Percentage of RN staff to other direct care staff, LPNs, and UAP.

social health Ability to relate to and interact with others.

sources of power Combination of conscious and unconscious factors that allow an individual to influence others to do as the individual wants.

spiritual distress Questioning of the purpose of life and its meaning, refusing to participate in one's usual religious practices, and seeking unusual assistance rather than the usual spiritual or religious support.

spiritual health Human capacity to find strength from within; results from a connection with a higher being or power (Chilton, 1998).

staffing pattern Plan that articulates how many and what kind of staff are needed, by shift and day, to staff a unit or department.

stakeholder Provider, employer, customer, patient, or payer who may have an interest in, and seek to influence, the decisions and actions of an organization.

stakeholders Vested interest groups.

stakeholder assessment A systematic consideration of all potential stakeholders to ensure that the needs of each of these stakeholders are incorporated into planning.

strategic plan The sum total or outcome of the processes by which an organization engages in environmental analysis, goal formulation, and strategy development with the purpose of organizational growth and renewal.

strategic planning A process that is designed to achieve goals in dynamic, competitive environments through the allocation of resources.

structure elements of quality Elements that identify what structures must be in place in a health care system/unit to deliver quality health care. Structure elements consist of such things as a well constructed hospital, quality patient care standards, quality staffing policies, environmental standards, and the like.

substitutes for leadership Variables that may influence or have an effect on followers to the same extent as the leader's behavior.

SWOT analysis A tool that is frequently used to conduct environmental assessments. SWOT stands for Strengths, Weaknesses, Opportunities, and Threats.

system Interdependent group of items, people, or processes with a common purpose.

team Small number of people with complementary skills who are committed to a common purpose, performance goals, and approach for which they hold themselves accountable (Katzenbach & Smith, 1993).

team nursing Care delivery model that assigns staff to teams that then are responsible for a group of patients.

teleology Theory stating that the value of a situation is determined by its consequences; the outcome of an action, not the action itself, is the criterion for measuring the goodness of that action.

tertiary health care Services that provide restorative or rehabilitation services for patients with chronic or irreversible conditions.

Theory X View that in bureaucratic organizations, employees prefer security, direction, and minimal responsibility; coercion, threats, or punishment are necessary because people do not like the work to be done.

Theory Y View that in the context of the right conditions, people enjoy their work, they can show self-control and discipline, are able to contribute creatively and are motivated by ties to the group, the organization, and the work itself; belief that people are intrinsically motivated by their work.

time management Set of related common-sense skills that helps you use your time in the most effective and productive way possible (Mind Tools, n.d.-b).

tort A private or civil wrong or injury, including action for bad faith breach of contract, for which the court will provide a remedy in the form of an action for damages.

total patient care Care delivery model in which nurses are responsible for the total nursing care for their patient assignment for the shift they are working.

traditional IRA Individual retirement account.

transcultural nursing Comparative study and analysis of different cultures and subcultures in the world with respect to their caring behavior, nursing care and health-illness values, beliefs, and patterns of behavior with the goal of developing a scientific and humanistic body of knowledge to provide culture-specific and culture-universal nursing care practices (Leininger, 1997).

transformational leader Leader who is committed to a vision that empowers others.

union Formal and legal group that works through a collective bargaining agent and within the context of the National Labor Relations Board to bring forth workers' requests to management.

values Personal beliefs about the truth of ideals, standards, principles, objects, and behaviors that give meaning and direction to life.

variable costs Costs that vary with volume and will increase or decrease depending on the number of patients.

variance Difference between what was budgeted and the actual cost.

veracity The obligation to tell the truth.

verbal communication Aspect of communication that relies on spoken words to convey a message.

vertical integration Occurs when different parts of health care are linked and delivered by one agency.

visual Pertaining to seeing.

voting block Group that represents the same political position or perspective.

vulnerable population groups Sub-groups of a community that are powerless, marginalized, or disenfranchised and are experiencing health disparities.

whistle-blowing Act in which an individual discloses information regarding a violation of a law, rule or regulation or a substantial and specific danger to public health or safety.

workplace advocacy Activities nurses undertake to address problems in their everyday workplace setting.

INDEX